P9-APG-614

Basic Life Support Skills

Baxter Larmon, PhD, MICP

Heather Davis, MS, NREMT-P

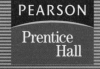

PEARSON

Prentice Hall

Upper Saddle River, New Jersey 07458

Library of Congress Cataloging-in Publication Data

Larmon, Baxter.
    Basic life support skills / Baxter Larmon, Heather Davis.
       p. ; cm.
    ISBN 0-13-093865-3 (alk. paper)
  1. Emergency medicine. 2. Life support systems (Critical care) 3. Medical emergencies.
4. First aid in illness and injury. 5. Emergency medical technicians.
    [DNLM: 1. Cardiopulmonary Resuscitation—methods—Examination Questions. 2. Emergency
Medical Technicians—education—Examination Questions. 3. Emergency Treatment—methods—
Examination Questions.   WG 18.2 L432b 2005] I. Davis, Heather.   II. Title.

    RC86.7.L367 2005
    616.02'5—dc22

                                                                    2004012996

Publisher: Julie Levin Alexander
Publisher's Assistant: Regina Bruno
Executive Editor: Marlene McHugh Pratt
Assistant Editor: Monica Moosang
Development Editor: Triple SSS Press Media Development
Senior Marketing Manager: Katrin Beacom
Channel Marketing Manager: Rachele Strober
Marketing Coordinator: Michael Sirinides
Director of Production and Manufacturing: Bruce Johnson
Managing Editor for Production: Patrick Walsh
Production Liaison: Julie Li
Production Editor: Emily Bush, Carlisle Publishers Services
Media Editor: John Jordan
Manager of Media Production: Amy Peltier
New Media Project Manager: Stephen J. Hartner
Manufacturing Manager: Ilene Sanford
Manufacturing Buyer: Pat Brown
Creative Director: Cheryl Asherman
Senior Design Coordinator: Christopher Weigand
Interior Designer: Mary Siener
Cover Designer: Christopher Weigand
Cover Photo: Getty Images
Composition: Carlisle Publishers Services
Printing and Binding: Von Hoffman Press
Cover Printer: Phoenix Color Corporation

Pearson Education LTD.
Pearson Education Singapore, Pte, Ltd
Pearson Education, Canada, Ltd
Pearson Education—Japan
Pearson Education Australia Pty, Limited

Pearson Education North Asia Ltd
Pearson Educación de Mexico, S.A. de C.V.
Pearson Education Malaysia, Pte. Ltd
Pearson Education, Upper Saddle River, New Jersey

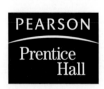

10 9 8 7 6 5 4 3 2 1
ISBN 0-13-093865-3

DEDICATION

In loving memory of my parents.
—Baxter Larmon

To Baxter, for encouraging my growth and professional development even when it was painful to let me go.
—Heather Davis

Contents

THE AUTHORS

Baxter Larmon, PhD, MICP

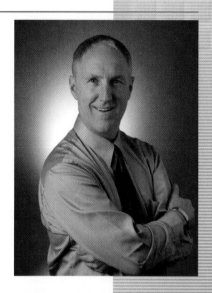

Dr. Larmon is a Professor of Medicine at the University of California at Los Angeles (UCLA) School of Medicine and is the Director of the UCLA Center for Prehospital Care. He has more than 30 years of experience with emergency medical services (EMS). He is the founding director of the Prehospital Care Research Forum and served on the founding board of directors of the National Association of EMS Educators (NAEMSE). Dr. Larmon is both nationally and internationally recognized as an EMS educator. He has spoken at more than 400 EMS conferences and has written more than 60 publications in emergency medicine.

Heather Davis, MS, NREMT-P

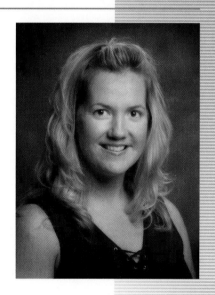

Heather Davis is the Education Program Director for the Los Angeles County Fire Department where she manages the primary EMT and continuing education programs for over 3,000 EMTs and paramedics. Her previous position was as the Clinical Coordinator for the UCLA Center for Prehospital Care, where she continues to lecture and be active in primary paramedic education. Heather has been involved in patient care and education activities in rural Iowa, suburban New York, and the Rocky Mountains of Colorado. She has worked in disaster response, critical incident management, and tactical EMS. Heather serves on the Board of Directors for NAEMSE and is the Prehospital Trauma Life Support State Coordinator for California. She holds a master of science degree from New York Medical College and is a published author and national speaker.

PREFACE

Congratulations! By purchasing this book you have demonstrated a commitment to acquiring the technical expertise associated with being an emergency medical technician (EMT). The actual job of providing emergency prehospital care is complex and dynamic, but gaining and maintaining excellence in the fundamental skills of the job will improve your confidence and competence as you provide care to patients in emergency situations.

This book is intended to be your resource for skills and procedures common to the practice of emergency medical services (EMS). This book covers EMT basic life support (BLS) skills. Hundreds of photos illustrate the proper procedural steps for each skill. A video/CD-ROM package is also available that supports this book. The videos actually demonstrate each skill in real time.

Each skill has several features that will enhance your use of this book:

▶ The *assessment* and *ongoing assessment* features precede and follow, respectively, each *step-by-step procedure* and will assist you in gathering pertinent information from the patient prior to and after engaging in the skill. In most cases, the assessment actually helps you determine whether or not that particular skill is indicated for your patient. The ongoing assessment helps you with the proper follow-up to make sure your use of the skill has been successful.

▶ More than 250 photos throughout the text help you visualize the step-by-step procedures.

▶ The *rationales* imbedded into the procedural steps help you understand why each step is to be done in the way it is described or why the step is important.

▶ Also, pay particular attention to the *problem-solving* section. For every procedure there exist possible complications or pitfalls to correctly completing the skill. The problem-solving section should help you develop alternative approaches when problems pop up.

▶ *Pediatric and geriatric notes* highlight particular issues and potential pitfalls with these populations.

▶ And finally, each chapter has a *case study* with chapter *review questions* to help you tie it all together.

These skills are presented using the most generic or broad-based equipment possible. When an EMS system chooses a particular piece of equipment, you should follow the manufacturer's instructions for use to ensure your safety and the safety of your patient. In some cases, specific manufacturer instructions could alter the steps presented here. Your EMT instructor or training officer is a good resource whenever a discrepancy arises. He or she should be familiar with national standards, state or local protocol, or the procedure set forth by your medical director.

ACKNOWLEDGMENTS

Reviewers

Rhonda J. Beck, NREMT-P
Central Georgia Technical College
Macon, GA

Tony Crystal, EMS Director
Lake Land College
Mattoon, IL

Barry Flores
Captain, Metro Fire
Sacramento, CA

Robert M. Hawkes, BA, BS, NREMT-P
South Portland, ME 04106

Jon Politis
Synergism Associated, Ltd.
Albany, NY 12212

Case Studies Writers

John L. Beckham
Nina Hand
Christopher Jones
William Krost
Ehren Ngo
Gail Weinstein

Section Review Questions Writer

Tony Crystal
Lake Land College
Mattoon, IL

Photo Shoot Coordination

Thank you to these special people from Town of Colonie EMS, Colonie, NY, who allowed Brady to use their facilities and who modeled for us:

MB Baker
John Daderian
Earl Evans
Ron Goodman
Dale Hebert
Calvin Krom
Tim LeBlanc

Joe Monaghan

Donna Palazynski

Aimee Peletier

John Qi

JeanAnn Riedell

Calvin Saylors

Denise Schultz

John Schultz

Jennifer Waterbury

Thank you to Denise Schultz, EMT-P, for coordinating the location and the equipment for the photo shoot.

SECTION 1

AIRWAY MANAGEMENT AND VENTILATION

Maintaining an airway, ensuring adequate ventilations, and providing supplemental oxygen are essential and basic components of emergency care. Without a clear and open airway, adequate ventilations, and/or sufficient oxygenation, all other treatment is futile.

Understanding when a patient needs airway and/or ventilation management must be made quickly. Mastering these skills is an essential part of being an Emergency Medical Technician. Without timely assessment and intervention a patient can have a poor outcome.

These chapters cover skills that the EMT may be able to do or will be able to assist another health care provider in performing. Check with local Medical Control to see what skills are within the scope of practice.

CHAPTER 1
Head-Tilt/Chin-Lift Maneuver

KEY TERMS

Altered level of
  consciousness
BSI equipment
Eye protection
Gag reflex
Head-tilt/chin-lift
  maneuver
Hyperextended
Supine position

OBJECTIVE

The student will successfully demonstrate how to perform the head-tilt/chin-lift maneuver.

INTRODUCTION

Providing an open airway is essential in patients who cannot maintain their own airway.

You will perform this skill primarily on the unresponsive patient with an **altered level of consciousness** or altered mental status, or respiratory or cardiac arrest. You should not perform this procedure on patients with actual or suspected head, neck, or spinal trauma.

The airway in these patients may be partially obstructed by the loss of muscle tone, which allows the tongue and lower jaw to obstruct airflow into and out of the lungs. The **head-tilt/chin-lift maneuver** opens the airway by tilting the head back while simultaneously pushing the chin forward, which brings the tongue forward, opening the air passage.

▶ EQUIPMENT

You will need the following body substance isolation, or **BSI, equipment:**

▶ Mask

▶ Gloves

▶ Eye protection

ASSESSMENT

The patient may be unresponsive or may be unconscious with an altered level of consciousness or altered mental status. The patient may also be in respiratory arrest or cardiac arrest. The patient should not have a mechanism of injury suggesting potential trauma to the head, neck, or spine. If the patient does have this type of injury, you should open his airway using the jaw-thrust maneuver instead of the head-tilt/chin-lift maneuver (see Chapter 2).

PROCEDURE: Head-Tilt/Chin-Lift Procedure

1. Apply BSI precautions.
   Rationale: Gloves and **eye protection** are required at a minimum, and a gown may be needed if large amounts of blood or fluid are present to prevent exposure to infectious diseases.

2. Place the patient in the supine position.
   Rationale: Although you can do this skill on a patient in any position, the **supine position** is the best position in which to place the patient.

3. Position yourself to the side of the patient if possible (Figure 1.1).
   Rationale: Although this skill can be performed in any position, it is easier to perform if you are at the patient's side.

4. Place the palm of one hand on the patient's forehead. Place the fingers of your other hand under the bony part of the lower jaw near the chin (Figure 1.2).

5. While applying pressure down on the forehead, simultaneously use the fingers of the other hand to lift the jaw upward, bringing the chin forward. Continue this until the teeth of the lower mouth almost touch the teeth of the upper (Figure 1.3).
   Rationale: Bringing the chin forward allows for the tongue to come off the back of the throat, opening the airway.

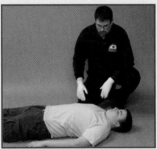

Figure 1.1

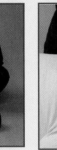

Figure 1.2

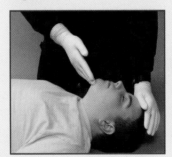

Figure 1.3

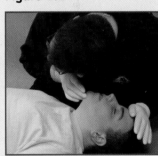

Figure 1.4

6. While maintaining the head-tilt/chin-lift maneuver, assess for breathing and ventilate as needed (Figure 1.4). Apply oxygen as needed.

7. Document findings.
   Rationale: It is extremely important to document your findings in order to have a history of facts and events that occurred at the scene.

Constantly monitor for changes in the patient's status. If no **gag reflex,** is present, consider using an airway adjunct and ensure the patient has a pulse.

▶PROBLEM SOLVING

▷ Use only the bony part of the jaw under the chin during this maneuver. If you use the soft tissue under the chin, an obstruction could occur during this maneuver.

▷ Do not place your finger into the patient's mouth during this maneuver; you may get bitten.

▷ Try not to completely close the mouth during this maneuver.

▷ Be careful not to push on the tongue when grasping the jaw.

▷ An airway adjunct can be used in conjunction with this maneuver.

 PEDIATRIC NOTE:

Note that on a child the airway does not need to be **hyperextended,** just extended (Figure 1.5). If hyperextended, the airway can be occluded or damaged.

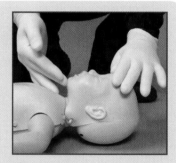

Figure 1.5

▶CASE STUDY

You arrive at the residence of a 53-year-old male. His wife said that he has had a headache all day. When she came into the living room to tell him dinner was ready, she could not wake him up. He is lying on the sofa and is unresponsive even when you shake him. His lips are blue. You and your partner move the patient to the floor. You position yourself at the patient's side and open his airway using the head-tilt/chin-lift maneuver. Then you look, listen, and feel to assess his breathing. He is breathing at 18 times per minute and his heart is beating at 98 times per minute. Your partner then puts the patient on oxygen with a nonrebreather mask at 15 liters per minute (lpm).

The patient's color begins to improve, and he is now responding to pain. You maintain the head-tilt/chin-lift maneuver while transporting the patient to the emergency department. ■

REVIEW QUESTIONS

1. To properly apply the head-tilt/chin-lift maneuver, you should place one hand on the forehead and the other hand:
   a. under the neck.
   b. on the bony part of the chin.
   c. on the soft tissue under the chin.
   d. behind the angle of the jaw.

2. When applying the head-tilt/chin-lift maneuver on a child, it is important not to hyperextend the neck because:
   a. it may cause the tongue to reocclude the airway.
   b. it can cause trauma to the cervical spine.
   c. it is not necessary due to the shape of the airway.
   d. it can cause the trachea to collapse on itself.

3. The head-tilt/chin-lift maneuver would be appropriate for which of the following patients?
   a. a 34-year-old male who is unresponsive after falling from a ladder
   b. a 72-year-old male who slipped in the shower and is unresponsive
   c. a 20-year-old female who is unresponsive with a low blood sugar
   d. a 54-year-old female who is extremely disoriented and confused

CHAPTER 2
Jaw-Thrust Maneuver

KEY TERMS

Angle of the jaw

BSI precautions

Inferior

Jaw-thrust maneuver

Lateral

Neutrally aligned position

Orbits

Unresponsive patient

OBJECTIVE

The student will successfully open the airway with little or no movement to the head or neck.

INTRODUCTION

Securing a patent airway is essential in patients who cannot maintain an open airway for themselves. Such patients are primarily the **unresponsive,** the respiratory arrest, or the cardiac arrest patient.

The airway in these patients is usually obstructed as a result of the loss of muscle tone, which allows the tongue and lower jaw to impede the entry of air into the lungs. The **jaw-thrust maneuver** is the recommended procedure for opening the airway of an unresponsive patient with a suspected head, neck, or spine injury. This is accomplished by lifting the jaw, thus bringing the tongue forward to open the airway, while limiting the movement of the head or neck during the procedure.

►EQUIPMENT

You will need the following BSI equipment:

► Mask
► Gloves
► Eye protection

ASSESSMENT

The patient should be unresponsive and have a suspected head, neck, or spinal injury. In addition, the patient may also have an altered mental status and be suffering from respiratory or cardiac arrest.

PROCEDURE: Jaw-Thrust Maneuver

1. Apply **BSI precautions.**

   Rationale: Gloves and eye protection are required at a minimum, and a gown may be needed if large amounts of blood or fluid are present to prevent exposure to infectious diseases.

2. The patient should be in the supine position. If she is not, carefully keep the patient in a **neutrally aligned position** and roll her as a unit into the supine position.

   Rationale: Although this maneuver can be done in any position, the supine position is the best position.

3. Position yourself at the top of the patient's head, if possible.

   Rationale: This position allows you the best access for the maneuver.

4. Without moving the head and neck, carefully place one hand on either side of the patient's head near the **orbits** (Figure 2.1).

   Rationale: Any movement of the head defeats the purpose of this maneuver.

5. Place your thumbs just **inferior** to the eyes and **lateral** to the nose. Using your fingers, place them at the **angle of the jaw** below the ears (Figures 2.2 and 2.3).

   Rationale: The thumb position allows you to maintain the head position during the maneuver.

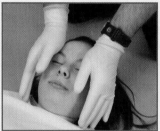 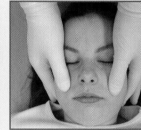

Figure 2.1   Figure 2.2

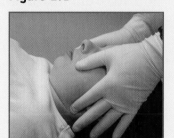 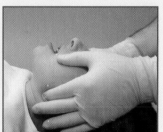

Figure 2.3   Figure 2.4

6. Without moving the head and neck and using your index and middle fingers, pull the angle of the jaw forward (Figure 2.4).

   Rationale: Again, any movement of the head will defeat the purpose of this maneuver. Jutting the jaw forward allows for the tongue to come off the back of the throat, opening the airway.

continued...

7. While maintaining the jaw-thrust maneuver and not moving the head, assess for breathing and ventilate as needed (Figure 2.5). Apply oxygen as needed.

   Rationale: Make certain that you do not push down on the jaw while ventilating the patient because the pressure can cause the lower jaw to be pushed posteriorly, causing the tongue to occlude the airway.

8. Document findings.

   Rationale: It is extremely important to document your findings in order to have a history of facts and events that occurred at the scene.

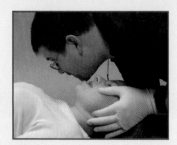

Figure 2.5

ONGOING ASSESSMENT

Constantly monitor for changes in the patient's status. If no gag reflex is present, consider using an airway adjunct and ensure the patient has a pulse.

▶PROBLEM SOLVING

▷ The jaw-thrust maneuver should be considered for a patient who needs an open airway and has a suspected head, neck, and/or spinal injury.

▷ Do not place your finger into the patient's mouth during this maneuver; you may get bitten.

▷ Try not to close the mouth during this maneuver.

▷ An airway adjunct can be used in conjunction with this maneuver.

▶CASE STUDY

You respond to an intersection where a 17-year-old female was hit by a car while riding her bicycle. The patient is lying supine on the ground and appears unresponsive. The patient had been wearing a helmet, but it fell off after she hit the pavement. You notice a large hematoma on the front of her head. She remains unresponsive when your partner attempts to use painful stimuli to wake her. Because of the trauma involved, you suspect that the patient could have a spinal injury. You position yourself at the head of the patient and open her airway using the jaw-thrust maneuver, being careful to keep the head and neck in a neutral position. The patient is breathing at 26 times per minute and has adequate chest rise and fall. You maintain the jaw-thrust maneuver while your partner applies a cervical collar and places the patient on oxygen with a nonrebreather mask at 15 lpm. The patient is "packaged" on the backboard and then transported to the emergency department. You maintain the jaw-thrust maneuver throughout the transport. ■

1. The correct position for placing the hands when performing the jaw-thrust maneuver is to:
   a. place your fingers under the angle of the jaw, and place your thumbs inferior to the bottom lip.
   b. place your fingers under the angle of the jaw, and place your thumbs on the cheeks.
   c. place your hand on the patient's forehead, and place your fingers under the angle of the jaw.
   d. place your thumbs in the patient's mouth, and place your fingers under the angle of the jaw.

2. The goal of the jaw-thrust maneuver is to:
   a. displace the tongue without moving the head or neck.
   b. stimulate the trauma patient, making him breathe.
   c. prevent the trauma patient from needing oxygen.
   d. secure the airway in a patient with suspected trauma.

3. The jaw-thrust maneuver would be most appropriate for which of the following patients?
   a. a 22-year-old male who was in an accident and is disoriented
   b. a 74-year-old female who is unresponsive in a wheelchair
   c. a 56-year-old male who fell down a flight stairs and is unresponsive
   d. a 38-year-old female who tripped and fell and is now complaining of neck pain

CHAPTER 3
Use of a Pocket Mask

KEY TERMS

Angle of the jaw

Aspiration

BSI precautions

Hyperventilation

Mandible

Nasopharyngeal airway

Oropharyngeal airway

Pocket mask

OBJECTIVE

The student will successfully apply a pocket mask when indicated.

INTRODUCTION

Various techniques are used to ventilate a patient. Mouth-to-mask ventilation is one of those options. The primary advantage of a **pocket mask** is its ability to be more accessible to the EMT-Basic when needed. Because pocket masks are small and compact, many EMT-Basics carry them with them when they are on or off duty.

Pocket masks are different than the shield barrier devices used in ventilation because they have a clear face mask with a one-way valve that allows for ventilation through the mask while preventing the patient's exhaled air from coming back through the valve and into the rescuer's mouth. Some pocket masks have a filter in addition to the one-way valve, which increases the barrier protection. Some pocket masks come with an oxygen inlet, which allows the EMT-Basic to significantly increase the concentration of oxygen delivered to the patient.

▶ EQUIPMENT

You will need the following equipment:

- ▶ BSI equipment
- ▶ Pocket mask with one-way valve
- ▶ Suction if available
- ▶ Oxygen extension tubing
- ▶ Oxygen tank and regulator

ASSESSMENT

Assess the airway by checking breathing rate, tidal volume, and quality. Check circulation and skin signs.

PROCEDURE: Application of a Pocket Mask

1. Apply **BSI precautions.**

   Rationale: Gloves and eye protection are required at a minimum, and a gown may be needed if large amounts of blood or fluid are present to prevent exposure to infectious diseases.

2. Position yourself at the head end of the patient if possible.

   Rationale: Although you can use a pocket mask from any position, the head end of the patient is the preferred position.

3. Open airway using the jaw-thrust maneuver.

   Rationale: Although you can use the head-tilt/chin-lift maneuver, the jaw-thrust maneuver is preferable.

4. Clear **oropharyngeal** and **nasopharyngeal airways** if necessary.

   Rationale: Ventilating a patient without a patent airway could cause an airway obstruction and/or **aspiration.**

5. Suction as necessary.

   Rationale: Ventilating a patient without a clear airway could cause an airway obstruction and/or aspiration.

6. Insert oropharyngeal (OP) or nasopharyngeal (NP) airway if available.

   Rationale: Using an OP or NP airway assists in maintaining an open airway. Refer to Chapters 5 and 6.

7. Connect oxygen tubing to pocket mask oxygen inlet (if available) (Figure 3.1).

   Rationale: Without oxygen attached, the concentration of oxygen would be approximately 17 percent. Attaching oxygen can significantly increase the concentration of oxygen.

8. Turn the oxygen regulator liter flow gauge to 15 liters per minute (or higher if available) (Figure 3.2).

   Rationale: Using the highest liter flow provides the patient with the maximum concentration of oxygen.

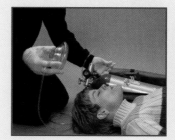

Figure 3.1

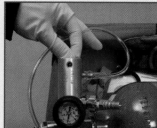

Figure 3.2

continued...

9. Center the pocket mask on the patient's face so the triangle is over the bridge of the patient's nose and the larger portion of the mask is placed between the lower lip and the chin (Figure 3.3).

   Rationale: This positioning provides the best seal for the mask.

10. While holding the mask firmly in place, place your thumbs over the top side of the mask and place your little, ring, middle, and index fingers on the patient's **mandible,** near the **angle of the jaw.** Some people may have to place their index and sometimes even middle fingers on the mask due to hand size. Simultaneously using the index, middle, ring, and little fingers, pull the jaw up toward the mask (Figure 3.4).

    Rationale: This continues to provide the best seal for the mask.

11. While continuing to make a seal between the mask and the patient's face, take a deep breath and exhale slowly into the one-way valve at the top of the mask (Figure 3.5).

    Rationale: You should feel no resistance during this ventilation. If you meet resistance, consider reopening the airway.

12. Adult ventilation should be delivered over a 1- to 2-second period, and the rate of ventilations should be at least one breath every 5 seconds. Watch for **hyperventilation.**

    Rationale: Ventilations at a lower rate could cause the patient to get hypoxic.

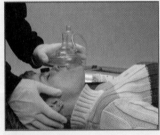
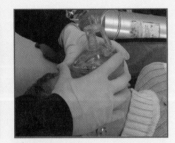

Figure 3.3   **Figure 3.4**

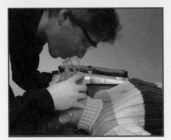
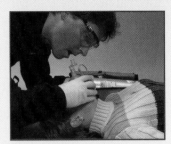

Figure 3.5   **Figure 3.6**

> **PEDIATRIC NOTE:**
>
> Children's and infant's ventilations should be delivered over 1 to 1.5 seconds, and the rate of ventilations should be at least one breath every 3 seconds.
>
> **Rationale:** Children and infants breathe faster than adults.

13. Remove your mouth from the one-way valve during each exhalation (Figure 3.6).

    Rationale: This allows for exhaled air to passively leave the mask.

14. If the patient does not have a pulse and both ventilations and compressions are necessary, perform CPR as usual. If alone consider using the attached head strap on the pocket mask to assist in maintaining alignment of the pocket mask on the patient.

    Rationale: The head strap, if available, maintains the mask in position over the patient's face. Although you need to make a seal each time, use of the head strap can reduce the time required to provide additional ventilations.

15. Document findings.

    Rationale: It is extremely important to document your findings in order to have a history of facts and events that occurred at the scene.

The patient should be constantly monitored during ventilations for chest rise and the lung compliance of each ventilation. The patient's condition should improve.

▶PROBLEM SOLVING

▶ Although the pocket mask has a one-way valve to reduce the chances of the EMT-Basic coming into contact with a patient's body fluids, the risk of such contact is still higher than with other forms of assisted ventilations. It is essential to maintain good BSI precautions when using a pocket mask. If there is any question that the patient could have a communicable disease, consult local policies and seriously consider using a bag-valve-mask unit and wearing a mask and eye shield.

▶ A mustache or beard on a patient should not interfere with the use of a pocket mask.

▶ If you notice fluids or vomit in the clear face mask during ventilation, immediately discontinue ventilations and clear the airway, including suctioning if necessary.

▶ Conserve energy while using a pocket mask—you never know how long you may have to continue to ventilate the patient.

 PEDIATRIC NOTE:

Pocket masks are usually sized for adult patients. A pocket mask may not make a tight seal on pediatric patients.

▶CASE STUDY

You are with your family at the mall when an elderly female in the store collapses. You go to the patient and find that she is unresponsive and is not breathing, but she does have a pulse. Fortunately, your wife carries a pocket mask in her purse. You remove the pocket mask from the case and assemble the one-way valve. You open the patient's airway with the head-tilt/chin-lift maneuver and place the pocket mask on the patient. You proceed to administer one breath every 5 seconds.

A security guard approaches with an automatic external defibrillator and oxygen. You hook the oxygen up to the pocket mask and continue to ventilate the patient, ensuring adequate chest rise and fall with each ventilation. Shortly after, members of the fire department arrive and begin to ventilate the patient with a bag-valve-mask unit. The patient is still not breathing on her own, but her color has improved. A firefighter secures the airway and packages the patient for transport to the emergency department, thanking you for your help prior to leaving. ■

(continued)

1. When delivering ventilations through a pocket mask, ventilations should be:
   a. delivered over 1 to 2 seconds.
   b. delivered over 1 to 1.5 seconds.
   c. delivered forcefully to ensure chest rise and fall.
   d. delivered at the same time as chest compressions.

2. Use of a pocket mask ensures that there is no cross-contamination between the patient and the rescuer.
   a. true
   b. false

3. Which of the following is *not* a feature of a pocket mask?
   a. one-way valve
   b. oxygen inlet
   c. filter
   d. airway adjunct

CHAPTER 4
Bag-Valve-Mask Ventilation, Two-Person Technique

OBJECTIVE

The student will be able to successfully perform bag-valve-mask ventilation.

INTRODUCTION

In most EMS systems, the bag-valve-mask (BVM) unit is the preferred method of ventilation over mouth-to-mouth, mouth-to-mask, and mechanical ventilation. The BVM consists of a self-inflating bag with a one-way **nonrebreather valve,** a face mask, and an attached oxygen supplemental **reservoir bag** or tube attached.

BVMs come in many brands and are available in both single-use and multiple-use modules. They come in many sizes but only one size BVM is used in adults; the volume of these adult bags is 1,600 mL. The volume generated by the BVM is directly related to the abilities of the EMS provider. If the BVM is attached to oxygen, the amount of volume needed to ventilate the average size adult patient is 500 mL, delivered over 1 to 2 seconds.

The BVM is not as easy to use as you might think. Trying to make a tight seal while simultaneously squeezing the bag may compromise ventilations. This is why, if possible, two EMS providers should be present when the BVM is being used. One provider makes the mask seal and the other provider squeezes the bag. The BVM can be used in conjunction with oral and nasal airways. The BVM can be used directly with advanced life support airways.

KEY TERMS

Bag-valve-mask ventilation

BSI precautions

Head-tilt/chin-lift
    maneuver

Jaw-thrust maneuver

Nasopharyngeal airway
    (NPA)

Nonrebreather valve

Oropharyngeal airway
    (OPA)

Reservoir bag

Spontaneous respirations

Supine position

▶ EQUIPMENT

You will need the following equipment and preferably two EMS providers:

- ▶ BSI equipment
- ▶ Oropharyngeal or nasopharyngeal airway (OPA) or (NPA)
- ▶ Suction
- ▶ Bag-valve-mask unit with attached oxygen reservoir
- ▶ Full oxygen tank and regulator

ASSESSMENT

The patient should be in a **supine position.** Assess respiratory rate, volume, and skin signs. If patient shows signs of anoxia, bradypnea, or hypoventilation, ventilation will be required. Inspect the patient for the proper size BVM. Inspect the BVM prior to usage for its integrity. Patients need to have a patent airway for the BVM to accomplish ventilations. If the airway is not patent, or if it is obstructed, the EMS provider must do airway obstruction maneuvers. If the airway has any fluids in it, suction should be accomplished prior to ventilations.

PROCEDURE: Bag-Valve-Mask Ventilation, Two-Person Technique

1. Apply **BSI precautions.**

   Rationale: Gloves and eye protection are required at a minimum, and a gown may be needed if large amounts of blood or fluid are present to prevent exposure to infectious diseases. This skill has great risks of exposure to body fluids. Complete BSI is a must when using a BVM.

2. Check patient for the proper size BVM.

   Rationale: In most cases the EMS provider has a choice between an adult, child, or infant BVM. The wrong size BVM could cause over- or underinsufflation.

3. Check bag for integrity.

   Rationale: If the BVM has been stored in a folded position for a long period of time, its integrity may be compromised. This may cause a reduction in the volume the BVM could deliver.

4. The patient should be in a supine position.

   Rationale: The only time you should attempt to ventilate a patient in any position other than the supine position is in cases of prolonged extrication.

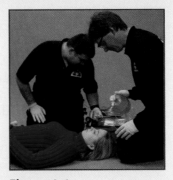

Figure 4.1

5. If possible, position yourself at the head of the patient. A second EMT may be at her side (Figure 4.1).

   Rationale: This position is the easiest position from which to open the airway and make a good seal with the BVM.

6. Open the airway (consider alternate maneuver for trauma).

   Rationale: Use the standard **head-tilt/chin-lift maneuver** to establish an airway. Consider the **jaw-thrust maneuver** in the suspected trauma patient.

7. Visualize the airway for materials and fluid (consider suction if needed).

   Rationale: Visualizing the airway is important. You do not want to ventilate a patient who has fluids or other materials in the upper airway because obstruction of the airway or aspiration of the fluid could occur. Suction of fluids is essential before placing the mask on the patient.

8. Insert an **oropharyngeal (OPA)** or **nasopharyngeal airway (NPA)** if available.

   Rationale: An OPA or NPA assists in maintaining an open airway and can make ventilation easier for the EMT. At no time should ventilations be delayed while accessing an oropharyngeal or nasopharyngeal airway. It is acceptable to initially ventilate a patient with a BVM and place the OPA or NPA at a later time.

9. The first EMT centers the mask on the patient's face so the triangle is over the bridge of the patient's nose, and the larger portion of the mask is placed between the lower lip and the chin. While holding the mask firmly in place, place your thumbs over the top side of the mask and place your little, ring, middle, and index fingers under the patient's jaw, near the angle of the jaw. Simultaneously using the index, middle, ring, and little fingers, pull the jaw up toward the mask (Figures 4.2 and 4.3).

   Rationale: Placing the hands in this position makes the best possible seal. Individuals with small hands might find that this is a little more difficult and may have to modify their hand position to find the best mask fit.

10. The second EMT begins squeezing the bag slowly at the desired breaths per minute. Ventilations should be delivered at a minimum of once every 5 seconds in adults and once every 3 seconds in children and infants. Each ventilation should be delivered over 2 seconds in adults (Figure 4.4).

    Rationale: It is *VERY* important for the EMT *NOT* to squeeze the bag too fast or too aggressively. The bag needs time to inflate and the patient needs time to expire air before trying to reinsufflate. Being too aggressive at squeezing the bag can cause the pressure in the upper airways to get too high. High pressure with a tight mask seal will cause air to go into the esophagus and then to the stomach. This may lead to vomiting and possibly to aspiration.

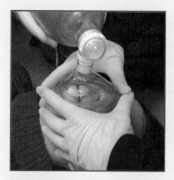 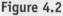 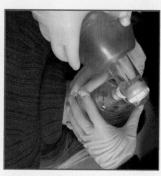

Figure 4.2   **Figure 4.3**

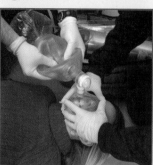

Figure 4.4

11. If not already attached, the BVM should be attached to the oxygen cylinder as soon as possible and placed at the highest possible liter flow.

    Rationale: Attaching the BVM to oxygen is important, but not as important as ventilating the patient. Initially it may be important to assist ventilations without oxygen and then, as soon as possible, connect the BVM to oxygen. Oxygen connected to a BVM reduces the required volume. This is *VERY* important when trying to ventilate large adults. Increasing the concentration of oxygen to a BVM also reduces hypoxia quicker. Make sure you connect the BVM to the oxygen reservoir correctly.

12. Visualize the chest for chest rise on each ventilation.

    Rationale: Each time you ventilate, you should see the chest rise. This visualization helps the EMT determine if the ventilations are being done properly.

continued...

13. Feel the compliance (ease of ventilation) of the bag on each ventilation (Figure 4.5).

Rationale: Each time you ventilate the patient, you should feel the compliance of the lungs (slight resistance). This is normal and ensures proper ventilations. If it is difficult to ventilate and you have to be too aggressive in squeezing the bag, consider the presence of an airway obstruction.

14. If no chest rise is observed during ventilation, consider the presence of an airway obstruction.

Rationale: Trying to forcefully ventilate an obstructed patient can make the obstruction worse. It is important to clear the obstruction before ventilating.

15. Continue to monitor the patient's airway, level of consciousness, and respiratory effort. Auscultation of the chest is advisable.

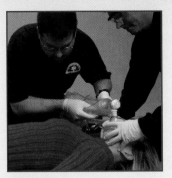

Figure 4.5

16. Document use and proper ventilations.

Rationale: It is extremely important to document your findings in order to have a history of facts and events that occurred at the scene.

ONGOING ASSESSMENT

Patients should be constantly monitored during ventilations for chest rise and the compliance of ventilations. If the patient responds with **spontaneous respirations,** reassess for adequacy of these respirations. An OPA or NPA should be inserted as soon as possible to assist the BVM in accomplishing proper ventilations. Constantly monitor for vomiting and oral secretions during ventilation. Suction as necessary.

▶PROBLEM SOLVING

▷ Use of a BVM should be a last resort. When one EMT tries to accomplish BVM ventilations alone, it is difficult to make a seal and squeeze the bag at the same time to get adequate volume. In some cases one, if not both, of these steps are compromised. This is even more dramatic when the EMS provider has small hands or the patient is large. Two EMS providers, however, can usually provide BVM ventilations efficiently.

▷ If you do not see chest rise or if you hear a leak in the mask, reposition the patient's head, again make a seal with the mask, and attempt to ventilate.

▷ Recent literature has described situations in which EMS providers may squeeze the bag at significantly high pressures. This is accomplished by squeezing the bag too vigorously.

PEDIATRIC NOTE:

Ventilate the infant once every 3 seconds for 1 to 1.5 seconds. Excess pressures can cause gastric distension, vomiting, and the possibility of aspiration (Figure 4.6).

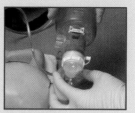

Figure 4.6

▶ Using a BVM is very difficult in the patient with a suspected spinal injury. Maintaining an open airway along with neutral alignment, while simultaneously using a BVM and ventilating, are extremely difficult. Using an OPA or NPA and having two EMS providers providing ventilations can make this process significantly more effective.

▶ Most BVMs have clear masks. These masks make it easy to visualize materials (for example, vomit) and fluids that may be in the airway. If the patient is ventilated, these materials and/or fluids can be aspirated. If this occurs, immediately remove the mask and suction the airway.

▶ Masks do not fit all patients, and you might experience difficulty ventilating certain patients. Patients with small or large faces, patients with mustaches and beards, patients with dental apparatus removed, trauma patients with C-collars applied, and facial trauma patients can present difficulties for BVM ventilation. Consider using a different size mask if possible or do your best at finding the best mask position that accomplishes the best ventilation.

▶ If you feel that the compliance of the bag during squeezing is difficult or is getting more difficult, consider the presence of an airway obstruction or increased pressure in the chest cavity in these patients.

▶ If you use a multiple-use BVM, make sure that the BVM is cleaned properly before reusing.

PEDIATRIC AND GERIATRIC NOTE:

In both the pediatric and the geriatric patient, the airways are more fragile and are more easily damaged with extensive pressure. Make sure that these patients are ventilated over 2 seconds with each compression of the bag. To avoid overventilation, monitor the chest rise during each ventilation. Make sure that you use the proper size BVM device for pediatric patients.

▶CASE STUDY

You respond to a residence where a 26-year-old female has taken an overdose of a prescription painkiller. The patient's family found her in bed and could not wake her up. You find the patient in the bed, unresponsive and cyanotic. The patient is breathing very shallow at 4 times per minute. You ask your partner for the bag-valve-mask unit while you open the patient's airway with a head-tilt/chin-lift maneuver. You place the mask on the patient and maintain a good mask seal with both hands as your partner begins to ventilate the patient every 5 seconds. Your partner ensures that there is adequate chest rise and fall with every ventilation. Your partner hooks the BVM to oxygen and continues to ventilate the patient at 20 times per minute. The patient's color begins to improve as does her mental status. You continue to ventilate the patient as a team until backup arrives to assist with the packaging and transport of this patient to the emergency department. ■

(continued)

1. Why is it preferable to utilize the two-person technique for bag-valve-mask ventilations?

   a. It allows for less strain on the person administering ventilations.

   b. It improves the quality of the face mask seal and ventilations.

   c. It allows for simultaneous ventilations and compressions.

   d. It allows for ventilations and manual airway maneuvers.

2. When using a bag-valve-mask device for ventilations, you know you have delivered enough air when:

   a. the BVM is compressed completely.

   b. it becomes difficult to ventilate the patient.

   c. the chest begins to rise.

   d. the patient begins to improve.

3. Which of the following is *not* necessary when administering ventilations with a BVM device?

   a. an oropharyngeal or nasopharyngeal airway

   b. BSI precautions

   c. manual airway maneuvers

   d. cervical spine immobilization

CHAPTER 5
Insertion of an Oropharyngeal Airway

OBJECTIVE
The student will successfully learn to insert the oropharyngeal airway.

INTRODUCTION

An **oropharyngeal airway (OPA)** or oral airway is a curved device, usually made of plastic. It has a flange that rests on the patient's lips. The rest of the device helps to hold the tongue away from the back of the throat. The OPA is considered an airway adjunct because it must be used in conjunction with manual airway maneuvers. The two commonly used oral airways are the Cathguide®, which is solid and has a hole through the center, and one that has channels on each side. OPAs are disposable and come in many sizes for adults, children, and infants. An entire set should be carried to ensure for quick proper selection.

The OPA may be used in conjunction with a bag-valve mask and is strongly suggested in any patient without a **gag reflex** in which assisted ventilations are necessary.

KEY TERMS
Angle of the jaw

Aspiration

BSI precautions

Cross-finger technique

Gag reflex

Oropharyngeal airway (OPA)

Painful stimulus

Tongue blade

Unresponsive

Upper airway

Uvula

▶ **EQUIPMENT**

You will need the following equipment:

▶ BSI equipment
▶ Full set of oropharyngeal airways
▶ Suction unit with a rigid suction catheter
▶ **Tongue blade** (optional)

ASSESSMENT

The use of an OPA should be considered in any patient who is not breathing or who is **unresponsive,** that is, where a gag reflex is not present. Use of a **painful stimulus** is a good technique to determine if the patient lacks a gag reflex. Insertion of an oral airway in a patient with a gag reflex can cause him or her to vomit, drastically increasing the chances of **aspiration.** It can also trigger spasms in the **upper airway.**

Examining the patient for the proper size is important. An improperly sized OPA can cause an airway obstruction. When measured, the airway should extend from the corner of the mouth to the bottom of the **angle of the jaw** or, if rotated, to the tip of the earlobe. If the patient starts to gag during insertion of the airway, immediately remove the airway.

PROCEDURE: Insertion of an Oropharyngeal Airway

1. Apply **BSI precautions.**
   Rationale: Gloves and goggles are required at a minimum, and a gown may be needed if large amounts of blood or fluid are present to prevent exposure to infectious diseases.

2. Place the patient in a supine position. If no spinal injury is suspected, the neck may be hyperextended. If there is the possibility of a spinal injury, the jaw-thrust maneuver should be used, making only the necessary movements to ensure an open airway.

   Rationale: Although an OPA can be inserted from any position, the supine position is the suggested position for this technique. If the patient has a suspected spinal injury, caution should be used to reduce cervical spinal movement. The jaw-thrust maneuver reduces spinal movement.

3. Determine if the patient has a gag reflex.
   Rationale: Use of a painful stimulus is a good technique to determine if the patient lacks a gag reflex. Insertion of an oral airway in a patient with a gag reflex can cause him or her to vomit, drastically increasing the chances of aspiration. It can also trigger spasms in the upper airway.

4. Select the proper size oral airway. Start by measuring the airway. When measured, the airway should extend from the corner of the mouth to the bottom of the angle of the jaw or, if rotated, to the tip of the earlobe (Figure 5.1).

   Rationale: The wrong size airway could cause an airway obstruction and/or not accomplish the opening of the airway.

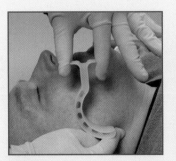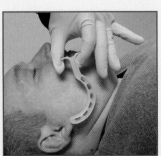

Figure 5.1

5. Open the patient's mouth using the **cross-finger technique.** To do this, cross the thumb and forefinger of one hand and place them on the upper and lower teeth at the corner of the patient's mouth. Spread your fingers apart to open the patient's jaws (Figure 5.2).

   Rationale: This technique is the best one for allowing the EMT to open the mouth of the patient while reducing injury to the patient and the EMT.

6. While doing the cross-finger technique, insert the airway with the tip pointing to the roof of the patient's mouth (Figure 5.3).

   Rationale: Although this seems to be the reverse of the way the airway should be inserted, this positioning allows the airway to be inserted without touching the tongue and possibly pushing it back where it can obstruct the airway.

7. Insert the airway and slide it along the roof of the mouth, past the **uvula** (soft tissue hanging down from the back), or until resistance is met against the soft palate. Be careful not to push the tongue back during this procedure (Figure 5.4).

   Rationale: Pushing the tongue back could obstruct the airway.

8. Gently rotate the airway 180 degrees. Continue to advance the oral airway until it lies flat on the top of the tongue. Stop advancing when the flange at the top of the airway rests against the patient's mouth. If the airway is too long or short, remove the airway and replace it with the correct size. Immediately stop and remove the airway if the gag reflex is stimulated. You do not need to rotate the device when removing it (Figures 5.5).

   Rationale: The flange keeps the airway in place and keeps it from moving down the airway. Stop insertion if the patient has a gag reflex to reduce the risk of vomiting and aspiration.

9. Place the mask you will use for ventilation over the airway adjunct you have inserted. If no barrier

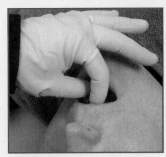

Figure 5.2

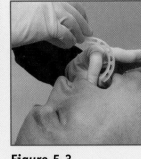

Figure 5.3

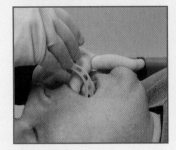

Figure 5.4

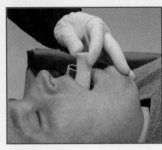

Figure 5.5

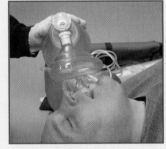

Figure 5.6

device is available, proceed with mouth-to-adjunct ventilation just as you would with mouth-to-mouth ventilation (Figure 5.6).

10. Reassess the patient's breathing and begin ventilations.

11. Document insertion of oral airway and any changes in the patient's condition.

   Rationale: It is extremely important to document your findings in order to have a history of facts and events that occurred at the scene.

ONGOING ASSESSMENT

Constantly assess patient respirations. Monitor for a gag reflex. If a gag reflex returns, immediately remove the airway.

▶ PROBLEM SOLVING

▶ If the patient's mental status improves and a gag reflex returns, the airway should be removed immediately. This can be accomplished by grasping the flange at the top of the airway and pulling it down toward the chin. Suction should be available during this process, because patients will often vomit during removal of an OPA.

 Improper oral airway sizing can obstruct the airway. It is imperative that you size each patient before inserting the airway.

 If you are aggressive during insertion of an OPA, you can cause trauma, spasms, and swelling in the upper airways. Remember to insert the airway gently. This is especially important in the suspected head trauma patient who may have fractures of the soft palate.

 An optional insertion technique using a tongue blade can be used. In this technique, the tongue blade is inserted in the patient's mouth and used to hold the tongue down while inserting the OPA. Rotation of the OPA is not necessary when using this technique.

 Suctioning may be difficult to perform with the airway in place. The OPA may obstruct vomitus from escaping from the mouth. Remove the airway to maintain a clear airway during vomiting.

 An oral airway might be used as a bite block in suspected seizure patients. Use only the tip of the airway to keep the teeth from coming together.

 In some cases, you will see an oral airway inserted after an endotracheal tube has been inserted. The airway is being used as a bite block to protect the endotracheal tube.

PEDIATRIC NOTE:

In pediatric patients, be sure to size the OPA properly. The wrong size airway could cause an obstruction (Figure 5.7). The rotational method of OPA insertion is not recommended in pediatric patients because of their relatively fragile airway structures.

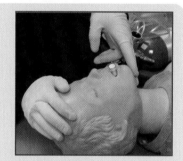

Figure 5.7

CASE STUDY

You and your partner respond to a patient in cardiac arrest. You arrive to find a 68-year-old unresponsive male. The patient is not breathing and does not have a carotid pulse. You open the airway with a head-tilt/chin-lift maneuver and and prepare to ventilate the patient with a bag-valve mask. You have some difficulty ventilating the patient. Your partner begins chest compressions. You hook the BVM to oxygen and reposition the patient's head in preparation for the next cycle of ventilations.

You still have some difficulty ventilating the patient and choose to insert an oropharyngeal airway while your partner resumes chest compressions. You size an OPA and elect to insert it using a tongue blade. You displace the tongue and insert the airway until the flange rests on the teeth. You reposition the head using the head-tilt/chin-lift maneuver and begin to ventilate. The patient ventilates easily, and you notice adequate chest rise and fall. You continue alternating compressions and ventilations until advanced life support personnel arrive. The patient remains easy to ventilate throughout the call. ■

1. An oropharyngeal airway should be considered in which of the following patients?

   a. a 37-year-old female who responds to painful stimuli

   b. a 28-year-old male who is going in and out of consciousness

   c. a 66-year-old female diabetic with decreased responsiveness

   d. a 70-year-old male who is unresponsive following a seizure

2. Which of the following is considered an acceptable method for inserting an oropharyngeal airway?

   a. Insert the airway in the correct anatomical position, while opening the airway with the jaw-thrust maneuver.

   b. Insert the airway in the correct anatomical position, using a tongue blade to provide for easy insertion.

   c. Insert the airway with the tip pointing up, using a tongue blade to displace the tongue while rotating the airway.

   d. Insert the airway with the tip pointing to the roof of the mouth, gently rotating the airway 360 degrees.

3. Which of the following would be the most appropriate action when a patient vomits while an oropharyngeal airway is in place?

   a. Suction the airway before removing the airway to prevent aspiration.

   b. Remove the airway, suction, then quickly reinsert the airway.

   c. Remove the airway, suction, consider alternative airway adjuncts.

   d. There is no need to suction because the airway adjunct reduces the risk of aspiration.

CHAPTER 6
Insertion of a Nasopharyngeal Airway

OBJECTIVE
The student will be able to successfully insert a nasopharyngeal airway.

INTRODUCTION

The **nasopharyngeal airway**—more commonly called the nasal airway or NPA—is a disposable, uncuffed plastic or soft rubber tube. Varying from 17 to 20 cm in length, its diameter ranges from 20 to 36 French. At the **proximal** end, a funnel-shaped projection and ring help prevent the tube from slipping inside the patient's nose. The beveled **distal** end makes it easier to insert the tube, and the airway's slightly curved design allows it to follow the natural curvature of the **nasopharynx.** When in place, the NPA rests between the tongue and the posterior **pharyngeal** wall, thus maintaining an open airway.

The nasal airway is considered an airway adjunct, because it *must be* used in conjunction with manual airway maneuvers. Although still secondary in use to oropharyngeal airways (OPAs), the nasal airway has gained in popularity. Some EMT-Basics prefer the NPA over the OPA because it does not stimulate a **gag reflex.**

The nasal airway may be used in conjunction with BVM ventilation. It is strongly recommended in any patient who requires assisted ventilations.

► EQUIPMENT

You will need the following equipment:

- ▶ BSI equipment
- ▶ Nasopharyngeal airway
- ▶ **Water-soluble lubricant**
- ▶ Suction equipment

ASSESSMENT

Nasal airways should be used in any unresponsive patient where a gag reflex is not present with insertion. As mentioned, the nasal airway is less likely to cause a gag reflex than an oral airway. If, however, while inserting a nasal airway in a patient, a gag reflex occurs, be aware that this can cause vomiting and dramatically increase the chances of **aspiration** or spasms of the upper airway. Patients who are not breathing should always be considered candidates for nasal airway usage.

Be careful to select the proper length nasal airway. A tube that is too small may not extend past the tongue, causing airway obstruction. A tube that is too long could enter the esophagus and cause gastric distention and/or inadequate ventilation. When measured, the airway should extend from the tip of the nose to the earlobe. Choosing the correct length will also ensure the proper diameter. If the patient should start to gag during insertion of the airway, immediately stop the insertion. Caution should be used when inserting the airway in a patient with suspected facial trauma. If you meet resistance during the insertion process, withdraw and gently try again or switch to the other nares. Do *NOT* push or force the airway; considerable trauma could result.

PROCEDURE: Insertion of a Nasopharyngeal Airway

1. Apply **BSI precautions.**

   Rationale: Gloves and eye protection are required at a minimum, and a gown may be needed if large amounts of blood or fluid are present to prevent exposure to infectious diseases.

2. Place the patient preferably in a supine position.

   Rationale: Although the NPA can be inserted in any position, the supine position is the suggested position for this technique.

3. Assess the level of responsiveness.

   Rationale: Although the NPA sometimes can be inserted in a patient with a slight gag reflex, it is best accomplished in the unresponsive patient.

4. Select the proper size nasal airway. The airway should extend from the tip of the nose to the earlobe (Figure 6.1).

   Rationale: The wrong size airway could cause an airway obstruction and/or not accomplish the opening of the airway.

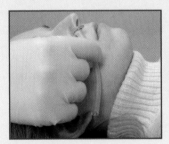

Figure 6.1

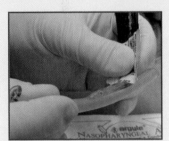

Figure 6.2

5. Apply a water-soluble lubricant to the NPA before inserting (Figure 6.2).

   Rationale: Water-soluble lubricant allows for easier insertion of the airway and reduces injury to the nasal passage.

   continued...

6. Gently insert the airway with the bevel (angled portion at the tip) pointing toward the base of the nostril or toward the **septum** (wall that separates nostrils) (Figure 6.3).

   Rationale: Gentle insertion reduces nasal trauma.

7. Slowly push the airway into the nostril. By slightly rotating the airway from side to side, you may make insertion easier (Figure 6.4). *You should never force the airway into the nostril.* If you meet resistance, remove the airway, apply new lubrication, and try inserting it into the other nostril. If the patient begins to gag at any stage of this procedure, immediately stop advancing the airway and remove it.

   Rationale: The slight rotation allows for easier insertion and reduces nasal trauma. Sometimes one nostril can be obstructed; trying the other nostril will make insertion easier and reduce trauma. Any forced insertion can cause nasal trauma, which can cause bleeding and aspiration.

8. Stop advancing the airway when the proximal ring has come in contact with the end of the nostril (Figure 6.5).

9. Assess the patient's breathing. Apply supplemental oxygen or begin ventilations as necessary.

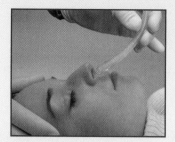

Figure 6.3

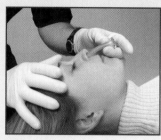

Figure 6.4

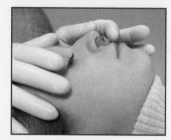

Figure 6.5

10. Document insertion of nasal airway.

    Rationale: It is extremely important to document your findings in order to have a history of facts and events that occurred at the scene.

ONGOING ASSESSMENT

Constantly assess patient respirations. Monitor for gag reflex. If a gag reflex occurs, immediately remove the airway. Because improper insertion can cause bleeding in the nostril, be sure to examine the posterior pharynx for any bleeding that may have occurred and suction if necessary.

▶ PROBLEM SOLVING

▶ If the patient's level of consciousness improves and a gag reflex returns, the airway should be removed immediately. This can be accomplished by grasping the proximal end of the airway and pulling it directly out. Suction should be made immediately available during this process, because patients will often vomit during the removal process.

▶ Improper nasal airway sizing can cause an airway obstruction. It is imperative that you size each patient before inserting the airway.

▶ It is very important to lubricate the airway. Do not consider insertion without lubrication. Insertion without lubrication could cause trauma to the nostrils and bleeding in the upper airway.

▶ If you are aggressive during the insertion process, you can cause trauma, spasms, swelling, and/or bleeding to the upper airways. Remember, gently insert the nasal airway. This is very important in the suspected head trauma patient who could have facial fractures in the airway. It can be dangerous to insert in the head trauma patient with basular skull fractures because this could cause further injuries.

▶ The nasal airway may prevent vomitus from escaping from the mouth. Suctioning could be hampered with the airway inserted. Remove the airway to maintain a clear airway during vomiting.

 PEDIATRIC NOTE:
In most EMS systems, child and infant-sized NPAs are not available.

▶CASE STUDY

You are called to respond to the residence of a 25-year-old male who has reportedly had a seizure. On arrival, you find the patient lying on the couch on his left side. After speaking to his girlfriend, you realize that he has a seizure disorder and was lying on the couch when he began to seize. You determine that the patient does not have much risk for a cervical spinal injury and decide not to immobilize his spine.

Your assessment reveals the patient to be responsive to a deep sternal rub but not awake or arousable to verbal stimulation. He has snoring respirations and is breathing at a rate of 14 times per minute. His pulse is 84 and regular. You determine that the patient is most likely in a postictal state and that he needs to have his airway opened until he regains consciousness. After performing a head-tilt/chin-lift maneuver, the snoring ceases. Realizing that the patient needs continuous airway support during his state of altered mentation, you make the decision to insert an airway adjunct. You choose to insert a nasal airway to prevent stimulation of the patient's gag reflex.

After inserting the nasal airway, the patient's airway remains open with a manual airway maneuver, aided by the presence of the nasal airway. You then begin to transport the patient to the emergency department for evaluation. En route, the patient begins to wake up. As the patient's mental status improves, you vigilantly observe the patient for indications that the NPA will stimulate the gag reflex. On arrival at the emergency department, the patient is awake, confused, but cooperative. ■

(continued)

1. The nasopharyngeal airway would be the preferred airway adjunct in which of the following patients?

   a. a 63-year-old patient in cardiac arrest

   b. a 26-year-old patient experiencing an asthma attack

   c. a 43-year-old patient unresponsive with a low blood glucose level

   d. a 50-year-old patient with a severe head injury

2. To correctly size the nasopharyngeal airway, it should be measured:

   a. from the angle of the jaw to the corner of the nose.

   b. from the nare to the earlobe.

   c. from the chin to the earlobe.

   d. by comparing the NPA to the size of the nare.

3. The nasopharyngeal adjunct assists in maintaining the airway by:

   a. placing the tip of the NPA in the glottic opening.

   b. directing ventilations toward the trachea.

   c. blocking the esophagus, allowing ventilation through the mouth.

   d. preventing the tongue from occluding against the hypopharynx.

CHAPTER 7
Oral Suctioning

OBJECTIVE
The student will be able to successfully perform oral suctioning.

INTRODUCTION

Immediate removal of any aspirated materials and/or fluids in a patient's airway is essential. Many types of **suction** units are available to accomplish the job. Each unit consists of the following:

- a suction source
- a collection container
- thick-walled, nonkinking, wide-bore tubing
- rigid (hard) suction tips or flexible (soft) catheters

Unconscious patients sometimes regurgitate stomach contents—a mix of **hydrochloric acid** and partially digested food. The patients might then aspirate some of these caustic substances into their lower airways. It only takes about 1 ounce of stomach acid to cause a potentially lethal **pneumonia.** So make clearing the patient's airway your first priority!

Suctions units can be either mounted or portable. Mounted "on-board" suction units are installed in the ambulance, usually near the head of the stretcher. Portable suction devices can be taken almost anywhere. They may be electrically powered, manually powered, or powered by oxygen or air. Each device has its advantages and disadvantages. You should weigh each unit's pros and cons before deciding which unit works best for you.

Whatever suction device you choose, it must have enough vacuum pressure to suction both large amounts of fluids and chunk-sized materials. Tubing and catheters should also be able to accommodate large pieces of particulate materials.

You should also anticipate the use of suction well in advance of its actual use. Running for a suction unit when you decide it is needed will delay patient care and may result in a negative outcome for the patient. Equally critical is the use of proper suctioning techniques. Improper suctioning can cause trauma, swelling, spasming, **hypoxia,** and **aspiration.**

►EQUIPMENT

You will need the following equipment:

- ► BSI equipment
- ► suction unit
- ► suction tubing
- ► suction catheters and/or suction tips
- ► collection container
- ► sterile water or irrigation solution

Currently, the most popular type of suctioning uses the rigid **pharyngeal** tip, also called the tonsil tip, tonsil sucker, or Yankauer tip catheter. Most of these catheters have a hole in the hard tube that allows suction only when the hole is covered.

ASSESSMENT

Suctioning involves the removal of body fluids and materials. Patients may cough, spit, and spatter, sending the vomit or regurgitation your way. Therefore, you must take full body substance isolation (BSI) precautions.

Overestimate the possible use of suction. Always have a portable suction unit at the side of any patient who could vomit or have secretions in his airway. Be prepared to use the equipment. Listen and look for signs of aspirated materials. In unresponsive patients, you may hear a wet, gurgling sound in the airway. In some cases, you can see materials and/or fluids in the mouth. In other cases, you may hear a wrenching-type sound just prior to regurgitation. All of these are indications that the patient needs immediate suctioning.

PROCEDURE: Oral Suctioning

1. Apply full **BSI precautions.**
   Rationale: Gloves and eye protection are required at a minimum, and a gown may be needed if large amounts of blood or fluid are present to prevent exposure to infectious diseases.
2. Check equipment.
   Rationale: It is important to make sure that all equipment is present and functioning prior to attempting procedure. Missing and/or nonfunctioning equipment can result in a negative outcome for the patient.
3. Place yourself at the patient's head (Figure 7.1).
   Rationale: Although you can do this skill from other positions, positioning yourself at the head of the patient is preferred.
4. Turn on the suction unit.

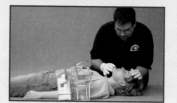 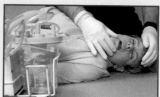

Figure 7.1   **Figure 7.2**

5. Place patient on her side, or turn head to the side if possible (Figure 7.2).
   Rationale: The patient can be placed in any position during this procedure.
6. Open the patient's mouth using a cross-finger technique.
   Rationale: This technique allows you to open the mouth with the best leverage.

7. Slowly insert the catheter into the mouth with the curved or distal part of the catheter pointing toward the jaw. Place the Yankauer so that the convex, or bulging-out, side is pointed toward the roof of the mouth. Insert the tip to the base of the tongue (Figure 7.3).

   Rationale: Careful insertion using this technique allows for reduction of trauma during insertion.

8. Insert *NO* further than the base of the tongue.

   Rationale: Insertion past the base of the tongue can increase the possibility of a gag reflex occurring during suctioning.

9. If a gag reflex begins, pull back slightly.

   Rationale: Causing a gag reflex can cause vomiting and an increase in aspirations.

10. Begin suctioning by placing your finger over the hole in the catheter tube (Figure 7.4).

    Rationale: Suction does not start until your finger is placed over the hole in the Yankauer.

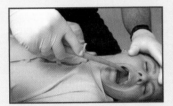
Figure 7.3

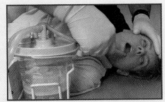
Figure 7.4

11. Move the suction catheter from side to side in the oral cavity (Figure 7.5).

    Rationale: Moving the suction catheter from side to side allows for removal of all matter in the oral pharynx.

12. Never suction for more than 15 seconds at a time. Instead of counting out 15 seconds, you can just take a breath and hold it before beginning to suction. When you need a breath, the adult patient probably does, too.

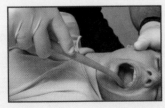
Figure 7.5

PEDIATRIC NOTE:
Do *NOT* suction more than 5 seconds in children and infants.

Rationale: Suctioning for move than 15 seconds can cause hypoxia. The technique of holding your breath can assist you in remembering that if you need a breath so does the patient.

13. If the catheter or tubing becomes clogged with materials, use sterile water or irrigation solution to clean or clear the catheter and/or tubing.

    Rationale: It is common for the suction tubing and the catheter to become clogged. Always having sterile water handy allows you to keep the catheter and the tubing clear. Material in the catheter and/or tubing can reduce or completely obstruct suction (Figure 7.6).

14. Allow a few seconds between suctions, giving the patient time to relax. If necessary, ventilate between suctioning attempts.

    Rationale: Continued suction attempts without periods of relaxation or ventilation can cause hypoxia.

15. Repeat the above technique as needed.

    Rationale: It is common to need multiple suctioning attempts to completely clear the airway.

16. Document your suction procedure.

    Rationale: It is extremely important to document your findings in order to have a history of facts and events that occurred at the scene.

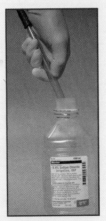
Figure 7.6

Constantly monitor for materials and/or fluids that may need to be removed. Monitor for signs of hypoxia during suctioning.

▶PROBLEM SOLVING

▸ If a gag reflex happens during suctioning, it is usually caused by a catheter that is placed beyond the base of the tongue.

▸ The placement of the catheter is important to monitor.

▸ Remove the catheter if a gag reflex is obtained.

▸ Make sure that you wear BSI protection when cleaning any suction equipment. Exposure while cleaning is a significant risk.

PEDIATRIC NOTE:

Be especially aware of vagal stimuli, which may cause vomiting in infants/children.

▶CASE STUDY

It is 0300 and your squad is called to the local bar to assist an unresponsive 32-year-old female. On arrival at the scene, you find the patient lying supine in the bathroom. Her friends state that she just had a little too much to drink and they need help getting her into their car. As you approach her, she begins to vomit. You quickly position her on her side and ask your partner to get the suction unit out.

As your partner pulls out the suction unit, she turns the pump on and you remove the Yankauer catheter from the wrapper. You ask your partner to hold the patient's mouth open using the cross-finger technique as you insert the tip of the catheter into the patient's mouth. While using a side-to-side sweeping motion, you notice that the suction unit does not appear to be working. You remove the suction tip and notice that it is full of large undigested pieces of food. Your partner gets out some sterile water and you attempt to clear the catheter without success. You then remove the catheter from the tubing and suck water into the tubing. After clearing the tubing, you reattach the catheter and determine that the obstruction within the catheter is cleared. You are now able to suction the patient again.

After the patient's airway has been cleared, you position her on your cot on her left side and begin to transport her with the suction unit at her side. While en route, the patient remains unconscious. A nasal airway is inserted and she is taken into the emergency department without any further changes. ∎

1. When applying suction to a patient, which of the following is most appropriate?
   a. Apply suction until the airway is clear of all secretions.
   b. Start suctioning as soon as the suction catheter is in the airway.
   c. Only apply suction while slowly withdrawing the catheter.
   d. Only use soft suction catheters to prevent damage to the mouth.

2. How far should the suction catheter be inserted into the mouth?
   a. The tip of the catheter should be inserted to the base of the tongue.
   b. The catheter should be inserted until the gag reflex is stimulated then removed.
   c. The catheter should only be inserted into the area between the teeth and lips.
   d. The catheter should be inserted until vagal stimulation causes bradycardia.

3. What is the most important factor when applying suction to a patient?
   a. Do not suction pediatric patients because of the potential for complications.
   b. Do not ventilate a patient between suction attempts to prevent aspiration.
   c. Only apply suction if the patient is lying on his side.
   d. Do not apply suction for longer than 15 seconds.

CHAPTER 8
Suctioning through an Endotracheal Tube

KEY TERMS

Carina

Endotracheal (ET) tube

Hypoxia

Soft suction catheter

OBJECTIVE

The student will successfully demonstrate the ability to suction a patient with an endotracheal tube.

INTRODUCTION

Suctioning through an **endotracheal (ET) tube** is necessary in both medical and trauma patients. See also Chapters 14 and 15. The goal is to clear the airway of unwanted materials and/or fluids. This should be done under the direction of an advanced life support (ALS) provider. A soft catheter is inserted down the ET tube beyond the tip to the level of the **carina,** the branching point of the trachea. A **soft suction catheter** is a hollow piece of plastic or rubber that has a hard plastic section, with a hole in it, located at the proximal end of the catheter. Once attached to the suction unit, suction is created when your thumb is placed over the hole of the hard plastic section.

▶ EQUIPMENT

You will need the following equipment:

- ▶ BSI equipment
- ▶ Suction unit
- ▶ Soft suction
- ▶ Sterile gloves
- ▶ Sterile water

ASSESSMENT

You will know that the patient needs suctioning if you hear gurgling sounds coming from the ET tube. You may visually see materials and/or fluids in the ET tube as well. Suctioning must be performed at the direction of an ALS provider. BSI precautions must be applied during this procedure because materials and/or fluids being suctioned are considered body fluids and exposure to them is highly likely.

See Chapters 14 and 15 regarding measuring of the ET tube. The length of the ET tube is critical to successful suctioning.

PROCEDURE: Suctioning through an Endotracheal Tube

1. Apply BSI precautions.

   Rationale: Gloves and eye protection are required at a minimum, and a gown may be needed if large amounts of blood or fluid are present to prevent exposure to infectious diseases.

2. Patient should be in a supine position.

   Rationale: Although the patient can be suctioned in other positions, supine is the recommended position.

3. Check and assemble equipment. Apply new, sterile glove to the dominant hand.

   Rationale: You don't want to be in a position to suction and find the equipment does not work. Care should be taken during suctioning that the newly gloved hand and suction catheter remain sterile to reduce the risk of contamination and introduction of infection to the airway.

4. Turn on suction, being sure to keep the dominant hand sterile. If electric suction is being used, place the control on the lower suction pressure. If your suction unit has a gauge, set it between 80 and 120 mm.

   Rationale: Suction at higher pressures can cause damage to the airway if the suction tip goes beyond the ET tube.

5. Hyperventilate patient prior to suctioning.

   Rationale: Patients can get hypoxic during the suctioning procedure. Hyperventilation reduces the chances of **hypoxia.**

6. Measure the distance the catheter will be advanced. Measure the distance from the nipple line to the patient's ear, then from the ear to the patient's lip line. Place a piece of tape at that point (Figures 8.1 and 8.2).

   Rationale: Measuring the distance ensures that the suction tip will not go below the ET tube, causing airway damage and complications.

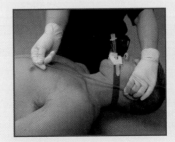
Figure 8.1

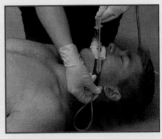
Figure 8.2

continued...

7. Using the sterile gloved hand, place the soft catheter into the ET tube (Figure 8.3).

   Rationale: Care should be taken during suctioning that the gloved hand remains sterile. A sterile gloved hand reduces the risk of contamination of the suction catheter. Contamination of the suction catheter can cause introduction of infection into the airway.

8. Advance the catheter slowly down the ET tube (Figure 8.4).

   Rationale: Fast insertion can increase the risk of gag and cough reflexes in the patient.

9. When the catheter has been advanced to the proper distance, place your thumb over the hard plastic hole and slowly withdraw the catheter using a semicircular motion. Never suction for more than 15 seconds (Figure 8.5).

   Rationale: Overinsertion of the catheter can cause injury to the airway. Placing your finger over the hole allows suctioning to begin; using a semicircular motion increases the sweep of the catheter, allowing more material to be suctioned. Suctioning for more than 15 seconds can cause hypoxia.

10. Clean the catheter in sterile water to remove materials and/or fluids (Figure 8.6).

    Rationale: In most cases the suction catheter will become clogged with material. Cleaning the catheter keeps it clear.

11. When setting the catheter down, make sure it is placed in a sterile environment.

    Rationale: A sterile environment reduces the risk of contamination of the suction catheter. Contamination of the suction catheter can cause introduction of infection into the airway.

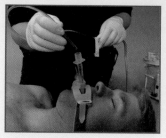
Figure 8.3

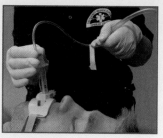
Figure 8.4

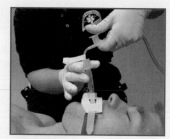
Figure 8.5

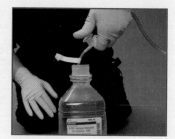
Figure 8.6

12. Hyperventilate the patient and repeat the procedure if necessary. Reglove if more suctioning is necessary.

    Rationale: Patients can become hypoxic during suctioning; hyperventilation reduces this risk. Regloving reduces the risk of introduction of an infection to the airway.

13. Document the procedure and outcome.

    Rationale: It is extremely important to document your findings in order to have a history of facts and events that occurred at the scene.

ONGOING ASSESSMENT

Assess the patient immediately after suctioning for signs of hypoxia. Constantly monitor the patient for possible repeat suctioning.

PROBLEM SOLVING

> Hypoxia can result if the suctioning procedure takes too long. Good preoxygenation and monitoring of the time it takes to do the procedure can eliminate the onset of hypoxia.

- If you do not measure the suctioning catheter and advance it too far, you can cause the coughing reflex, bronchospasms, arrhythmias, and injury to the mucosa of the lower airways.
- Suction pressure that is too high can also cause the preceding complications. Monitor the pressure you are using.
- If the catheter becomes clogged with materials, place the tip of the soft suction catheter into sterile water, put your thumb over the plastic hole, and draw water through the catheter. This will clean the catheter.

▶CASE STUDY

You are transporting a 43-year-old male who was involved in a single-car motor vehicle collision. The patient is unconscious and has massive facial trauma. While en route, your paramedic partner intubates the patient orally and advises you that the patient's airway was full of blood. She states that she is concerned that the patient still has blood in his airway.

As you begin to ventilate the patient, you note that ventilations are more difficult than usual. You report this difficulty to your partner. She auscultates for lung sounds and determines that the patient has equal sounds bilaterally. Your partner decides that since your transport time to the closest facility is still 15 minutes, she would like you to suction the patient's airway to help clear the ET tube to facilitate better ventilation of the patient. You prepare your equipment and don your eye shield and face mask.

You ask your partner to hyperventilate the patient and, after she has done so, the bag-valve device is removed from the end of the ET tube and you slowly insert the suction catheter through the end of the ET tube. Once you have reached your pre-measured depth, you cover the hole on the catheter with your thumb to apply suction. As you apply suction, you note that large amounts of bloody fluid are being removed from the patient's airway. After you complete suctioning of the patient, you ask your partner to hyperventilate the patient again. While she is hyperventilating the patient, she notes greater ease in bag compression. The patient is transported to the emergency department without further need for suctioning. ■

(continued)

1. It is important to measure the suction catheter prior to insertion because:
   a. you need to ensure that the tip does not extend past the tip of the endotracheal tube.
   b. you need to ensure that the suction catheter does not extend past the carina.
   c. you need to ensure that the suction catheter does not extend past the base of the tongue.
   d. you need to avoid stimulating the patient's gag reflex.

2. Why is it important to use sterile technique with ET tube suctioning?
   a. Sterile technique is no more important than with any other procedure.
   b. To prevent contamination from any other products that may be present in the ambulance.
   c. To prevent you from contracting any of the patient's illnesses.
   d. To prevent contamination that could cause further infection.

3. Why is it important to ventilate the patient between suction attempts?
   a. because ventilation can correct the hypoxia caused by suctioning
   b. because the patient still needs ventilation even though suctioning is necessary
   c. to help distribute the fluid throughout the lung, making ventilation easier
   d. so that you know when you have suctioned enough to not need further suctioning

CHAPTER 9
Oxygen Tank Assembly

OBJECTIVE
The student will successfully assemble an oxygen tank.

INTRODUCTION

Administration of oxygen is one of the most important treatments that an EMT-Basic can give to a patient. The earth's atmosphere provides about 21 percent oxygen—that's enough oxygen for a healthy person to function normally. As an EMT-Basic, however, you will come in contact with sick or injured people who often require **supplemental oxygen.** The delivery of oxygen begins with preparation of the oxygen tank.

You may either assemble the tank for use with an oxygen delivery device, or you may be asked to change an oxygen tank on scene. Keep in mind that most oxygen tanks and regulators have standard fittings and only work one way.

You must become familiar with several types of portable cylinders that are used in the field:

▶ A D cylinder contains about 350 liters of oxygen.

▶ An E cylinder contains about 625 liters of oxygen.

▶ An M cylinder contains about 3,000 liters of oxygen.

On-board tanks found in the ambulance (fixed system) include these types:

▶ A G cylinder contains about 5,300 liters of oxygen.

▶ An H cylinder contains about 6,900 liters of oxygen.

►EQUIPMENT

You will need the following equipment:

- ► Oxygen cylinder with yoke
- ► **Oxygen regulator,** (must be connected to cylinder to provide a safe working pressure of 30 to 70 psi)
- ► Flowmeter
- ► Oxygen key

On E-size cylinders, or smaller, the pressure regulator is secured to the cylinder valve assembly by a yoke assembly. This is called a **pin-index safety system.** This system prevents an oxygen delivery system from being connected to a cylinder containing another gas because the pin position varies for different gases.

Cylinders larger than the E size have a valve assembly with a threaded outlet. The inside and outside diameters of the threaded outlets vary according to the gas in the cylinder. This is to prevent an oxygen regulator from being connected to a cylinder containing another gas such as helium or nitrogen.

A **flowmeter** is used to regulate the flow of oxygen in liters per minute. It is connected to the pressure regulator, and most services keep the flowmeter permanently attached to it. There are three major types of flowmeters:

- ► Bourdon gauge flowmeter (useful for most portable units)
- ► Constant-flow selector valve (useful with any size oxygen cylinder)
- ► Pressure-compensated flowmeter (useful for fixed delivery systems)

ASSESSMENT

Whenever you are working with an oxygen tank, safety should be foremost in your mind. Therefore, it is very important that you inspect the tank and regulator for damage prior to assembly. Before assembling the tank, make sure that it contains medical-grade oxygen. Medical oxygen tanks are usually green or stainless steel with a green stripe at the top and are labeled "Oxygen U.S.P." In most cases, you will find a seal or plastic wrapper around a full tank. Remove this protective seal from the tank valve. Make sure the oxygen regulator has an O-ring, or washer, in the area where the oxygen regulator fits with the oxygen tank. Oxygen should be stored in or near room temperature. Exercise great caution if a tank is either too hot or too cold.

PROCEDURE: Oxygen Tank Assembly

1. Evaluate the tank and regulator for damage. Do *NOT* use a tank if you notice any damage (Figure 9.1).

   Rationale: Safety needs to be paramount. A damaged tank and/or regulator has the potential to cause an explosion and should *NEVER* be used.

2. To reduce the risk of injury, place the cylinder in a secure, upright position and stand to one side. If you are transporting a patient who is using an

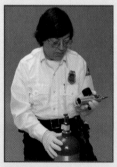

Figure 9.1

oxygen cylinder, be sure to lay the cylinder down and secure it to the stretcher.

Rationale: Again, safety first. A tank that falls or is dropped can cause injury to you, the patients, or others.

3. Remove the plastic seal or cap protecting the cylinder outlet or valve. Keep the plastic washer (Figure 9.2).

Rationale: A plastic seal or tape is placed on the cylinder outlet to identify the tank as being full of oxygen. It also keeps the outlet valve clean of debris. The plastic seal also ensures that an O-ring is in place on the outlet valve. If the O-ring falls off during removal of the seal, replace it.

4. Quickly open and close the valve. This will remove any dust or debris from the valve assembly.

Rationale: This step reduces the chances of clogging the regulator.

5. Select the correct pressure regulator and flowmeter. Then place the cylinder valve gasket on the oxygen regulator port.

6. Make sure the pressure regulator is closed. Now align the pins on the regulator's yoke, or thread by hand, so they fit into the spaces on the tank's valve (Figure 9.3).

Rationale: You will note that the regulator has a safety pin system that only allows for oxygen regulators to be applied. Note that it can only be assembled one way.

8. Place the oxygen key on the screw of the tank valve. Slowly open the valve to charge the oxygen regulator. One-half turn is usually all that is necessary (Figure 9.5).

Rationale: Open the valve slowly to avoid damaging the regulator.

9. Check the pressure gauge to see that an adequate amount of oxygen is present in the tank (Figure 9.6).

Rationale: If you are working with a tank that has been used previously, check the pressure gauge to ensure that an adequate amount of oxygen is present in the tank. Your service's standard operating procedures will list the required pressure limits that mandate when a used oxygen tank should be changed out for a new one.

10. Attach tubing and the oxygen delivery device of choice.

Rationale: The type of delivery system is based on the patient assessment.

11. Open the main valve and adjust the flowmeter to the desired liters per minute (Figure 9.7). Chapters 10 and 11 cover types of oxygen delivery systems.

Rationale: The desired liters per minute is based on the patient assessment.

12. Document the oxygen delivered to the patient.

Rationale: It is extremely important to document your findings in order to have a history of facts and events that occurred at the scene.

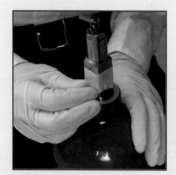 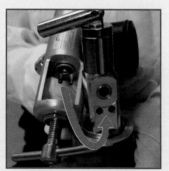 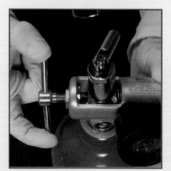 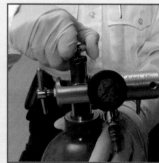

Figure 9.2   **Figure 9.3**   **Figure 9.4**   **Figure 9.5**

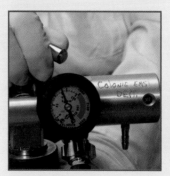 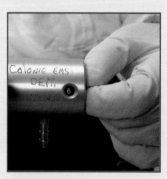

7. Hand tighten the T-screw on the pin yoke of the oxygen regulator, or tighten a threaded outlet with a nonferrous wrench (Figure 9.4).

Rationale: Hand tightening is all that is needed to complete the seal; any tighter and it maybe difficult to take off when needed.

Figure 9.6   **Figure 9.7**

The pressure gauge should be constantly monitored for pressure. If it is possible that the tank may need to be changed at the scene, have a tank ready prior to when it will be needed. Check your service's standard operating procedures for mandatory pressure limits to change out tanks after usage.

▶PROBLEM SOLVING

- ▶ If you notice damage to the tank or its valves, do not use it.
- ▶ Damaged oxygen regulator gauges can result in inaccurate readings on the gauges.
- ▶ If you open the tank valve with the regulator attached and you hear a leak, remove the oxygen regulator and check the O-ring for proper fitting, then reassemble and try again.

▶CASE STUDY

It has been a crazy day and you have just finished dropping your ninth patient off at the emergency department. As you are walking out, you notice that another squad from your department has arrived with a critical patient. Identifying the fact that they have been even busier than you, you ask the lead medic if there is anything you can help her with. "Change our portable O_2; that would be great," she responds.

You get into the squad and find the portable bottle of oxygen lying in the wheel well; it has about 200 psi remaining. You open the oxygen cabinet and pull a new bottle of oxygen out of the cabinet. You note that the new bottle still has an intact seal and does not appear to be damaged. You turn the near-empty bottle off and bleed out any remaining gas. You then remove the regulator from the old bottle, make sure the plastic seal is still intact and functional, and attach it to the new bottle. After attaching it to the new bottle, you notice that it is leaking. You retighten the regulator and the bottle still leaks. Realizing that the seal must be bad, you get a new plastic seal and replace it with the old one. After replacing the seals and reattaching the regulator, you turn the oxygen back on; no leak is heard or felt and the regulator reads 1,800 psi. You put the old bottle back in the oxygen cabinet and put the new bottle in the oxygen harness in the side compartment of the squad. ■

1. Which of the following is important to remember when changing an oxygen tank?

   a. Make sure the seal is replaced every time the regulator is changed.

   b. Make sure you do not open the valve prior to attaching the regulator.

   c. Crack the valve to remove any dust from the neck of the tank.

   d. Always make sure the new tank has greater than 2,000 psi.

2. You drop the spare oxygen tank while changing it out and notice a small dent. What should you do?

   a. Attach the regulator and use the tank as long as there are no leaks.

   b. Do not use this tank now, but put it aside to use later.

   c. Be very careful when handling the tank because it may explode.

   d. Use another tank and take the damaged tank out of service.

3. A full D cylinder holds how many liters of oxygen?

   a. 625 liters

   b. 350 liters

   c. 325 liters

   d. 3,000 liters

CHAPTER 10

Administration of Oxygen by a Nonrebreather Mask

KEY TERMS

Nonrebreather mask

One-way valve

Reservoir bag

OBJECTIVE

The student will be able to administer oxygen successfully by a nonrebreather mask.

INTRODUCTION

A **nonrebreather mask** provides the highest concentration of supplemental oxygen delivered during emergency medical service. This mask is indicated for patients who exhibit any of the following signs or symptoms:

▶ inadequate breathing

▶ cyanosis

▶ cool, clammy skin

▶ shortness of breath

▶ chest pain

▶ severe injuries

▶ altered mental status

The device delivers oxygen by means of an attached **reservoir bag** or by a reservoir tube connected to the mask with a **one-way valve.** The valve prevents the patient's exhaled air from mixing with the oxygen in the reservoir area. The mask also has rubber washers that cover the exhalation ports. These washers allow air to escape on exhalation while keeping oxygen inside the mask. Should the oxygen supply fail, recent mask designs feature an emergency port so the patient can still take in atmospheric air.

A nonrebreather face mask can be used in combination with oropharyngeal airways or nasopharygeal airways. The optimal oxygen flow rate should be 15 lpm. A nonrebreather face mask will provide concentrations of oxygen ranging from 80 to 100 percent.

▶ EQUIPMENT

To use a nonrebreather face mask, you will need the following equipment:

▶ Full oxygen tank and regulator
▶ Nonrebreather face mask

ASSESSMENT

The patient should be breathing at a good rate and volume for the nonrebreather face mask to be effective. Nonrebreather face masks come in different sizes, so make sure that you're using the proper size for the patient.

PROCEDURE: Administration of Oxygen by a Nonrebreather Face Mask

1. Apply BSI precautions.

   Rationale: Gloves and eye protection are required at a minimum, and a gown may be needed if large amounts of blood or fluid are present to prevent exposure to infectious diseases.

2. Introduce yourself to the patient, and explain the need for a nonrebreather face mask as well as the steps involved in applying the mask.

   Rationale: As with any oxygen mask, a nonrebreather face mask can cause a patient to feel claustrophobic, increasing her anxiety. The mask may also make it difficult for you to obtain a patient's history. Exercise caution when applying a mask to patients with altered mental status so that they do not aspirate secretions or vomit that may collect in the mask.

3. Make sure that the oxygen tank is full and that the pressure is within accepted limits. (Figure 10.1).

   Rationale: Although the tank should be checked at the beginning of a shift and changed after any

call where the tank pressure is not within acceptable limits, it should be rechecked during each usage. You never want to run out of oxygen on a call if it can at all be avoided.

4. Attach the nonrebreather face mask to the nipple of the oxygen regulator (Figure 10.2).

5. Set the flowmeter to 15 lpm or at the rate specified by medical direction.

   Rationale: Although you may be directed to deliver at lower rates, the highest liter flow is usually indicated.

6. If the mask has a reservoir bag, allow the bag to fill completely. To inflate the reservoir bag, use your finger to cover the exhaust port or the connection between the mask and the reservoir.

   Rationale: This allows the patient to immediately get the highest amount of oxygen.

continued...

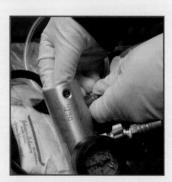

Figure 10.1

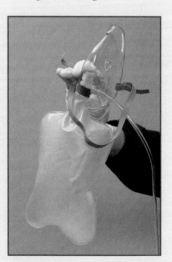

Figure 10.2

7. Instruct the patient to breathe normally while the mask is in place (Figure 10.3).

    Rationale: A face mask can cause a patient to feel claustrophobic, increasing her anxiety. Breathing rates that increase can inversely reduce volume. Normal respirations are preferred.

8. Position the mask over the patient's nose and mouth.

9. Next slip the elastic strap over the patient's head so that it rests above the patient's ear (Figure 10.4).

    Rationale: The elastic strap allows the mask to be held in place. Sometimes you can reduce the patient's feelings of claustrophobia by having her hold the mask on her face for a few minutes before applying the elastic strap.

10. Tighten the strap as needed.

11. Again coach the patient on how to breathe (Figure 10.5).

12. Document the use of a nonrebreather mask and the rate at which you delivered the oxygen.

    Rationale: It is extremely important to document your findings in order to have a history of facts and events that occurred at the scene.

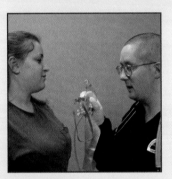

Figure 10.3

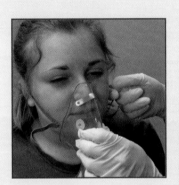

Figure 10.4

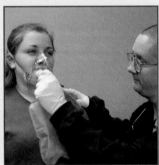

Figure 10.5

ONGOING ASSESSMENT

Remind the patient to breathe normally. Also, check the position of the mask to ensure comfort and effectiveness. Monitor the oxygen cylinder for a consistent pressure and flow rate. Make sure that blankets or sheets do not obstruct the valves on the nonrebreather mask.

Also watch the volume in the reservoir bag when the patient inhales from the mask. The bag should be at least half full. If this is not the case, the patient is over-breathing, and you will need to increase the flow rate slightly.

▶ PROBLEM SOLVING

▷ Constant reassurance will help reduce the feelings of claustrophobia associated with any oxygen mask.

▷ You might also have the patient hold the mask on her face, reducing claustrophobia even more.

▷ Be careful when using any mask if the patient has an altered level of consciousness. If not immediately removed during vomiting, the mask can cause aspiration.

►CASE STUDY

You are called to the residence of an 81-year-old male who is complaining of difficulty breathing. On arrival, you find the patient seated upright in a recliner with a nasal cannula in his nose. The patient states that he began having increased breathing difficulty during the last 4 to 5 hours. Your assessment reveals the patient to be alert and his responses are appropriate, with rapid respirations. The patient tells you that he has a history of emphysema and is normally on 4 liters of oxygen. He does not have any explanation for why his breathing got worse, but states he did not change his routine and has not been out of his recliner all day except to increase his oxygen to 6 liters. He states that he increased his oxygen level because he was short of breath.

As you obtain the patient's history, your partner obtains vital signs. He reports the vitals as follows: Pulse is 114, strong and regular; blood pressure is 162/90; respirations are 28 and appear labored; and his "pulse ox" is 92 percent on 6 liters. The patient tells you his blood pressure is slightly elevated from what it normally is, but he does have a history of hypertension and his pulse ox is generally about 96 percent while on oxygen.

You determine that the patient requires some additional oxygen support and since he is already on 6 lpm, he will have to be switched over to a nonrebreather mask. After explaining your intent to the patient, he agrees to use the mask. The patient is then lifted onto the cot and taken to the ambulance for transport to the hospital. While en route, the patient is still appearing to have difficulty in breathing but states he is feeling better. His pulse oximeter reading on 15 lpm is now 95 percent. The patient is taken to the emergency department without event. ■

(continued)

1. The appropriate liter flow for a nonrebreather mask would be:
   a. 6 lpm.
   b. 10 lpm.
   c. 15 lpm.
   d. 25 lpm.

2. The reservoir on the nonrebreather mask is deflating with each ventilation. Which of the following is not an appropriate action?
   a. Increase the liter flow on the nonrebreather.
   b. Tell your patient to stop breathing so deeply.
   c. Begin positive pressure ventilation.
   d. Make sure that the valve between the reservoir and mask is still intact.

3. A nonrebreather mask would be appropriate for which of the following patients?
   a. a 28-year-old with an ankle fracture from an auto accident
   b. a 74-year-old stroke patient with shallow respirations at 6/minute
   c. a 17-year-old patient who is hyperventilating
   d. a 53-year-old patient with chest pain who says it hurts to take a deep breath

CHAPTER 11

Administration of Oxygen by a Nasal Cannula

OBJECTIVE

The student will be able to successfully administer oxygen by a nasal cannula.

KEY TERMS

Low-flow oxygen

Nasal cannula

INTRODUCTION

A **nasal cannula** provides low concentrations of oxygen, ranging from 24 to 44 percent. Oxygen is delivered to the patient by two soft plastic tips, commonly referred to as nasal prongs, that are connected by thin tubing to the main oxygen source. The prongs rest a short distance inside the patient's nostrils.

The main indication for use of a nasal cannula is for a patient who feels "suffocated" by a nonrebreather face mask, despite your best coaching and reassurance. A nasal cannula may also be indicated for chronic obstructive pulmonary disease (COPD) patients with minimal respiratory distress and for patients who are experiencing nausea or vomiting.

You will find that many patients like nasal cannulas because of the device's comfort. A cannula also allows them to talk while receiving oxygen, making it a lot easier for you to gather a history. Even so, the nasal cannula is not the preferred method of oxygen delivery in the prehospital setting. Obviously, it is contraindicated for patients with nasal obstructions. A nasal cannula also should not be used with patients who exhibit chest pain, hypoxia, signs of shock, or other more serious problems that require higher concentrations of oxygen. However, if a patient refuses to wear a mask, the cannula is better than no oxygen at all.

▶ EQUIPMENT

You will need the following equipment:

- ▶ Full oxygen tank and regulator
- ▶ Nasal cannulas of various sizes, such as cannulas for adults and children

ASSESSMENT

For a nasal cannula to function effectively, a patient must exhibit adequate respirations and the ability to breathe through the nose. As previously mentioned, consider this method of oxygen delivery only for those patients who require low to moderate concentrations of oxygen.

After selecting a correctly sized cannula and placing the prongs in the patient's nostrils, set the flow rate at between 1 and 6 liters per minute (lpm). This is often referred to as **low-flow oxygen,** which ranges in concentration from 24 to 44 percent, depending on the patient's condition and orders from medical direction. At flow rates higher than 6 lpm, the cannula dries out nasal mucous membranes and increases patient discomfort.

PROCEDURE: Administration of Oxygen by a Nasal Cannula

1. Apply BSI precautions.

   Rationale: Gloves and eye protection are required at a minimum, and a gown may be needed if large amounts of blood or fluid are present to prevent exposure to infectious diseases.

2. Introduce yourself to the patient, and explain the need for a cannula as well as the steps involved in applying the mask (Figure 11.1).

   Rationale: As with any oxygen mask, a cannula mask can cause a patient to feel claustrophobic, increasing her anxiety. At this point, you might tell the patient that mouth breathing with a nasal cannula in place is OK. The patient will still get adequate oxygen delivery, assuming nasal passages are free of obstructions.

3. Make sure that the oxygen tank is full and that the pressure is within accepted limits.

   Rationale: Although the tank should be checked at the beginning of a shift and changed after any call where the tank pressure is not within acceptable limits, it should be rechecked during each usage. You never want to run out of oxygen on a call if it can at all be avoided.

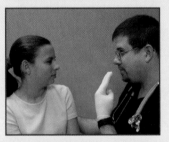

Figure 11.1

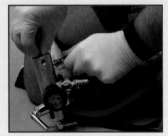

Figure 11.2

4. Attach the nasal cannula tubing to the nipple of the regulator (Figure 11.2). Set the liter flow between 1 and 6 lpm.

   Rationale: The flow rate will depend on the patient's condition, local protocols, or advice from medical direction. Keep in mind that the nasal cannula's low-flow system does not supply enough oxygen to provide the entire tidal volume during inspiration. Therefore, a large portion of the patient's inhalation consists of ambient air that is mixed with the oxygen supplied by the nasal cannula. It is important for you to instruct the patient to breathe as normally as possible while the prongs are in place.

5. Insert the two prongs into the patient's nostrils. Make sure the prongs curve downward toward the patient (Figure 11.3).

   Rationale: This makes the cannula feel comfortable to the patient.

6. If the patient's nostrils are blocked, you can place the prongs into the patient's mouth. Patients generally want to breathe through their noses, thinking that they will receive more oxygen. Assure them that they don't need to do this. They will receive plenty of oxygen if they breathe as normally as possible.

   Rationale: Although acceptable this is not the perfered technique for application of a nasal cannula. Advise the receiving facility of your placement and why this was done.

7. After you have placed the nasal cannula in the nostrils, position the tubing of the cannula over the patient's ears (Figure 11.4).

8. Bring the remainder of the tubing under the patient's chin, and secure the slip loop by gently sliding the plastic adjuster in place. Do not make the tubing too tight. If your unit carries nasal cannulas with elastic straps, instead of plastic tubing, follow the same general approach. Fit the strap over the patient's ears and tighten it comfortably under the patient's chin (Figure 11.5).

9. Coach the victim on how to breathe (Figure 11.6).

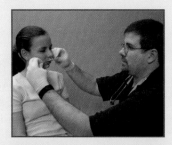

Figure 11.3

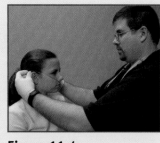

Figure 11.4

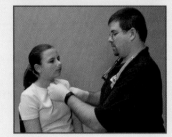

Figure 11.5

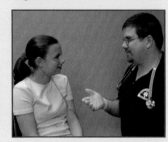

Figure 11.6

10. Remember to check the cannula position periodically to make sure that it does not become dislodged during extrication, moving, or transportation.

11. Document the use of a nasal cannula and the liter flow.

    Rationale: It is extremely important to document your findings in order to have a history of facts and events that occurred at the scene.

ONGOING ASSESSMENT

Monitor the patient during transport. Make sure that you monitor the pressure in the tank during transport. Change tanks if necessary.

▶ PROBLEM SOLVING

▷ Exercise caution whenever you move a patient with a nasal cannula in place. Nasal trauma could occur.

▶ CASE STUDY

You are called to the home of Mr. Jones, an elderly patient with a history of obstructive lung disease. Upon your arrival you find a thin 67-year-old male patient who is sitting up in his favorite chair. He explains that he has had a cold for the past few days and is a little more short of breath than normal today.

   He is alert and oriented to person, place, and time, and is answering your questions appropriately. Mr. Jones is able to answer almost all your questions with complete sentences, only occasionally having to stop for a breath. Your partner begins to assess baseline vital signs. She advises you that the patient has a heart rate of 110, is breathing 26 times per minute, and has a blood pressure of 156/92. She also advises you that the patient's skin is very warm. You apply the pulse oximeter and obtain a reading of 91 percent.

Your partner begins to prepare a nonrebreather mask for Mr. Jones, but as she starts to apply it, Mr. Jones refuses saying that masks make him more short of breath. While trying to convince Mr. Jones of the need for high-flow oxygen, he tells you about his claustrophobia. You then decide to administer oxygen with a nasal cannula so that you do not cause any unnecessary distress. After setting up the nasal cannula, you set the flow at 4 liters and apply the device. Mr. Jones thanks you for being so helpful. Your partner starts setting up the cot for transport while you complete your history and detailed physical exam.

During the ongoing assessment, en route to the local emergency department, Mr. Jones says that he is now breathing without difficulty. You recheck his pulse oximeter reading and find it to be 96 percent. You notify the emergency department regarding the patient's status, and complete the transport without further changes. ■

1. Which of the following patients would *not* be a candidate for nasal cannula use?
    a. a 22-year-old female complaining of abdominal cramping, but who is not in any obvious distress
    b. a 56-year-old unresponsive patient who is vomiting and has the potential for aspiration
    c. a 73-year-old patient with a history of COPD, complaining of mild shortness of breath
    d. a 42-year-old patient who fractured her arm and is becoming nauseated from the pain

2. Which of the following most accurately describes the administration of oxygen with a nasal cannula?
    a. A nasal cannula can provide more than 6 lpm as long as humidification is added.
    b. A nasal cannula can provide 100 percent oxygen because, at 6 lpm, the oxygen provided is the same as the patient's minute volume.
    c. A nasal cannula should only be used for patients who cannot tolerate a nonrebreather mask.
    d. A nasal cannula can be used whenever a patient needs oxygen, but is not in obvious distress.

3. A nasal cannula provides oxygen at which of the following?
    a. 24 to 44 percent
    b. less than 21 percent
    c. up to 10 liters per minute
    d. none of the above

CHAPTER 12
Nasogastric Intubation in Infants and Children

KEY TERMS

Anatomical disturbances

Artificial ventilation

Aspiration

Caustic solutions

Distal

Epiglottitis

Esophagus

French (unit of measure)

Gastric distension

Gastric extension

Hydrocarbons solutions

Nares

Nasogastric (NG) tube

Nasopharynx

Nostril

Proximal

Water-soluble lubricant

Xiphoid process

OBJECTIVE

The student will successfully demonstrate the ability to insert a nasogastric (NG) tube in an infant or child.

INTRODUCTION

Infants and children have smaller airways than adults, so they are adversely affected by the high ventilation pressures used during **artificial ventilation.** It is common for air to enter the **esophagus** and be forced into the stomach in infants and children who need to be ventilated. The air in the stomach pushes the less developed diaphragm up, compressing the chest cavity; this reduces the ability of the lungs to expand, making ventilation difficult to impossible at times. Air in the stomach also increases the risk of vomiting and **aspiration** of gastric contents.

Insertion of a **nasogastric (NG) tube** has other indications but is reserved for the EMT-Basic to use in infants and children to reduce air in the stomach during artificial ventilation. This skill is controversial and is reserved as an optional skill based on your local policies and procedures or medical direction. Although air can also enter the stomach in adults, it causes a much more serious problem in infants and children than in adults.

The primary indication for use of an NG tube in infants or children is if you are unable to ventilate due to **gastric extension.** It is also used as a preventive measure in certain cases to reduce the risk of **gastric distension** in the patient infant or child being ventilated.

Nasogastric tube insertion is contraindicated in infants and children with facial, head, or spinal trauma; **epiglottitis,** croup, or other airway diseases; and in any infant or child with **anatomical disturbances.** NG tube placement is also contraindicated in infants or children who may have ingested **caustic** or **hydrocarbon solutions.**

The NG tube is inserted through the **nares, nasopharynx,** esophagus, and into stomach of the infant or child. NG tubes come in a variety of sizes and are measured in units called **French.** Infants usually take a 8.0 French; toddlers and preschool children take a 10 French; school-aged children take a 12 French.

▶ EQUIPMENT

You will need the following equipment:

- ▶ BSI equipment
- ▶ BVM, with reservoir attachment
- ▶ oxygen cylinder
- ▶ suction and catheter
- ▶ tape to secure the tube
- ▶ stethoscope
- ▶ NG tube, proper size
- ▶ 20-cc syringe
- ▶ **Water-soluble lubricant**

ASSESSMENT

This procedure is indicated for unconscious infants or children with no gag reflex who need assisted respirations.

Assess for gastric distension:

- ▶ inability to ventilate or difficulty ventilating and have *NO* airway obstruction
- ▶ visible gastric distension
- ▶ rigid abdomen

Assess for contraindications:

- ▶ facial, head, or spinal trauma
- ▶ signs or symptoms of epiglottitis, croup, or other airway diseases
- ▶ any anatomical disturbances
- ▶ possible ingestion of caustic or hydrocarbon solutions

Assess for the **nostril** that appears to be most patent (clear of debris). If materials and/or fluids are present, they must be suctioned at once. BSI must be applied during NG tube insertion; exposure to body fluids is highly likely during intubation.

PROCEDURE: Nasogastric Intubation in Infants and Children

1. Apply BSI precautions.
   Rationale: Gloves and eye protection are required at a minimum, and a gown may be needed if large amounts of blood or fluid are present to prevent exposure to infectious diseases.

2. Prepare and assemble the equipment.
   Rationale: Equipment should be kept in a clean environment in order to ensure it remains sterile.

continued...

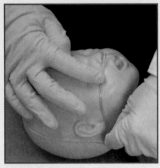
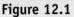

Figure 12.1

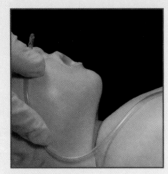

Figure 12.2

3. Measure the tube by holding the **distal** end of the NG tube at the tip of the nose, then around the nose, and extending the tube until it is just below the **xiphoid process** of the infant or child. Mark the **proximal** end of the tube with a piece of tape (Figures 12.1 and 12.2).

   Rationale: This measurement determines the proper distance for the tube to be inserted. The tube will not be inserted further than the taped mark on the tube.

4. Lubricate the NG tube 6 to 8 inches at the distal end of the tube with water-soluble lubricant. (Figure 12.3).

   Rationale: Lubrication makes insertion easier and reduces the risk of causing trauma.

5. Place the patient in a supine position.

6. You may wish to hyperventilate the patient prior to placement of the NG tube.

   Rationale: Because the infant or child will not be breathing during the procedure, hyperoxygenating the patient reduces the risk for hypoxia developing during the procedure.

7. Remove the oral or nasal airway if inserted.

   Rationale: Removal of an airway device may make insertion of the NG tube easier.

8. Choose the nostril that is most clear of debris.

9. Insert the lubricated tube gently in the nostril (Figure 12.4).

10. Advance the NG tube gently straight back toward the infant or child's ear. Continue to gently advance until you come to the tape marker on the NG tube (Figure 12.5).

    Rationale: Gentle insertion is important to reduce any risk of trauma. *STOP* any insertion if you meet any resistance during insertion. *NEVER* force the NG tube.

11. Check NG tube placement by attaching the 20-cc syringe to the tube. Pull back on the plunger, aspirating gastric contents (Figure 12.6).

    Rationale: Proper tube placement is essential. Knowing that the tube is placed in the stomach needs to be the first priority after insertion. Improper placement could cause injury or hypoxia.

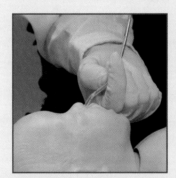

Figure 12.4

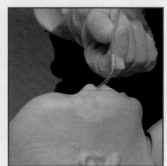

Figure 12.5

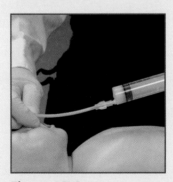

Figure 12.3

Figure 12.6

12. Immediately place your stethoscope over the infant's or child's epigastric area (just under the left intercostals area), and inject 10 to 20 cc of air into the tube. You should hear a gurgling sound with your stethoscope (Figure 12.7).

    Rationale: If no sound is heard, immediately remove the tube and consider reinsertion.

13. Once placement of the NG tube in the stomach is verified, gently pull back on the syringe to remove most of the air.

    Rationale: Removing most of the air in the stomach should make ventilations easier.

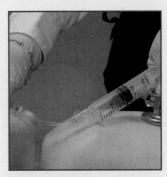 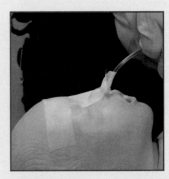

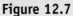

Figure 12.7   **Figure 12.8**

14. Secure the tube using tape to the infants or child's nose or forehead (Figure 12.8).

    Rationale: Securing the NG tube reduces the risk of the tube becoming dislodged.

15. Keep the syringe on the tube.

    Rationale: This reduces the risk of foreign material entering the NG tube.

16. Constantly monitor the tube for proper placement.

17. Document the procedure.

    Rationale: It is extremely important to document your findings, in order to have a history of facts and events that occurred at the scene.

ONGOING ASSESSMENT

After insertion of the NG tube, ventilation of the infant or child should be easier. If ventilation becomes difficult after insertion, check tube placement. If it is properly positioned in the stomach, consider removing more air from the stomach. Constantly monitor the tube for proper placement. Closely reassess the infant or child after each time he moves.

▶ PROBLEM SOLVING

▷ Because the NG tube is inserted in infants and children who are proving difficult to ventilate, it is very important that you first check to make sure there is no airway obstruction present. Insertion of a NG tube in an infant or child who has an airway obstruction could complicate the airway obstruction further.

▷ Gentle insertion of the NG tube is extremely important. Forcing the NG tube can cause injury to the upper airway, possibly resulting in an obstruction or aspiration of blood.

▷ You should use every precaution to keep the NG tube as clean as possible during insertion to reduce the possibility of infection.

▷ Insertion of the NG tube must be avoided in any infant or child who has any of the contraindications listed earlier. Insertion could cause further complications in such cases.

▷ Make sure the NG tube is properly positioned. Insertion of the tube in the lungs could cause serious complications. If the tube curls up in the pharynx, it could cause an airway obstruction.

▷ Securing the NG tube is essential to make sure it does not dislodge and cause complications.

►CASE STUDY

You are called to a possible drowning. En route to the scene, dispatch advises you that the patient is 6 months old and was in the bathtub. The babysitter went to get a towel and returned to find the baby under the water. After removing the baby from the water, she noticed that he was not breathing.

You and your partner are met at the door by the hysterical babysitter. You take the cyanotic infant and proceed to the ambulance to start care, while your partner obtains the infant's history from the babysitter. You place the patient on the cot, open the airway, and check for breathing. The patient is apneic, so you grab the BVM and administer two breaths. The ventilations enter the chest and cause visible chest rise and fall. Next, you check for a pulse and find a slow, weak pulse. Your partner returns to the ambulance to give you a hand and relay the history and mechanism of injury from the babysitter. He asks what you need. You update him on the patient's condition. He suggests insertion of a nasogastric tube to help ensure ease in ventilation and to prevent gastric insufflation. You agree and start to prepare the equipment while he takes over ventilations.

As you are preparing the equipment, your partner hyperventilates the patient. You measure the NG tube and your partner stops ventilating the patient. You insert the NG tube and confirm placement. Your partner advises you that ventilations are easier. Your backup arrives and transports you to the hospital. En route, the patient's heart rate increases. You call the emergency department and advise them of the patient's condition and your estimated time of arrival. After transferring care to the ED staff, the doctor compliments you on inserting the NG tube, because it definitely contributed to the patient's positive disposition. ■

1. Which of the following is *Not* a cause of gastric distension in infants?
   a. overfeeding
   b. appropriate artificial ventilation
   c. aggressive ventilation
   d. hyperventilation

2. Which of the following is *Not* a contraindication for NG tube insertion in an infant?
   a. possible cervical spinal injury from a fall
   b. possible ingestion of bleach
   c. asphyxia from drowning
   d. a patient who had a barking cough prior to apnea

3. What is the correct method for confirming placement of the NG tube?
   a. Inject 20 cc of air while listening over the lungs for the absence of breath sounds.
   b. Inject 20 cc of air while listening for gurgling in the epigastrium.
   c. Withdraw 20 cc, looking for gastric contents.
   d. Hook the patient up to low-pressure suction and monitor the pulse oximeter.

CHAPTER 13
Sellick's Maneuver

OBJECTIVE

The student will successfully apply Sellick's maneuver in patients who do not have a gag reflex.

INTRODUCTION

You may sometimes hear **Sellick's maneuver** referred to as the "application of cricoid pressure." The maneuver presses the **cricoid cartilage** against the **esophagus,** which in turn blocks the esophagus. The technique may be useful for the EMT-Basic who does not have the training or authorization to intubate, but who needs to protect the airway by temporarily reducing the risk of vomiting and/or **aspiration.**

Sellick's maneuver has other applications as well. By blocking the esophagus, the technique allows a rescuer to ventilate a patient without causing gastric distension. The maneuver can also be used to assist in endotracheal **intubation.** By closing off the esophagus, vomiting is suppressed. At the same time, the maneuver helps bring the vocal cords into view for the intubator. Finally, while applying cricoid pressure, you can feel the endotracheal tube pass, allowing you to confirm correct placement.

According to recent studies, use of Sellick's maneuver increases the success rate of intubation. The technique has also proven beneficial for trauma patients who need to be intubated but have a suspected cervical spinal injury. In such cases, visualization of the **glottic opening** and vocal cords can be difficult, and movement of the neck could cause further spinal cord injury.

To use Sellick's maneuver, it is imperative that you know the exact anatomy and location of the cricoid cartilage—the only cartilage in the neck that completely surrounds the trachea. This technique can seriously injure the airway if you apply pressure to the wrong spot.

▶EQUIPMENT

You will need the following equipment:

▶ BSI equipment

ASSESSMENT

Sellick's maneuver should be used in unresponsive patients who do not have a gag reflex. It may be used as a temporary technique while rolling patients to their side or getting suction equipment. When performing the maneuver, the patient should be **supine** with the head in a neutral position.

The cricoid cartilage is located inferior to the **thyroid cartilage,** or Adam's apple. To find it, palpate the thyroid cartilage with the tip of your finger until you find a slight depression. This depression is the cricothyroid membrane. Just inferior to the cricothyroid membrane is the solid ring of cartilage known as the cricoid cartilage.

PROCEDURE: Sellick's Maneuver

1. Apply BSI precautions.

   Rationale: Gloves and eye protection are required at a minimum, and a gown may be needed if large amounts of blood or fluid are present to prevent exposure to infectious diseases.

2. Ensure that the patient is in a supine position.

   Rationale: Although this maneuver can be done in any position, the supine position is the best position.

3. Place the head in the neutral position. Place yourself to the side of the patient (Figure 13.1).

   Rationale: The neutral position places the anatomy in the proper position for the maneuver to work.

4. Find the cricoid cartilage. To find it, palpate the thyroid cartilage with the tip of your finger until you find a slight depression. This depression is the cricothyroid membrane. Just inferior to the cricothyroid membrane is the solid ring of cartilage known as the cricoid cartilage (Figure 13.2).

   Rationale: The landmark of the cricoid cartilage is the best location for this maneuver to work; any other area could cause injury or not accomplish the objectives.

5. Place the thumb and index finger on the lateral sides of the cricoid cartilage (Figure 13.3).

6. Using the thumb and index finger of one hand, apply pressure to the anterior and lateral aspects of the cricoid cartilage, just next to the midline. Apply firm, but gentle **posterior** pressure (Figure 13.4).

   Rationale: This pressure needs to be enough to cause the cricoid cartilage to press against the

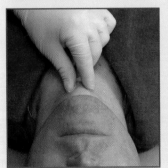

Figure 13.1

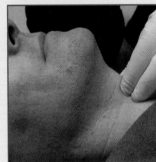

Figure 13.2

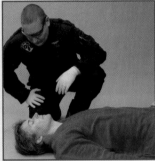

Figure 13.3

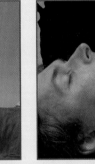

Figure 13.4

esophagus. You will not feel any closing of the esophagus. Too much pressure can cause injury to the cricoid cartilage, causing injury to the airway.

7. Document that the maneuver was performed.

   Rationale: It is extremely important to document your findings in order to have a history of facts and events that occurred at the scene.

Watch for signs of swelling (or other trauma) around the cricoid cartilage after the maneuver is performed.

▶ PROBLEM SOLVING

▶ The most significant problem that you may encounter when performing Sellick's maneuver is not having enough EMS providers available to perform this procedure while accomplishing other procedures.

▶ When you use this technique during bag-valve-mask ventilation and endotracheal intubation, a second rescuer is required, and you must remember that the patient is likely to regurgitate when you release cricoid pressure.

▶ Ideally, once you have applied Sellick's maneuver, you must maintain it until endotracheal intubation is confirmed and personnel are ready to suction the oropharynx or place a **nasogastric tube** to decompress the stomach.

PEDIATRIC NOTE:

Remember that it may be very hard to find the cricoid cartilage in some patients—most notably in infants, children, small adults, and patients with short or fat necks or neck deformities. Also, with pediatric patients, excessive pressure on the relatively soft cartilage may cause tracheal obstruction or disruption. The use of Sellick's maneuver in children should be limited and used as a last resort (Figure 13.5).

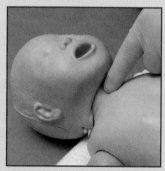

Figure 13.5

▶ CASE STUDY

You are called to assist a patient who is having difficulty breathing. Once on scene, you find the patient in cardiac arrest. You call for backup while your partner begins to treat the patient. Your partner begins artificial ventilation while you initiate chest compressions. You observe gastric distension increasing with ventilations.

When your backup arrives, one of them begins to set up equipment for intubation. You ask the other to apply cricoid pressure to help prevent further gastric distension. Your partner begins to hyperventilate the patient prior to the intubation attempt. During the hyperventilation, you observe no further increase in the gastric distension. You tell the EMT applying cricoid pressure to continue because he is doing a good job. Your partner is then ready to intubate the patient. She is able to obtain rapid visualization of the glottic opening due to the cricoid pressure and quickly places the endotracheal tube. She confirms the tube placement and then secures the ET tube while cricoid pressure is released.

You continue to treat the patient as the other crew prepares your cot for transport. You load the patient and begin a rapid transport to the local emergency department. You notify the hospital of your patient. After arriving at the emergency department your partner transfers care to the emergency physician and helps you restock the supplies. ■

1. Cricoid pressure should be applied on which of the following patients?
   a. a 53-year-old patient with respiratory distress who is receiving positive pressure ventilation
   b. a 17-year-old patient who is unresponsive from a head injury and actively vomiting
   c. a 46-year-old patient with a deformity to the cervical spine who is in cardiac arrest after a motor-vehicle collision
   d. a 32-year-old overdose patient who is in respiratory arrest and experiences dry heaves with attempted intubation

2. Which of the following most accurately describes the application of Sellick's maneuver?
   a. gentle pressure on the trachea at the cricoid ring
   b. firm posterior pressure inferior to the thyroid cartilage
   c. firm depression of the larynx against the esophagus
   d. application of pressure only when administering ventilations

3. Which of the following is *not* a goal of Sellick's maneuver?
   a. prevent air from entering the stomach
   b. aid in successful nasogastric intubation
   c. aid in the visualization of the glottic opening
   d. feel for the passage of the tube during successful intubation

CHAPTER 14

Assisting with Endotracheal Intubation

KEY TERMS

Aspiration

Distal

Endotracheal (ET) intubation

Gag reflex

Gastric distension

Hypoxia

Laryngoscope

Pharynx

Pulse oximetry

Sellick's maneuver

Stylet

OBJECTIVE

The student will successfully demonstrate how to assist with endotracheal intubation.

INTRODUCTION

Endotracheal (ET) intubation is a skill performed by advanced life support (ALS) personnel. In many cases you will be asked to assist the ALS provider in performing or maintaining an endotracheal tube.

The ET tube is the preferred device for maintaining the airway of an unconscious patient. Although the ET tube is usually used in situations where the patient does not have a **gag reflex,** patients may be given a medication to remove the gag reflex so that an ET tube can be placed. The ET tube allows for complete control of the airway and provides a direct route for ventilations to the lungs. Once the ET tube is in place, the position of the head is irrelevant.

The ET tube is designed to isolate the trachea from the **pharynx** and eliminates the risks of materials and/or fluids entering the trachea, thus reducing the risk of **aspiration.** It also allows for reduced chances of **gastric distension.** The ET tube allows for the best artificial method of oxygenation and ventilation to the lungs. If needed, a suction catheter can be placed directly down the ET tube to suction the air passages (see Chapter 8). In addition, some cardiac resuscitation drugs can be passed through the ET tube if vascular access is not available.

The ET tube is placed directly into the trachea using a direct visualization technique by way of a **laryngoscope.** The laryngoscope has a light on it to make visualization easier. Two types of blades are used in the prehospital setting, straight and curved blades. Laryngoscope blades come in many sizes, depending on the size of the patient.

The ET tube is a slightly curved tube that has a cuff at the **distal** end. An opening, distal to the cuff, allows for ventilations. If the tube is placed into the trachea, the distal cuff seals the trachea and does not allow for materials and/or fluid to enter the airway passage, reducing the risks of aspiration. In most cases the ET tube is used in conjunction with a stylet. A **stylet** is a piece of pliable coated metal that is inserted into the ET tube to allow the ET tube to be molded into the desired position for insertion.

Some studies show that **Sellick's maneuver** can be used to increase successful intubation attempts. In trauma patients, a modified intubation technique is recommended. Intubation is not difficult, but it is technical. With proper assistance the technique can be made considerably more easy.

▶ EQUIPMENT

You will need the following equipment:

- ▶ BSI equipment
- ▶ BVM, with reservoir attachment
- ▶ Oxygen cylinder
- ▶ Suction and catheter
- ▶ ET tube (properly sized)
- ▶ Stylet
- ▶ Laryngoscope handle
- ▶ Laryngoscope blades (straight, curved)
- ▶ Water-soluble lubricant
- ▶ 10-cc syringe
- ▶ Towel
- ▶ ET tube securing device (tape)
- ▶ Stethoscope

ASSESSMENT

Unconscious patients with no gag reflex are the primary patients who require ET intubation. In cases where patients have a gag reflex and signs of **hypoxia,** or have pending respiratory failure, ET intubation may be required. In some cases a medication may be given in those cases to reduce, or eliminate, the gag reflex.

If the patient has a suspected spinal injury, cervical immobilization must be maintained at all times. If materials and/or fluids are present, they must be suctioned at once. BSI must be applied during ET intubation because, exposure to body fluids is highly likely during intubation.

 PROCEDURE: Assisting with Endotracheal Intubation

1. Apply BSI precautions.

   Rationale: Gloves and eye protection are required at a minimum, and a gown may be needed if large amounts of blood or fluid are present to prevent exposure to infectious diseases.

2. Place patient in the supine position.

   Rationale: If the patient is breathing, intubation may be attempted in another position; in most cases, however, the patient will be placed in the supine position.

3. Assist in gathering endotracheal intubation equipment.

   Rationale: The ALS personnel may be busy with other tasks, so setting up the equipment for them may save time. Knowing the equipment and how the ALS personnel like it placed are essential.

4. Assist with ventilations.

   Rationale: Because the patient is not breathing in most cases, he needs assisted ventilations while he is prepared to be intubated.

continued...

5. Assuming there is no concern about trauma, place a towel under patient's head.

   Rationale: This action places the head in a neutral position, which allows the airway to be placed in a more anterior position, making the vocal cords more visible.

6. Begin to keep track the time it takes to do the intubation.

   Rationale: The person doing the intubation may get so caught up in the intubation process that she forgets how long the procedure is actually taking.

7. Hyperventilate the patient, prior to intubation (Figure 14.1).

   Rationale: Because the patient will not be breathing during the procedure, hyperoxygenating the patient reduces the risks for hypoxia during the procedure.

8. Remove the oral or nasal airway if inserted.

   Rationale: Visualization of the vocal cords is not as easy with an airway in place.

9. Hand requested equipment to the ALS provider.

   Rationale: The ALS provider needs to concentrate on the visualization of the vocal cords. If she looks away to retrieve equipment, she can lose sight of the vocal cords. You must be sure you hand the ALS provider the proper equipment in the correct anatomical direction.

10. Apply Sellick's maneuver—slight pressure using two fingers over the cricoid cartilage—if requested (Figure 14.2).

    Rationale: Sellick's maneuver can assist in aligning the vocal cords within the sight of the ALS provider. Sellick's maneuver can also reduce the risk of stomach contents interfering with the intubation and can reduce the risk of aspiration.

11. Utilize the BVM and hyperventilate the patient for 2 minutes when requested, or re-ventilate the patient using the BVM if placement of the ET tube is not sucessful (Figures 14.3 and 14.4).

    Rationale: After the tube has been placed, the ALS personnel will ask you to ventilate the patient on her request. The ALS provider will be

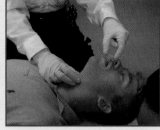

Figure 14.1

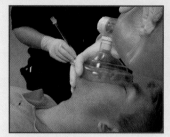

Figure 14.2

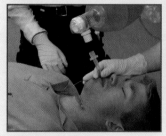

Figure 14.3

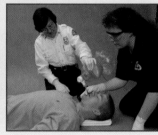

Figure 14.4

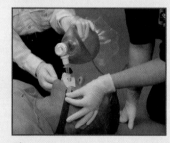

Figure 14.5

auscultating the chest and abdomen to confirm tube placement. If the tube has not been successfully placed, the ALS provider will request that you replace the oral or nasal airway and hyperventilate the patient, while she prepares for a second attempt.

12. Assist in securing the ET tube (Figure 14.5).

    Rationale: It is easy to dislodge an ET tube. The securing system reduces the risk of a dislodged tube.

13. Document your findings.

    Rationale: It is extremely important to document your findings in order to have a history of facts and events that occurred at the scene.

It is the responsibility of the person placing the ET tube to confirm placement of the tube. Once the tube has been placed, be very careful not to move the tube until it is secured. In many EMS systems a confirmation device that ensures proper tube placement may be used. This will entail a syringe or bulb aspiration technique, or the use of a colorimetric end-tidal CO_2 device.

After the tube has been placed, **pulse oximetry** may also be used to monitor continued tube placement. During initial ventilations you should monitor the compliance of ventilations; if the ventilations become more difficult to accomplish, notify the ALS provider immediately. Movement of the patient has the greatest likelihood of causing ET tube displacement. Closely reassess the patient after each movement.

PROBLEM SOLVING

▶ A dislodged ET tube is the most common problem facing the EMT. If you notice that the tube has moved or dislodged, do *NOT* try to replace the tube. Consult with the ALS provider immediately.

▶ Hypoxia can occur during the intubation process. The person performing the intubation may be so involved with the process of the intubation that he might not notice the exceeded time. If you notice that the time seems excessive or you notice signs of hypoxia, consult with the ALS provider to reoxygenate the patient. Hyperventilation or preoxygenation prior to an intubation attempt can also reduce the risks of hypoxia.

▶ Patients may have physiologic problems that can make giving ventilations difficult. If you notice that you are having a difficult time ventilating the patient, consult with the ALS provider immediately.

▶ You may be requested to suction the ET tube. See Chapter 8 for the steps that should be followed to perform tracheal suctioning.

CASE STUDY

You and your paramedic partner are responding to back up a basic life support crew that is working on a patient in cardiac arrest. Once on scene, your partner gets the report from the EMT in charge. You begin preparing the equipment for your partner to intubate the patient after she is done with her initial assessment. You ask her what equipment she will need. She advises that she wants an 8.0 ET tube and a #4 curved blade. You secure this equipment. While setting up the supplies, you also remove a 10-cc syringe, an end-tidal CO_2 detector, and a commercial tube holder.

Your partner completes the rest of her assessment while the EMT hyperventilates the patient. Your partner assembles the laryngoscope blade, and asks you to apply Sellick's maneuver while she attempts visualization. She reaches for the tube and you hand it to her so she can maintain visualization. After passing the ET tube, you attach the BVM and the end-tidal CO_2 detector and ventilate the patient while she is confirming ET tube placement. You then help your partner in securing the ET tube. You continue with ventilations as the patient is prepared for transport.

The patient is being transported to the emergency department. En route, you hear gurgling from the ET tube. You help your partner suction the ET tube. Once ventilations are resumed, you observe that the gurgling is no longer present. Your partner notifies emergency department personnel that you will arrive in 5 minutes. Upon arrival, patient care is transferred to the emergency personnel without any further changes. ■

1. Which of the following is not recommended equipment for intubation?
   a. oxygen tank
   b. suction unit
   c. bulb syringe
   d. tube holder

2. Correct placement of the ET tube will put the distal tip at which of the following locations?
   a. just inferior to the vocal cords
   b. superior to the carina
   c. with the cuff above the glottic opening
   d. as far as possible

3. Confirmation of the placement of the ET tube can be accomplished through all of the following *Except*:
   a. listening for bilateral breath sounds.
   b. visualizing the tube pass through the cords.
   c. applying an esophageal detection device.
   d. visualizing condensation in the ET tube.

CHAPTER 15

Insertion of the Esophageal Tracheal Combitube®

OBJECTIVE

The student will be able to successfully insert an Esophageal Tracheal Combitube®.

INTRODUCTION

In some EMS systems, the **Esophageal Tracheal Combitube® (ETC)** or Combitube® cannot be used by EMT-Basics. In most states, local medical direction may or may not authorize training and protocols for its use.

The Combitube® is the primary backup airway in most ALS systems. The device offers several major advantages. First, it uses a "blind" insertion technique that does not require visualization of the trachea. Second, the Combitube® may prevent vomit from entering the trachea, thus protecting the airway. Third, the Combitube® allows for rapid intubation of the patient independent of the patient's position. This is especially helpful for trauma patients for whom limited movement of the cervical spine is necessary. Despite these advantages, the Combitube® is not as easy to use as you might think.

The Combitube® comes in two sizes, and as mentioned, requires no visualization during the insertion process. It is a double lumen airway in which the two lumens are separated by a partition wall. The Combitube® was developed to be placed in either the trachea or the esophagus. The **distal** end of the Combitube® has a cuff that is used to seal either the trachea or the esophagus, depending on where the airway is placed. The **proximal** end has a cuff used to seal the **pharynx.**

The #1 tube is a little longer than the #2 tube and has a closed end. It delivers ventilations through small holes in the tubing between the distal cuff and the pharynx cuff. The perforations are just proximal to the **glottic opening.**

When the Combitube® is placed in the esophagus, the distal cuff will block the esophagus and the pharynx cuff will seal the mouth. During ventilations, the tube's sealed end prevents oxygen from entering the esophagus and stomach. Ventilations flow out of the small holes into the pharynx and are diverted into the trachea and lungs. Esophageal placement is best achieved with the Combitube®.

The #2 tube has an open end similar to an endotracheal tube. If the Combitube® is placed into the trachea, the distal cuff will ensure that ventilations are delivered directly into the trachea.

▶ EQUIPMENT

You will need the following equipment:

- ▶ BSI equipment
- ▶ Oxygen cylinder
- ▶ BVM and reservoir
- ▶ Suction equipment
- ▶ Combitube
- ▶ Water-soluble lubricant
- ▶ Large 100-cc syringe
- ▶ Small 20-cc syringe
- ▶ Stethoscope

ASSESSMENT

Use of the Combitube® is indicated when:

- ▶ patients are unconscious and lack a **gag reflex.**
- ▶ **endotracheal intubation** is not allowed or cannot immediately be performed, even though strongly indicated.
- ▶ endotracheal intubation is unsuccessful after two attempts.
- ▶ **in-line immobilization** of the patient prevents endotracheal intubation.
- ▶ bleeding, vomiting, or a patient's anatomy obstructs the direct visualization required for endotracheal intubation.

Use of the Combitube® is contraindicated when:

- ▶ patients are younger than 16 years of age.
- ▶ patients are less than 5 feet tall or over 7 feet tall.
- ▶ esophageal disease is present.
- ▶ patients are conscious with a gag reflex.
- ▶ patients have swallowed a **caustic substance.**

Use the Combitube® with caution in any patient who has facial trauma. The anatomy may have been altered with the trauma, and insertion can be difficult at times.

PROCEDURE: Insertion of the Esophageal Tracheal Combitube®

1. Apply BSI precautions.

   Rationale: Gloves and eye protection are required at a minimum, and a gown may be needed if large amounts of blood or fluid are present to prevent exposure to infectious diseases.

2. Place the patient in the supine position.

   Rationale: Maintaining proper anatomical alignment is important in this procedure. The Combitube® was developed to be placed in a patient only in the supine position but is sometimes used otherwise in trauma patients for whom limited movement of the cervical spine is necessary.

3. Position yourself at the patient's head.

   Rationale: This location is the best position for placement of the tube. If this position is not available, you may try from the side of the patient.

4. Confirm patient for proper age and size.

   Rationale: The Combitube® is contraindicated in patients who are less than 16 years, or less than 5 feet tall or over 7 feet tall.

5. If needed, suction any materials and/or fluids that might be obstructing the airway.

   Rationale: Aspiration of materials and/or fluid into, the upper airway could happen if materials are not suctioned.

6. Assemble and check equipment, noting any air leaks in the cuffs (Figure 15.1).

   Rationale: Checking equipment now is essential to make sure that a problem does not occur during the insertion procedure. Later is not the time to find out that you have an equipment failure. Make sure that you maintain equipment in a clean environment. Foreign material on the Combitube® could cause an infection. Controversy surrounds whether the syringes should be attached to the Combitube® during insertion. Some individuals feel that it may make insertion more difficult with syringes attached.

7. Lubricate the distal end of the tube (Figure 15.2).

   Rationale: Lubrication of the tube allows for easier insertion and reduces the risk of trauma during insertion.

8. Keep the patient supine, with the head in a neutral, in-line position.

   Rationale: Maintaining the head in neutral alignment is important to maintain proper anatomical alignment.

9. **Hyperventilate** the patient for a few minutes prior to inserting the Combitube® (Figure 15.3).

   Rationale: Patients can become hypoxic during this procedure. Hyperventilating the patient before insertion reduces this risk. It is important to note to yourself how long it is taking to perform the Combitube® insertion.

10. Perform a **jaw-lift maneuver** (Figure 15.4).

    Rationale: This allows easy access to the oral cavity to insert the Combitube®. Be careful in performing this maneuver if the patient has experienced facial trauma.

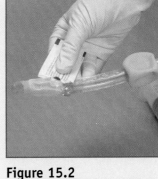
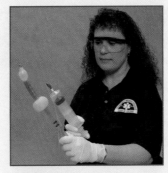

Figure 15.1   **Figure 15.2**

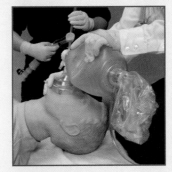
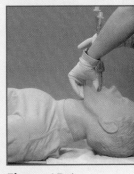

Figure 15.3   **Figure 15.4**

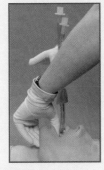
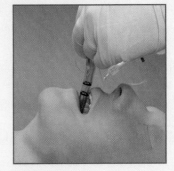

Figure 15.5   **Figure 15.6**

11. Place the Combitube® into the patient's mouth and gently insert the airway. If resistance is met, do not force the tube (Figure 15.5).

    Rationale: Trauma to the upper airway could be caused by forceful insertion of the Combitube®.

12. Insert the Combitube® until the airway's black rings meet the level of the patient's teeth (Figure 15.6).

    Rationale: This is the point at which the Combitube® has been seated for proper positioning in the patient's airway.

continued...

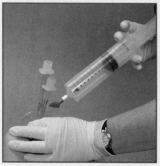

Figure 15.7

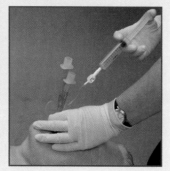

Figure 15.8

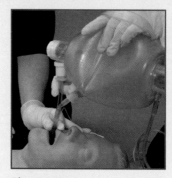

Figure 15.9

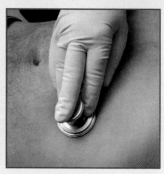

Figure 15.10

13. Using the large syringe, inflate the pharyngeal cuff with 100 cc of air (Figure 15.7).

14. Using the smaller syringe, inflate the distal cuff with 10 to 15 cc of air (Figure 15.8).

15. Attach the BVM to tube #1 and slowly begin ventilations (Figure 15.9).

16. Place a stethoscope over the patient's stomach and **auscultate** for gurgling sounds (Figure 15.10).

    Rationale: Because you have blindly inserted the Combitube® into the airway, you need to do an assessment to confirm the tube's location.

17. If no sounds are heard over the patient's stomach, watch for chest rise, and auscultate the chest for breath sounds bilaterally. If the chest rises with each ventilation and you hear breath sounds, continue ventilations. Consider hyperventilation for 2 minutes after insertion and then resume normal ventilations.

    Rationale: Signs of chest rise, breath sounds, and *NO* stomach gurgling confirm the location of the Combitube® in the esophagus. Consider hyperventilation because your patient might have become slightly hypoxic during the procedure.

18. If gurgling sounds are present and you do not see chest rise and/or cannot hear breath sounds, your Combitube® is located in the trachea. Immediately

stop ventilations through tube #1 once you are convinced the tube is located in the trachea.

Rationale: Additional ventilations into the stomach will increase the risk that the patient will vomit. Also prolonged ventilations into the stomach can cause **gastric distension,** resulting in pressure on the diaphragm and making ventilations of the lungs difficult.

19. Slowly begin ventilations through tube #2 (Figure 15.11).

20. Auscultate the stomach for gurgling sounds. Also look for chest rise, and auscultate the chest for bilateral breath sounds (Figure 15.12).

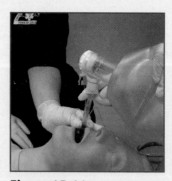

Figure 15.11

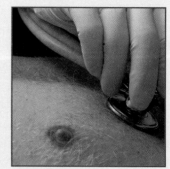

Figure 15.12

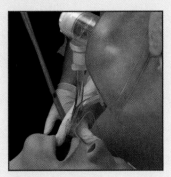

Figure 15.13

stomach gurgling confirm the location of the Combitube® in the trachea. Consider hyperventilation because your patient might have become slightly hypoxic during the procedure.

21. If there are *NO* epigastric sounds and if you see chest rise and/or hear breath sounds, continue ventilations. Consider hyperventilation for 2 minutes after insertion and then resume normal ventilations (Figure 15.13).

    Rationale: When ventilating through tube #2, these signs of chest rise, breath sounds, and *NO*

22. Although controversial, if at anytime you are confused or unsure of the location of the Combitube®, consider removing the tube, hyperventilating the patient for a few minutes and trying again.

    Rationale: Being unsure of the placement of the Combitube® is not acceptable. Ventilating a patient through the wrong tube could result in death or severe disability. You are better off starting over than being unsure of the Combitube's® location.

23. Document your findings.

    Rationale: It is extremely important to document your findings in order to have a history of facts and events that occurred at the scene.

ONGOING ASSESSMENT

Constantly monitor chest rise. Watch for gastric distension. Monitor the pilot balloon on the end of each syringe tube. Each balloon should retain air pressure if the cuffs are adequately inflated. Re-evaluate lung sounds after every movement of the patient. Visualize the airway for materials and/or fluids.

▶ PROBLEM SOLVING

▶ If during the insertion process you meet resistance, do not force the tube. Forcing the tube could cause trauma to the upper or lower airways or to the esophagus.

▶ The major complication of the Combitube® is a failure to determine where the tube has been placed. You *MUST* assess the patient to make sure proper ventilations are being accomplished. If you are unsure of tube placement, remove the Combitube®, hyperventilate, and try again.

▶ Use care when inserting the Combitube® in patients who have sustained facial trauma.

▶ If you suspect cervical trauma, do not **hyperextend** the head during insertion of the Combitube®.

▶ **Hypoxia** can result if too much time is spent inserting the airway. If you suspect an extended time, remove the Combitube®, hyperventilate the patient, and try insertion again.

▶ You must maintain adequate air pressure in both the pharynx and distal cuffs. Improper inflation can allow aspiration and/or cause air to leak from the tube. Monitor distal balloon pressure to ensure proper inflation.

▶ If the patient regains consciousness or demonstrates a gag reflex, remove the Combitube®. (Remember, vomiting almost always follows **extubation.**) For extubation, that is, to remove the Combitube®, take these steps:

1. Apply BSI precautions.
2. Have suction ready.
3. Place the patient on his side.
4. Deflate the pharynx cuff.
5. Deflate the distal cuff.
6. Remove tube gently.
7. Reassess the patient.

▶CASE STUDY

You are called as backup for a crew on scene with an intoxicated patient. When you arrive you find the original crew suctioning the patient. The patient is unresponsive, has vomited, and the crew is preparing to secure his airway. The patient remains un-responsive even with painful stimuli. During suctioning, the paramedic noticed that the patient did not have a gag reflex. He elects to insert an oropharyngeal airway. The patient accepts the airway without difficulty.

The paramedic begins positive pressure ventilation, while his partner maintains cricoid pressure. The patient's level of responsiveness has not changed, so the para-medic decides to insert an advanced airway. Unfortunately, after two attempts, the paramedic is unable to intubate the patient successfully. Your partner suggests the Combitube®. The paramedic agrees, and your partner begins to prepare the equip-ment while the patient is being hyperventilated. The paramedic takes the Com-bitube® and inserts it gently. You assist him by inflating the cuffs. You begin ventilating the patient through tube #1 while he listens over the epigastrium. He hears nothing, and proceeds to listen over the lungs. He gives you a thumbs up on the placement of the tube, and he begins to secure it. You continue ventilating the patient as the remaining providers package the patient for transport. Ventilations are continued through the Combitube® during transport, and the patient remains well oxygenated. Upon arrival at the emergency department the patient care is trans-ferred to the emergency staff. ■

1. Which of the following is *not* an indication for Combitube® use?
   a. when tracheal intubation is not successful after two attempts
   b. when immobilization of a trauma patient prevents successful intubation
   c. when the patient is vomiting and you want to minimize exposure risks
   d. when endotracheal intubation cannot immediately be performed

2. Which of the following is true of the Combitube®?
   a. The Combitube® does not require direct visualization of the epiglottis.
   b. The Combitube® is properly placed regardless of its location.
   c. The Combitube® can be used on anyone without a gag reflex.
   d. The Combitube® can be used by all providers without medical direction.

3. Which of the following patients would qualify for Combitube® use?
   a. a patient who is 14 years old and 5 feet, 8 inches tall
   b. a patient who has a history of esophageal varices
   c. a patient who is apneic after ingesting cleaning solution
   d. a patient in cardiac arrest who is trapped in a vehicle

CHAPTER 16

Artificial Ventilations of a Stoma Breather

KEY TERMS

Agonal respirations

Artificial ventilations

Head-tilt/chin-lift
   maneuver

Jaw-thrust maneuver

Laryngectomy

Mucous plugs

Pharynx

Stoma

OBJECTIVE

The student will be able to perform successfully artificial ventilations of a stoma breather.

INTRODUCTION

Stomas are surgical openings in the neck that allow a patient to breathe. These airways may be created when a patient suffers a trauma or illness that prevents normal breathing through the mouth and nose.

When you find patients with stomas in severe respiratory distress or respiratory arrest, you may provide ventilations through the stoma. As with other uses of the bag-valve mask, two rescuers are recommended for effective ventilations.

▶EQUIPMENT

You will need the following equipment:

▶ BSI equipment

▶ Suction

▶ Bag-valve mask with attached oxygen reservoir

▶ Pediatric mask

▶ Full oxygen tank and regulator

ASSESSMENT

Mucous plugs often obstruct the stoma, causing respiratory distress. You should check for this condition first, and clear the stoma as necessary. Suctioning through the stoma may be necessary with a suction catheter. Attempt to ascertain information about the stoma such as the reason it was placed, when it was placed, and whether the patient relies entirely on the "neck breather." In the case of a partial **laryngectomy,** for example, the patient may be able to take in some air by mouth and/or nose.

PROCEDURE: Artificial Ventilations of a Stoma Breather

1. Apply BSI precautions.

   Rationale: Gloves and eye protection are required at a minimum, and a gown may be needed if large amounts of blood or fluid are present to prevent exposure to infectious diseases.

2. Remove any items of clothing, such as scarves or ties, from the area of the stoma.

   Rationale: You need complete access to the area. Clothes and other objects can hinder your access.

3. Clear the stoma of obvious mucous plugs or secretions (Figure 16.1).

   Rationale: Remove any obvious materials from around the stoma opening. In many cases this may be all that is necessary for the patient to breathe more comfortably.

4. Leave the patient's head and neck in a neutral position. You do not need to perform a **head-tilt/chin-lift** or **jaw-thrust maneuver** on a patient with a stoma. You already have a direct route into the trachea.

   Rationale: The stoma is a direct opening to the trachea. Specific positioning is not required in these patients.

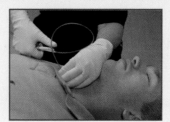 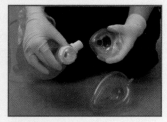

Figure 16.1   **Figure 16.2**

5. Select a mask, most often a pediatric mask, that fits securely over the stoma and can be sealed against the neck (Figure 16.2).

   Rationale: A pediatric mask, because of its size, works well in making a seal over the stoma and the neck. Soft masks or masks that have less air in their bladders sometimes work better than a large mask as well.

6. Hold the mask seal with your hand. If two people are available, one partner makes a seal with both hands around the mask, while the other ventilates. **Artificial ventilations** should be delivered at a minimum of once every 5 seconds in adults and once every 3 seconds in children

continued...

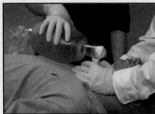

Figure 16.3

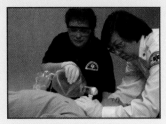

Figure 16.4

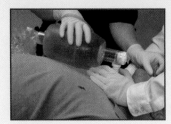

Figure 16.5

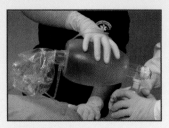

Figure 16.6

and infants (Figures 16.3). Each ventilation should be delivered over 2 seconds in adults.

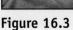
> **PEDIATRIC NOTE:**
>
> Each ventilation should be delivered over 1 to 1.5 seconds in children and infants.

7. Assess effectiveness of ventilations. Watch for chest rise and fall. Feel to be sure the air is escaping back through the stoma upon exhalation (Figure 16.4).

   Rationale: If the patient is being ventilated properly, the chest should rise and you should be able to auscultate for breath sounds on the patient.

8. If the chest does not rise, suspect a partial laryngectomy. Seal the nose and mouth with one hand by placing the palm over the lips and pinching the nose between the third and fourth fingers (Figure 16.5). Repeat ventilations.

   Rationale: Patients with partial laryngectomies have a stoma, but also have an intact upper airway. In this case the patient can be ventilated through either the stoma or the mouth/nose. The stoma is the preferred technique. Closing of the mouth and nose allows air to flow to the lungs.

9. If unable to artificially ventilate through the stoma, consider sealing the stoma and ventilating through the mouth/nose (Figure 16.6).

   Rationale: Although not the preferred technique, it is acceptable to ventilate in a normal fashion except you need to block off the stoma opening.

10. If still not able to ventilate, consider an obstruction to the stoma. Suctioning must be immediately considered.

11. Document your findings.

    Rationale: It is extremely important to document your findings in order to have a history of facts that occurred at the scene.

ONGOING ASSESSMENT

Constantly assess the stoma for mucous obstruction. Multiple suctioning attempts may be necessary to maintain a patent airway. Assess the effectiveness of ventilations (e.g., mask seal, chest rise/fall, lung sounds, skin color, and pulse oximetry).

▶ PROBLEM SOLVING

▶ If mucus is too thick to suction, and the materials are available to you, consider injecting 3 to 5 cc of normal saline through stoma to break up the plug and aid in its removal.

▶ As stated earlier, if ventilation through the stoma is unsuccessful, consider sealing the stoma and ventilating through mouth/nose. Use of this technique depends on whether the trachea is directly attached to the stoma or still attached to the mouth, nose, and **pharynx.**

▶ An endotracheal tube can be inserted through the stoma into the trachea. Follow local protocols when performing this procedure.

▶CASE STUDY

You are called to a nursing home to transport a geriatric patient in respiratory distress. Upon arrival, you find a patient in obvious distress with central cyanosis. During your assessment, you find that the patient has a stoma. Your partner finds the nurse, and determines that the patient has had a complete laryngectomy. You inspect the stoma and find that it has a lot of mucus around it. You attempt to suction it, but have difficulty removing anything. Your partner injects some saline into the stoma and you attempt to suction again. You are able to remove a thick mucous plug from the airway. Then you assess the patient's respiratory status. The patient has only **agonal respirations.**

Your partner goes to the truck to get a pediatric mask, while you prepare the BVM for positive pressure ventilations. When your partner returns, he holds a mask seal while you attempt to ventilate the patient. The ventilations cause chest rise and fall, and the cyanosis slowly disappears. You call for backup so you can have an extra set of hands available during transport. When backup arrives, you package the patient and transport him to the emergency department. The transport concludes without any further changes in the patient condition. ■

1. How would you assess for an airway obstruction in a patient with a stoma?
   a. Attempt to ventilate the patient while maintaining a modified jaw-thrust maneuver.
   b. Ensure a good mask seal around the stoma and attempt ventilation.
   c. Listen for breath sounds while ventilating through the mouth and nose.
   d. Advance a suction catheter through the stoma to ensure patency.

2. Which of the following best describes the location of a stoma?
   a. superior to the sternal notch
   b. inferior to the cricoid cartilage
   c. at the location of the cricoid cartilage
   d. proximal to the larynx

3. Which of the following could affect your ability to ventilate through a stoma?
   a. not inserting an airway adjunct prior to ventilating
   b. failing to adequately open the airway with a jaw-thrust maneuver
   c. not maintaining a good head-tilt/chin-lift maneuver
   d. losing air through the mouth and nose

CHAPTER 17
Pulse Oximetry

OBJECTIVE
The student will be able to successfully measure oxygen levels using a pulse oximeter.

KEY TERMS
Acetone wipe

Anemic patients

Bronchodilator therapy

Hemoglobin

Hypoperfused patients

Hypoxia

Oxygen saturation percentage

Pulse oximeter

INTRODUCTION

A **pulse oximeter** is a photoelectric device that measures the level of oxygen circulating in a patient's blood vessels. It consists of a portable monitor and a sensing probe.

An oximeter's sensor is most commonly clipped onto a fingertip, toe, earlobe, or, in the case of an infant, the distal foot. Once activated, the device sends different colors of light into the tissue and measures the amount of light that returns. It records the results as the **hemoglobin** saturation percentage and, in the case of oxygen, may be recorded as SpO_2. The measurements are affected by the percentage of any molecule bound to hemoglobin. In most cases, this is a measure of oxygen.

Normally, the SpO_2 is around 95 to 99 percent. **Oxygen saturation percentages** below 95 percent may represent varying levels of **hypoxia.** Be aware, however, that some patients may present normally with a SpO_2 of less than 95 percent. A good example would be a chronic obstructive pulmonary disease (COPD) patient.

Instead of relying solely on the pulse oximeter, incorporate it into your overall clinical assessment. Any patient who complains of respiratory difficulty or who exhibits an altered mental status should be assessed with a pulse oximeter. This is a noninvasive device without any notable complications except when it distracts you from other indications of the patient's condition. Treat the patient—not the device.

Each device comes with a manual on how to operate that particular device. It is essential for you to become familiar with the workings of that particular device. These procedures will make you familiar with the generic procedures of a pulse oximeter.

► EQUIPMENT

You will need the following equipment:

▷ Pulse oximeter

▷ Various sizes of probes (adult, pediatric, infant)

▷ Extra batteries

▷ **Acetone wipes** (to remove fingernail polish)

ASSESSMENT

Do not delay your initial assessment or the administration of oxygen to apply the pulse oximeter. A pulse oximeter is most useful in two situations:

▷ when used to evaluate the effectiveness of any interventions you may perform, such as artificial respirations, oxygen therapy, **bronchodilator therapy,** or bag-valve-mask ventilations

▷ when used to alert you to a deterioration of the patient's oxygen saturation

When using a pulse oximeter, keep in mind that readings will not be accurate in all patients. For example:

▷ Patients exposed to carbon monoxide (CO), including chronic cigarette smokers, may have falsely high readings because CO binds to hemoglobin, producing the red color read by the device.

▷ **Anemic patients** and patients who have ingested certain kinds of poisons may also have falsely high SpO_2 readings.

▷ **Hypoperfused patients,** including patients in shock or hypothermic patients, do not have enough blood flowing through their capillaries for accurate readings.

▷ Patients with an injured extremity on which the probe is placed will give inaccurate readings.

PROCEDURE: Pulse Oximetry

1. Apply BSI precautions.

   Rationale: Gloves and eye protection are required at a minimum, and a gown may be needed if large amounts of blood or fluid are present to prevent exposure to infectious diseases.

2. Connect the sensor lead to the monitor and clip the sensor probe to the patient's fingertip on a noninjured extremity (Figure 17.1). Determine the patient's pulse rate.

   Rationale: Although other types of probes are available, finger probes seem to be the most comfortable and nonintrusive to patients. In most cases the finger probe is a reusable device. An injured extremity may give a false or no reading.

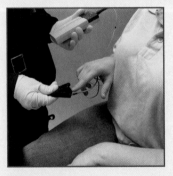

Figure 17.1

3. Turn on the pulse oximeter.

4. Observe for the SpO$_2$ and heart rate. Make sure the heart rate displayed on the monitor screen is the same as the patient's pulse rate (Figure 17.2).

   Rationale: It may take a few seconds for the device to get a reading. The patient's pulse and the heart rate on the pulse oximeter should be the same. If they are not, consider moving the probe to another finger.

5. Some pulse oximeters may display a pulsatile waveform, which should correspond with the patient's pulse rate.

6. Once you get an accurate reading, check the oximeter reading every 5 minutes, or if the patient suddenly becomes more short of breath or shows signs of hypoxia. A convenient time to do this is when you check the patient's vital signs (Figure 17.3).

   Rationale: It is important that, if you have placed a pulse oximeter on the patient, you constantly

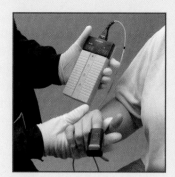
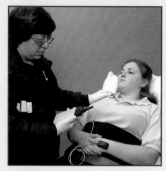

Figure 17.2   **Figure 17.3**

monitor the readings. Changes in oximetry readings should be documented and reported to ALS providers. Some oximeter devices have alarms that can be set if the pulse oximetry reading drops below a preset level.

7. Document the SpO$_2$ measurement.

   Rationale: It is extremely important to document your findings in order to have a history of facts and events that occurred at the scene.

ONGOING ASSESSMENT

Constantly check to make sure that the sensor probe is still attached to the patient. Movement of the patient, either voluntarily or involuntarily, may dislodge the probe. You might turn on the pulse oximeter's alarm, which will alert you if the probe becomes dislodged. Also, note that some models turn themselves off after a period of inactivity.

▶ PROBLEM SOLVING

▷ If you think the sensor probe may become easily dislodged, consider securing it in place with tape.

▷ If you're unable to obtain a reading or if you get poor waveforms or a "trouble" indicator, consider repositioning the sensor probe or moving it to an alternate site. Check to ensure that the batteries are functioning; if they are not, change batteries.

▷ In patients with poor peripheral perfusion, the earlobe may a preferable site for monitoring SpO$_2$.

▷ Some fingernail polish and fingernail embellishments, such as acrylic nails and decals or stones placed on the nail, can interfere with pulse oximeter measurements. If present, acetone wipes should be used before attaching the sensor probe. Acetone wipes should be stored with the pulse oximeter.

▶ CASE STUDY

You have been called to the home of a 30-year-old male who is having difficulty breathing. When you arrive, you find him sitting in a chair in the kitchen. The patient is wheezing loudly and has a history of asthma. The patient stated that the difficulty in breathing started approximately a half hour before calling for help. He states that he used his inhaler once with no relief.

On your initial assessment, his skin is warm and dry and he has a strong pulse. Your partner obtains baseline vital signs. The patient is breathing at 32 times per minute, has a heart rate of 96, and a blood pressure of 132/76. You place the pulse oximeter on the patient's finger and his initial SpO_2 on room air is 92 percent. You place a nonrebreather mask at 15 liters on your patient. On auscultation, you hear wheezing. You assist the patient in administering another dose of his inhaler.

With the inhaler and the high-flow oxygen, the patient begins to feel some relief. You recheck the patient's pulse oximeter reading, and obtain an SpO_2 of 98 percent. You place the patient on the cot and begin transport to the local emergency department. En route, the patient starts to complain of more wheezing. You notice that the pulse oximeter reading is at 94 percent. You assist with the third dose of the inhaler. As the patient feels relief, his pulse oximeter reading hits 97 percent. You continue the transport without any further changes. ■

1. Which of the following patients would have an accurate pulse oximetry reading?
   a. a 23-year-old patient suffering from smoke inhalation
   b. a 42-year-old patient who was found lying in the snow
   c. a 16-year-old trauma patient who is hypovolemic
   d. a 54-year-old patient with chest pain and hypotension

2. A pulse oximeter operates through which of the following principles?
   a. It detects the amount of oxygen in the red blood cells.
   b. It uses light to determine the oxygen dissolved in plasma.
   c. It detects the amount of bound hemoglobin in the blood.
   d. It uses light to determine the arterial concentration of oxygen.

3. The pulse oximeter is recommended for all of the following *except:*
   a. evaluating the effectiveness of bronchodilator therapy.
   b. checking the patient's heart rate.
   c. monitoring the oxygenation of an intubated patient.
   d. establishing a baseline for future therapy.

SECTION 1

AIRWAY MANAGEMENT AND VENTILATION

1. A nonrebreather mask provides concentrations of oxygen ranging from:
    A. 12 to 24 percent.
    B. 24 to 44 percent.
    C. 40 to 60 percent.
    D. 80 to 100 percent.

2. Major advantages of the Combitube® include which of the following?
    A. It is a blind technique that does not require tracheal visualization.
    B. It allows for rapid intubation independent of the patient's position.
    C. It may prevent vomitus from entering the trachea.
    D. all of the above.

3. When ventilating a pediatric patient with a pocket mask, you should:
    A. deliver ventilations over 1 to 1.5 seconds at a rate of 1 breath every 5 seconds.
    B. deliver ventilations over 1 to 2 seconds at a rate of 1 breath every 5 seconds.
    C. deliver ventilations over 1 to 1.5 seconds at a rate of 1 breath every 3 seconds.
    D. deliver ventilations over 1 to 2 seconds at a rate of 1 breath every 3 seconds.

4. When suctioning with a catheter that is inside an endotracheal tube, you should insert the suction catheter to the level of the:
    A. cricoid cartilage.
    B. carina.
    C. thyroid cartilage.
    D. vocal cords.

5. _____ is a safety system to ensure proper regulators are used on the proper compressed gas tanks.
    A. Threaded outlets
    B. Yoke-indexing
    C. Pin-indexing
    D. None of the above

6. Oropharyngeal airways should be used in a patient who is:
    A. not breathing or unresponsive with a gag reflex.
    B. not breathing or unresponsive without a gag reflex.
    C. breathing or unresponsive with a gag reflex.
    D. breathing or unresponsive without a gag reflex.

7. A nasogastric tube is used for:
   A. ensuring a direct pathway into the trachea.
   B. relieving gastric distension.
   C. isolating the stomach from overventilation.
   D. none of the above.
8. The jaw-thrust maneuver is the preferred technique for opening the airway in:
   A. any patient.
   B. a patient with suspected head or spinal injury.
   C. a patient without suspected head or spinal injury.
   D. cardiac arrest patients without suspected head or spinal injury.
9. While attempting to suction thick mucus from a patient with a stoma, you should consider:
   A. injecting 3 to 5 cc of normal saline and using a Yankauer (rigid) suction catheter.
   B. injecting 3 to 5 cc of normal saline and using a French (soft) suction catheter.
   C. injecting 5 to 10 cc of normal saline and using a Yankauer (rigid) suction catheter.
   D. injecting 5 to 10 cc of normal saline and using a French (soft) suction catheter.
10. Which of the following statements is *incorrect* regarding the accuracy of a pulse oximeter reading?
   A. Patients exposed to carbon monoxide (CO) may have falsely high readings because CO binds to hemoglobin.
   B. Patients exposed to carbon monoxide (CO) may have falsely low readings because CO binds to hemoglobin.
   C. Hypoperfused patients, including patients in shock or hypothermic patients, do not have enough blood flowing through their capillaries for accurate readings.
   D. If the probe is placed on an injured extremity, the resulting readings may be inaccurate.
11. Which of the following is *not* a type of oxygen flowmeter?
   A. Bourdon gauge
   B. pressure-compensated flowmeter
   C. DeLee gauge
   D. constant-flow selector valve
12. You should suction an adult patient no longer than:
   A. 5 seconds.
   B. 10 seconds.
   C. 15 seconds.
   D. 20 seconds.
13. Ideally, you should maintain Sellick's maneuver until:
   A. an oropharyngeal airway is in place.
   B. a nasopharygeal airway is in place.
   C. an endotracheal tube is in place.
   D. a Combitube® is in place.

14. The preferred technique in maintaining the airway of an unconscious patient is to use a(n):
    A. Combitube®.
    B. oropharyngeal airway.
    C. endotracheal tube.
    D. nasopharyngeal airway.
15. Which of the following is *not* a portable oxygen tank?
    A. C cylinder
    B. D cylinder
    C. E cylinder
    D. H cylinder
16. A nasal cannula provides concentrations of oxygen ranging from:
    A. 12 to 24 percent.
    B. 24 to 44 percent.
    C. 40 to 60 percent.
    D. 80 to 100 percent.
17. The head-tilt/chin-lift maneuver opens the airway by:
    A. pushing the tongue backward, thus opening the air passage.
    B. pushing the tongue laterally, thus opening the air passage.
    C. lifting the tongue superiorly, thus opening the air passage.
    D. bringing the tongue forward, thus opening the air passage.
18. A bag-valve-mask device with supplemental oxygen should provide an adult patient:
    A. 500 mL volume delivered over 1 to 1.5 seconds.
    B. 500 mL volume delivered over 1 to 2 seconds.
    C. 1,000 mL volume delivered over 1 to 1.5 seconds.
    D. 1,000 mL volume delivered over 1 to 2 seconds.
19. The cricoid cartilage is located
    A. superior to the thyroid cartilage.
    B. anterior to the thyroid cartilage.
    C. inferior to the thyroid cartilage.
    D. posterior to the thyroid cartilage.
20. When inserting a nasopharyngeal airway, the bevel should be facing:
    A. toward the septum.
    B. away from the septum.
    C. away from the base.
    D. in any direction.

SECTION 2
PATIENT ASSESSMENT

Good assessment skills are the most powerful tools an EMT has with which to treat a patient. The assessment holds the key to unlocking the problem suffered by the patient, and helps define how EMS may be of service to him. The information discovered in the patient assessment will help the EMT determine a treatment plan, a mode of transportation, and a proper receiving facility for the needs of the patient. In this way, the EMT can work with the other members of the health care team to provide safe, effective, and compassionate care to those who call EMS.

EMTs can provide the highest quality care to patients by knowing the order of the assessment and understanding which assessment to use for each patient. When the EMT gets interrupted or confused by the patient or scene, reliance on a systematic approach to every patient will assist in regaining focus and composure. Extensive practice on simulated patients is required to feel comfortable with the order and elements of the different assessments. The following chapters will give you those tools step-by-step so you can feel confident in different situations.

The EMT should remember that a patient who calls EMS is experiencing some sort of crisis that has overwhelmed his coping mechanisms. EMTs can do a wealth of good for this patient by appearing calm and confident in emergency situations. In order to extract the important information needed from patients, EMTs must listen first to the needs of the patient, then ask for information in a kind and compassionate manner. Only when the patient feels comfortable and trusting of EMS will they divulge personal information needed by the EMT.

CHAPTER 18

Body Substance Isolation Precautions

KEY TERMS

Airborne particles

BSI precautions

Eye protection

Gloves

Gown

Infection control plan

Infectious diseases

Mask

Pathogens

OBJECTIVE

The student will understand the importance of body substance isolation precautions and be able to ensure that the proper equipment is used on each call.

INTRODUCTION

Body substance isolation precautions, or **BSI precautions** reduce the chances of the EMT-Basic coming into contact with **pathogens,** which are the organisms that cause infections. Pathogens can be spread through the air or by contact with blood and other body fluids. The most common entryways for pathogens to the EMT-Basic are through open wounds or sores; being stuck with a needle or sharp object; or through your eyes, nose, or mouth.

It is difficult to impossible to identify patients who might be carrying **infectious diseases** or exactly what that wet substance is when you go to lift the patient in a dark area. Because of this, standard BSI precautions should be applied for all patients who have a chance of exposing you to body fluids. Forgetting to take appropriate precautions can increase your risk and your family's risk of exposure to disease. In addition, you need to be aware of reducing the risk of infecting the patient with your illnesses.

BSI personal protective equipment includes protective latex or vinyl **gloves, eye protection, masks,** and **gowns.** When you should wear these items may depend on the different types of patient situations you may encounter and the risk of exposure associated with those situations. Consult your agency's policies and exposure control plan for specific requirements for application of personal protective equipment. Consider, however, the following guidelines for appropriate BSI equipment:

- ▶ **Gloves:** Wear at any time your hands could come into contact with body fluids.
- ▶ **Eye protection:** Wear at any time when the possibility exists that body fluids may come into contact with the eyes or where **airborne particles** could be present.

▶ **Mask:** Wear any time when the possibility exists that body fluids could get into the mouth or where airborne particles may be present. Consider the use of a surgical mask for patients who have a history of respiratory infection. A specific type of mask may be needed in certain cases such as a high-efficiency particulate air (HEPA) mask or a OSHA-approved (Occupational Safety and Health Administration) mask (N-95) for tuberculosis exposure.

▶ **Gowns:** Wear in situations where significant amounts of body fluids are present or in situations where you need to protect clothing and base skin from body fluids.

The Occupational Safety and Health Administration (OSHA) has issued strict guidelines for employers and employees to reduce your exposure to pathogens. Your employers must have a written **infection control plan** and must provide you with the proper annual training, immunizations, and personal protective equipment. Recent legislation also requires your agency to assign a person to coordinate your infection control plan, called an infection control liaison. This legislation requires EMT-Basics to be notified if they have potential for exposure as a result of contact with an infected patient. An exposure report form should be available to you to document any potential risk of exposure.

▶EQUIPMENT

You will need the following equipment:

▶ Gloves, latex or vinyl

▶ Eye protection

▶ Mask, appropriate particulate protection available

▶ Gowns

▶ Hand-washing solution

ASSESSMENT

The type of personal protective equipment that the EMT-Basic may wear depends on the assessment conducted by the EMT-Basic. You should ask yourself the following questions when determining which BSI precautions to take:

▶ Is there any blood or body fluids present, or is there any risk of exposure to blood or body fluids that are not currently present?

▶ Is there a risk of the patient spitting or vomiting?

▶ Is the patient coughing?

▶ Is urine or feces present?

▶ Am I going to need to suction the patient?

▶ Am I going to need to place my fingers in the patient's oral cavity?

▶ Are there objects at the scene that may have to be touched that could have blood or body fluids on them?

▶ Will I need to clean equipment at the end of the call?

PROCEDURE: Body Substance Isolation Precautions

1. Explain to the patient the reasons for taking BSI precautions.

   Rationale: Understand that BSI precautions can alienate you from the patient. Explaining the reasons for BSI precautions can reduce some of those feelings of alienation.

2. Apply gloves (Figure 18.1).

3. Apply eye protection (Figure 18.2).

4. Apply mask, if appropriate (Figure 18.3).

5. Apply gown, if appropriate (Figure 18.4).

6. Provide appropriate assessment and treatment.

7. Gather any contaminated materials from the scene and place them in the appropriate disposal bag or container (Figure 18.5).

8. Remove personal protection only after any possibility of exposure has passed.

   Rationale: Because cross-contamination can occur during this process, remove yourself from the exposure prior to removing the personal protective equipment.

9. Dispose of all contaminated materials, gloves, masks, and gowns in proper infection control waste disposal containers.

10. Wash your hands as soon as possible with any approved infection control soaps or solutions (Figure 18.6).

    Rationale: Washing hands has been shown to be one of the most important techniques for reducing the risk of pathogen exposure.

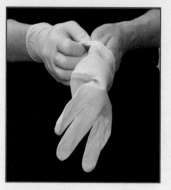

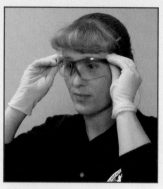

Figure 18.1   **Figure 18.2**

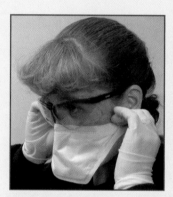

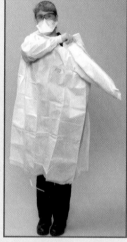

Figure 18.3   **Figure 18.4**

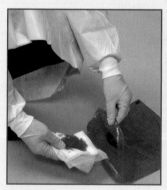

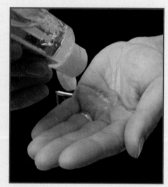

Figure 18.5   **Figure 18.6**

Constantly monitor your risks for exposure. Monitor the integrity of your personal protective equipment. If you find tears or breaks, or your equipment becomes soaked, consider removing it and reapplying a fresh set.

▶PROBLEM SOLVING

▶ If at any time you feel you could have been exposed to blood or body fluids, fill out the appropriate forms provided by your agency. Contact your infection control liaison. If you have been directly exposed, seek medical attention immediately. Consult your agency's exposure control plan.

▶ Reduce touching equipment at the scene with contaminated gloves. Cross-contamination can occur to your equipment. Also be careful about any items you touch in the ambulance with contaminated gloves.

▶ Be very careful at the scene to reduce your chances of getting stuck by needles or glass or getting cut by any object that could be contaminated.

▶ If you are treating multiple patients, consider changing gloves when you approach a new patient, to avoid cross-contamination of that patient.

▶ By applying gloves prior to starting to assist the patient, especially before carrying equipment, you could get a hole or small tear in your gloves that you might not notice before you make contact with the patient.

▶ It is *NOT* necessary for the driver to protect himself from the steering wheel.

▶ Consider wearing all personal protective equipment during the cleaning of equipment and the ambulance. Consider wearing heavy-duty gloves during cleaning.

▶ Change a contaminated uniform or personal clothing as soon as possible. Your EMS agency should have facilities for laundering uniforms that have been soiled. These clothes should not be taken home and mixed with your family's laundry.

▶ Some individuals consider personal glasses to be BSI eye protection. Proper eye protection should come into contact with all sides of the face and should have side ports. Some EMT-Basics wear goggles, which may have the problem of fogging.

▶ If you place a mask on the patient, constantly monitor the patient's respiratory efforts because the mask can hinder your assessment.

▶CASE STUDY

Your ambulance and engine are dispatched to aid a 5-year-old boy who fell through a glass window. Upon your arrival you find a screaming babysitter who is very upset. She tells you that the boy is outside in the backyard. Walking toward the back door, you notice that the glass is broken out of the lower half of the door. You exit the house onto the back patio where you see a young boy lying on the ground.

The boy is just lying there and does not seem to react to your presence. You notice the patient has a long laceration to the right arm that is spurting blood. Your partner opens the trauma bag and grabs a trauma dressing while you apply your gloves and eye protection. Because the patient is showing signs of shock, and appears to have lost a large amount of blood, you quickly apply direct pressure to the wound through a bulky dressing. After handing you the dressing, your partner assumes manual C-spine control. The engine crew arrives on scene and asks if you need any equipment. You direct them to bring the cot and backboard to the backyard. You also ask them to bring gowns with them. When they come into the backyard, they take over bandaging the extremity and obtaining baseline vital signs while you and your partner don the gowns for transport.

The patient has a blood pressure of 70/36 with a heart rate of 138. The patient is breathing at 32 times per minute and has an altered mental status and appears hypoxic. You place the patient on high-flow oxygen, apply a cervical collar, and log roll the patient onto the backboard. After securing the patient, you place him on the cot and begin transport to the emergency department. En route, you control the bleeding, and the patient's vital signs remain unchanged. The patient is quickly transferred to the emergency staff as you and your partner disinfect the ambulance and make sure that each other has not been contaminated. ■

1. Which of the following is *not* a part of *routine* BSI precautions?
   a. gown
   b. HEPA mask
   c. gloves
   d. eye protection

2. BSI precautions are utilized for all of the following *except*:
   a. preventing cross-contamination during a multiple casualty incident.
   b. reducing the risk of infecting you with the patient's illnesses.
   c. eliminating the need to clean your hands following each patient contact.
   d. reducing the risk of you infecting the patient with your illnesses.

3. Which of the following is true of contaminated equipment?
   a. It can be reused as long as there are no visible signs of contamination.
   b. It can be cleaned by rinsing it in the sink and drying with paper towels.
   c. It should be taken out of service until diseases are no longer communicable.
   d. It should be thoroughly cleaned with an appropriate disinfectant.

CHAPTER 19
Lifting and Moving

KEY TERMS

Body mechanics

Lifting devices

Nonurgent moves

Power grip

Power lift

Urgent moves

OBJECTIVE

The student will successfully demonstrate moving a patient in a safe manner.

INTRODUCTION

Nearly every emergency medical run requires a patient to be moved from where he sits or lies to the stretcher and then to the ambulance. Safe lifting and moving of the patient involves both patient and rescuer safety. Proper **body mechanics** and proper use of **lifting devices** are essential to safe patient handling.

▶ EQUIPMENT

You will need the following equipment:

- ▶ Blanket
- ▶ Stretcher
- ▶ One, two, or three rescuers

ASSESSMENT

Be sure to manage any scene hazards before engaging in this skill. If it is impossible to manage the scene hazards, then an emergency movement of the patient should be initiated. Ideally, all threats to airway, breathing, or circulation should be managed on scene, before the patient has been moved. However, in the presence of danger, the patient should be moved to safety *first,* then assessed and managed appropriately.

PROCEDURE: Lifting and Moving

1. Apply BSI precautions.

   Rationale: Gloves and eye protection are required at a minimum, and a gown may be needed if large amounts of blood or fluid are present to prevent exposure to infectious diseases.

2. Observe the following proper body mechanics principles (Figure 19.1).

   A. Position feet on a firm surface, shoulder width apart.

   B. Use legs, not back, to lift by bending at the knees and keeping head up.

   C. Keep back straight.

   D. Keep patient's weight close to body.

   E. Do not twist while lifting.

   F. Avoid reaching more than 20 inches in front of your body.

   G. Push, rather than pull, an object when possible.

   H. Keep elbows bent and arms close to sides.

   I. Use the **power lift** and **power grip** whenever possible.

   Rationale: These principles should be observed to minimize the risk of musculoskeletal injury to the EMT.

3. Differentiate between the need for an **urgent** or **nonurgent move.**

   Rationale: Most scenes are not dangerous and a nonurgent move will be appropriate.

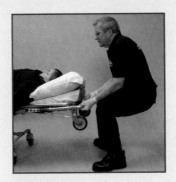

Figure 19.1

4. Select the most desirable move given the circumstances. See the discussion following in this procedure about the different types of moves.

5. Perform the move, placing the patient on the stretcher. Be sure the patient is secured to the stretcher using straps, belts, or tape.

   Rationale: Securing the patient prevents further injury to the patient.

6. Reassess patient for stability of condition and comfort.

   Rationale: The lift or move itself may have caused a change in the patient's condition. Treat as indicated if a change is observed.

7. Move patient on stretcher to the ambulance for transport.

continued...

NONURGENT MOVES

One-Rescuer Assist (Figure 19.2)

1. The EMT places the patient's arm around his neck.
2. Grasp the patient's hand.
3. Place other arm around the patient's waist.
4. Help the patient to walk to safety or to the stretcher.

Two-Rescuer Assist (not pictured)

1. One EMT stands on each side of the patient.
2. Each EMT places one of the patient's arms around his neck and shoulder.
3. Each EMT grips the patient's hands.
4. Both EMTs help the patient walk to safety or the stretcher.

Extremity Carry (Figure 19.3)

1. With patient on her back, with knees flexed, position one EMT at the patient's head and the other at the patient's feet.
2. The rescuer at the patient's feet grasps the patient's wrists to pull the patient's torso off the floor in order for the other rescuer to slip her arms under the patient's armpits.
3. The rescuer at the head should grasp the patient's wrists to provide stability and prevent the patient's arms from flailing.
4. The rescuer at the feet grasps the patient's legs around the knees, either facing toward or away from the patient.
5. Both EMTs should stand at the same time, moving as a unit while carrying the patient to safety or to the stretcher.

Direct Carry (Figure 19.4)

1. Two rescuers align themselves alongside the patient, one at the head and torso and one at the hips and feet.
2. The rescuer at the head slides his or her arms under the patient's neck and back.
3. The rescuer at the hips should slide one arm under the patient's hips, and one under the thighs or calves.
4. Both rescuers slide the patient to the edge of the bed or couch.

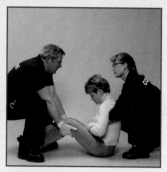
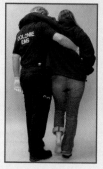

Figure 19.2   **Figure 19.3**

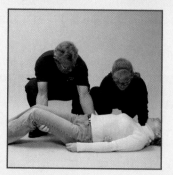

Figure 19.4

5. Both rescuers lift the patient by curling the patient toward their chests while moving to a standing position.
6. The patient is then moved to safety or to the stretcher.

 PEDIATRIC NOTE:

A small child will be able to be picked up and carried by rescue personnel or a parent. It is appropriate to carry a small child in the arms of the rescuer if doing so is more convenient, safer, or quicker than the above-described lifts and carries.

URGENT (EMERGENCY) MOVES

Firefighter's Drag (Figure 19.5)

1. Place patient in the supine position.
2. Tie the patient's hands together with something that will not cut the skin, such as soft restraints.
3. Straddle the patient, facing her head.
4. Crouch and pass your head through the patient's trussed arms.

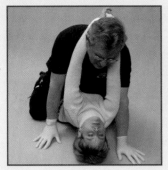
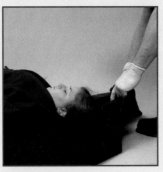
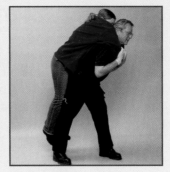
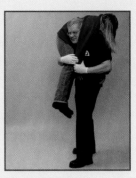

Figure 19.5 **Figure 19.6** **Figure 19.7** **Figure 19.8**

5. Rise up until the patient's head, neck, and trunk are barely off of the ground.

6. Crawl on hands and knees dragging the patient to safety.

Blanket Drag (Figure 19.6)

1. Lay a blanket on the ground next to a supine patient.

2. Gather half of the blanket up against the side of the patient.

3. Roll the patient toward you and pull the blanket in behind her.

4. Roll the patient back onto the blanket.

5. Move to the head of the patient, gathering the excess blanket near the head and shoulders.

6. Drag the patient to safety using the rolled blanket, keeping the head near the ground.

Pack Strap Carry (Figure 19.7)

1. Assist the patient to a standing position.

2. Turn your back to the patient, bringing her arms over your shoulders and then cross them over your chest.

3. Keep the patient's arms as straight as possible, and her armpits over your shoulders.

4. Hold the patient's wrists, pulling the patient onto your back.

5. Move the patient to safety.

Piggyback Carry

1. Assist the patient to a standing position.

2. Turn your back to the patient, bringing his arms over your shoulders and then cross them over your chest.

3. While the patient holds onto you with his arms, you crouch down and grabs the patient's legs under his thighs.

4. Use a lifting motion with your legs to move the patient onto your back.

Firefighter's Carry (Figure 19.8)

1. Stand toe to toe with the patient.

2. Bend at the waist and flex your knees.

3. Hold the patient by one wrist and pull the wrist across your shoulder.

4. Use your free arm to reach between the patient's legs and grasp her thigh.

5. Lift the weight of the patient and let it fall onto your shoulders.

6. Stand up, transferring your grip on the patient's thigh to her wrist.

Once the patient has been moved to safety or to the stretcher, repeat the initial assessment, verifying that airway, breathing, and circulation are still intact. Treat any life-threatening situations now that the patient has been moved to safety.

Patients placed on the stretcher should be secured with straps, belts, or tape. The patient should not be left unattended when the stretcher is in an upright position because many stretchers can tip on uneven surfaces or when the patient readjusts his weight.

Communication between partners is essential when lifting and moving a patient. Should one rescuer feel unsteady or overwhelmed with the patient's weight, he should speak up immediately to ensure the safety of both patient and rescuers. A patient who is dropped could receive a serious injury or could hurt the rescuer. In addition, such a situation creates a legal liability for the rescuer or service.

▶PROBLEM SOLVING

▶ The most common problem experienced when lifting and moving patients is attempting to move patients who are too heavy for the strength of the rescuers. When rescuers are unsure of their ability to lift a patient, additional help should be called *before* the lift is attempted to avoid injury to the patient and rescuers.

▶ When transferring an obese patient, consider alternate methods of transport such as the Stokes' basket or double-wide backboard. Some manufacturers now offer stretcher's with widths that are nearly twice that of a regular stretcher and weight capacity tolerances up to 1,000 pounds, nearly twice as much as a traditional stretcher.

▶CASE STUDY

You are called to the residence of an elderly female. Dispatch advises you that the patient has been complaining of flu-like symptoms for 3 days and has been unable to take her medications. Upon arriving at the house, you and your partner are met by the patient's granddaughter who says they found her like this today, but she did not seem so bad before. You enter the house and see a frail, elderly female lying supine on the sofa. During your initial assessment, you notice that the patient has a high fever and appears to be very dehydrated. The patient is so weak that she is barely able to complete simple tasks such as squeezing your hand.

While you are completing your assessment, you partner obtains baseline vital signs. He reports that the patient has a blood pressure of 96/64, a heart rate of 126, and a respiratory rate of 28 and shallow. You obtain a sample history as your partner prepares the cot.

You determine that the best way to move the patient will be the direct carry. You line up at the patient's head and torso as your partner does the same at the hips and legs. You position the patient's arms on her chest and then begin to count to three. On three, you and your partner gently lift the patient off the sofa. You then proceed to take a few steps backward so that you have the patient in line with the stretcher. Again you begin to count so that you and your partner can lower the patient in unison. After securing the patient to the stretcher, you wheel her to the ambulance where your partner loads the stretcher. En route to the hospital, you continue to monitor the patient's vital signs and also complete the detailed physical and the ongoing assessment. After arriving at the emergency department you transfer patient care to the charge nurse. ∎

1. Which of the following would be an acceptable method for lifting a patient?
   a. using the extremity lift to rotate the patient from the bed to the cot
   b. lifting the patient from the floor to the cot using the elbow-knee lift
   c. using only one person to do a direct carry on a 7-year-old
   d. using the blanket drag foot first down three stairs

2. Which of the following should *Not* be attempted when performing a lift?
   a. Always lift with your legs.
   b. Push/pull no more than 36 inches from your body.
   c. Keep your back straight and chin up.
   d. Have your feet shoulder width apart.

3. Which of the following carries could be used when a single patient who is alert and able to ambulate with assistance needs to be moved by a single rescuer?
   a. the backpack carry
   b. the direct carry
   c. firefighter's drag
   d. the blanket drag

CHAPTER 20
Obtaining Vital Signs

KEY TERMS

Antecubital fossa

Apnea

Baseline vital signs

Brachial pulse

Bradycardia

Carbon monoxide poisoning

Carotid pulse

Cyanosis

Diastolic blood pressure

Dorsalis pedal pulse

Dysrhythmia

Femoral pulse

Hyperventilation

Hypotension

Hypoventilation

Jaundiced skin

Palpated blood pressure

Pulse

Radial pulse

Rales

Respiration

Serial vital signs

Sphygmomanometer

Stridor

Systolic blood pressure

Tachycordia

Tachypnea

Tripod positioning

Wheezing

OBJECTIVE

The student will successfully demonstrate obtaining a complete set of vital signs including pulse, respirations, blood pressure, skin color, and pupil appearance.

INTRODUCTION

Following your initial patient assessment and control of any life-threating problems, you should obtain a set of **baseline vital signs** as soon as possible. Vital signs are measurable items that include **pulse; respirations;** blood pressure; skin color, temperature, and condition; and pupil appearance.

The baseline vitals—the first readings that you record—will give you a foundation on which to make health care decisions and to judge the impact of these decisions. As you retake vital signs, you will compare the readings to your previous findings. These subsequent readings are called **serial vital signs.** Serial vital sign assessments allow you to note trends in the patient's condition, such as a declining blood pressure or increasing respiratory rate.

▶ EQUIPMENT

You will need the following equipment:

- ▶ BSI equipment
- ▶ Documentation form
- ▶ Pen
- ▶ Stethoscope
- ▶ **Sphygmomanometer** or blood pressure cuff
- ▶ Watch with a second hand
- ▶ Penlight

ASSESSMENT

Be sure to manage any scene hazards before engaging in this skill. Additionally, all threats to airway, breathing, or circulation should already have been managed during the initial assessment. Vital sign assessment should be completed after the initial assessment. A complete set of vital signs should be obtained on every patient encountered by EMS personnel regardless of whether or not the patient was transported, released at the scene, or refused medial care against medical advice.

 PEDIATRIC NOTE:

It may be impossible to assess blood pressure in infants and children if properly sized equipment is not available. Often, agencies, due to the cost and infrequency of pediatric calls, will not have a full range of blood pressure cuffs available. In this case, it is appropriate to skip the blood pressure measurement and assess pulse, respiration, skin signs, and pupils instead.

PULSE

A patient's pulse is the rhythmic beats felt as the heart pumps blood through the arteries. When taking a patient's pulse you should be concerned with the pulse rate, rhythm, and strength. Many disorders can be related to variations in pulse rate, rhythm, and strength.

Rate

The pulse rate is the number of beats per minute. The number you count will allow you to decide if the patient's pulse is normal, rapid, or slow. The normal rate for an adult at rest is between 60 and 100 beats per minute. Any pulse rate above 100 beats per minute is rapid. A rapid pulse is called **tachycardia.** Any pulse rate below 60 beats per minute is slow. A slow pulse is called **bradycardia.**

Rhythm

Pulse rhythm reflects regularity. A pulse is said to be regular when the intervals between beats are constant. When the intervals are not constant, the pulse is said to be irregular.

Strength

Pulse strength refers to the pressure of the pulse wave as it expands the artery. Normally the pulse should feel as if a strong wave has passed. When the pulse feels weak and thin, the patient has a "thready" pulse.

PROCEDURE: Taking a Pulse

1. Apply BSI precautions.

   Rationale: Gloves and eye protection are required at minimum, and a gown may be needed if large amounts of blood or fluid are present to prevent exposure to infectious diseases.

2. Locate the **radial pulse** on the lateral part of the patient's wrist (Figure 20.1). If the radial pulse is absent or difficult to assess, you might also use the **carotid** (Figure 20.2), **brachial** (Figure 20.3), **femoral** (Figure 20.4), and **dorsalis pedal pulses** (Figure 20.5).

3. Assess the heart rate by counting the number of pulses you feel in 1 minute.

   Rationale: This method is usually very accurate. It may be more convenient, however, to count the number of beats over a shorter time period such as 30 seconds and then multiply by 2 or 15 seconds multiplied by 4 to determine the rate per minute.

4. Pay close attention to any irregular patterns, or rhythms, in the pulse. A regular rate means that the beats are spread evenly over 1 minute.

   Rationale: Irregular heart rates are a sign of cardiac **dysrhythmias** and can be life threatening.

5. Note the quality of the pulse. It should be strong and easily palpated.

   Rationale: Any pulse that is thready, or hard to feel, can be an indication of shock or other medical problems.

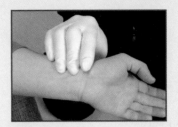

Figure 20.1

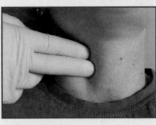

Figure 20.2

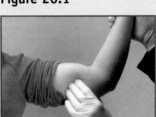

Figure 20.3

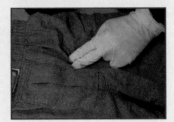

Figure 20.4

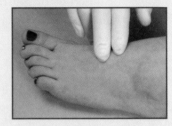

Figure 20.5

6. Document the rate and quality of the pulse, as well as the time of assessment, on the prehospital care report.

   Rationale: Serial vital signs establish a pattern over time; therefore, the time at which vitals were assessed is important to note.

PROBLEM SOLVING

▷ Be familiar with normal pulse rates so that you can immediately note whether your findings indicate a possible problem.

▷ The 15 seconds multiplied by 4 or 30 seconds multiplied by 2 method of counting a pulse works in many cases. But sometimes a full 60-second count is indicated. When the pulse is very irregular or the rate is very slow, you will need to count for one full minute in order to be accurate.

▷ Avoid pressing too hard on the pulse point during assessment. Too much pressure can occlude the arterial blood flow, causing the pulse to seemingly disappear.

 GERIATRIC NOTE:

Many geriatric patients take medication that causes their heart rate to be slow or irregular. Although this is usually normal for the patient, medication-induced bradycardia or an irregular beat still has the potential to cause **hypotension** and cause the patient to be dizzy or weak.

RESPIRATION

The act of breathing is called respiration. For the determination of vital signs you are concerned with four factors regarding respiration: rate, depth, rhythm and pattern, and quality.

Rate

The respiration rate is the number of breaths a patient takes in 1 minute. The rate of respiration is classified as normal, rapid, or slow. The normal respiration rate for an adult at rest is between 12 and 20 breaths per minute.

Depth

The depth of respiration can be defined as:
1. normal: deep, even movement of the chest
2. shallow: minimal rise and fall of the chest and abdomen
3. deep: the rib cage expands fully, and the diaphragm descends to create a maximum capacity

Rhythm And Pattern

Rhythm and pattern are described as follows:
1. Regular: exhalations twice as long as inhalations
2. Irregular

3. **Hypoventilation:** slow and shallow respirations
4. **Hyperventilation:** sustained increased rate and depth of respiration
5. **Sigh:** deep inhalation followed by a slow audible exhalation
6. **Apnea:** temporary absence of breathing
7. **Tachypnea:** increased respiration rate, usually 24 or more breaths per minute

Quality

The quality of a patient's breathing may fall into any of four categories:
1. Normal: effortless, automatic, regular rate; even depth, noiseless, and free of discomfort
2. Dyspnea: difficult or labored breathing
3. **Wheezing** or whistling sound
4. Rhonchi or rattling
5. Rales, bubbling, or crackling

PROCEDURE: Measuring Respiration Rate

1. Apply BSI precautions.

   Rationale: Gloves and eye protection are required at minimum, and a gown may be needed if large amounts of blood or fluid are present to prevent exposure to infectious diseases.

2. Look for the presence of breathing by watching for chest rise and fall. In the absence of chest rise and fall, or if ventilations are inadequate, begin rescue breathing (Figure 20.6).

   Rationale: The patient can survive periods of apnea of only 4 to 6 minutes before cardiopulmonary arrest will ensue.

3. Observe the patient's position.

   Rationale: Most patients in respiratory distress prefer to be seated upright or standing. Hunching forward is called **tripod positioning** and indicates severe respiratory distress.

4. Note any abnormal noises during breathing.

   Rationale: A high-pitched noise like **stridor** can indicate upper airway obstruction. Whistling or wheezing sounds may indicate lower airway constriction. Bubbling, wet, or crackling sounds, known as rhonchi or **rales,** can indicate fluid in the airway.

5. Watch to see how hard the patient works to breath.

   Rationale: Signs of labored breathing include use of accessory muscles, nasal flaring, and retractions above the collarbones or between the ribs.

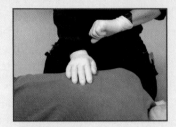

Figure 20.6

6. Note any respiration patterns.

   Rationale: Respirations that are very fast, very deep, or interrupted (apnea) can be signs of serious medical conditions.

7. Determine the respiratory rate by counting the number of times the patient breathes in 1 minute. One breath includes an inspiration and an expiration.

   Rationale: This method is usually very accurate. It may be more convenient, however, to count the number of respirations over a shorter time period such as 30 seconds and then multiply by 2 or 15 seconds multiplied by 4 to arrive at the number of respirations in 1 minute.

8. Document the respiratory rate, quality, and any rhythms that you might observe as well as the time on the prehospital care report.

   Rationale: It is extremely important to document your findings in order to have a history of facts and events that occurred at the scene. Serial vital signs establish a pattern over time; therefore, the time at which vitals were assessed is important to note.

▶PROBLEM SOLVING

▷ Avoid telling the patient that you are counting his respirations. Patients will sometimes alter their respiratory rate or pattern when they know that you are watching.

▷ Be familiar with normal respiratory rates so that you can immediately note whether your findings indicate a possible problem.

▷ At times, it may be difficult to count a respiratory rate due to patient movement or talking. Respiratory assessment is important, and accuracy is vital. Politely ask the patient to be quiet for a few moments if you are experiencing difficulty counting.

▷ When the respiratory pattern is very irregular or the rate is very slow, you will need to count for 1 full minute in order to be accurate. The 15 seconds times 4 or 30 seconds times 2 method works in many cases, but sometimes a full 60-second count is indicated.

BLOOD PRESSURE

When measuring blood pressure, a piece of equipment called a **sphygmomanometer** is used. The sphygmomanometer is a blood pressure cuff and gauge. You can collect readings by auscultating, or listening to, the characteristic clicking or tapping sounds with a stethoscope. Or you can palpate, or feel, the radial or brachial pulse with your fingertips after you have positioned the cuff on the patient.

To report blood pressure readings, use a blood pressure fraction. The top or first number reported is the **systolic blood pressure.** This is the pressure created when the heart contracts and forces blood into the arteries. The bottom or second number is the **diastolic blood pressure.** It measures the pressure remaining in the arteries when the left ventricle relaxes and refills or the residual pressure in the system.

As already noted, assess vital signs right after your initial assessment and management of the ABCs. Even when you find yourself without a stethoscope or an environment quiet enough for auscultation, blood pressure can still be taken by palpation. Palpation is less accurate than auscultation, because you can only approximate the systolic pressure. But it is vital that blood pressure be measured—even in noisy situations—so the health care team can determine appropriate patient care.

PROCEDURE: Measuring Blood Pressure

1. Apply BSI precautions.

   Rationale: Gloves and eye protection are required at minimum, and a gown may be needed if large amounts of blood or fluid are present to prevent exposure to infectious diseases.

2. Select the appropriate size blood pressure cuff.

   Rationale: Proper size selection helps ensure accuracy of the results. The cuff should measure two-thirds of the length of the upper arm, from elbow to shoulder. Additionally, it should be long enough to fasten the Velcro securely when the cuff is placed circumferentially around the arm.

3. Remove or roll clothing to expose the bare skin (Figure 20.7).

   Rationale: Be sure that sleeves, when rolled, do not occlude the arteries of the arm, preventing blood flow.

4. Place the cuff on the bare arm, following the instructions on the cuff for putting it over the artery.

5. With your fingertips, locate the brachial pulse on the medial upper arm near the **antecubital fossa,** or the crease of the elbow.

6. Place the diaphragm, or bell, of the stethoscope over this pulse point.

7. With the bulb valve closed, inflate the cuff until the pulse is no longer heard or felt.

8. Listen for the sound of the pulse returning as the pressure in the cuff is slowly released. Note the

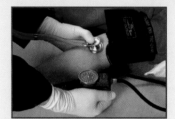

Figure 20.7

number on the cuff's gauge as soon as you hear the first pulse beat (Figure 20.7). This is the systolic pressure or the top number of the blood pressure fraction.

9. Continue to deflate the cuff, this time listening for the point at which the beats fade. Again note the figure indicated on the gauge. This is the diastolic blood pressure or the blood pressure fraction's bottom number.

10. Let the cuff deflate rapidly. Record measurements and the time.

   Rationale: It is extremely important to document your findings in order to have a history of facts and events that occurred at the scene. Blood pressure is reported in even numbers. If the blood pressure reading falls between two lines on the gauge, pick the bigger number. Serial vital signs establish a pattern over time; therefore, the time at which vitals were assessed is important to note.

PALPATED BLOOD PRESSURE

As already mentioned, you may find yourself in a situation where it is impossible to hear an auscultated blood pressure due to external noises on scene or in the back of the ambulance. In such cases, an estimated blood pressure can be obtained by palpation. Because **palpated blood pressure** is usually lower than actual blood pressure, an auscultated blood pressure should be taken as soon as you possibly can.

The steps for palpating blood pressure are basically the same as those used for auscultation. The obvious difference is that you do not rely on a stethoscope to hear the presence or absence of a pulse beat.

PROCEDURE: Palpating Blood Pressure

1. Apply BSI precautions.

   Rationale: Gloves and eye protection are required at minimum, and a gown may be needed if large amounts of blood or fluid are present to prevent exposure to infectious diseases.

2. Select the appropriate size blood pressure cuff.

   Rationale: The cuff should measure two-thirds of the length of the upper arm, from elbow to shoulder. Additionally, it should be long enough to fasten the Velcro securely when the cuff is placed circumferentially around the arm.

3. Remove or roll clothing to expose the bare skin.

   Rationale: Be sure that sleeves, when rolled, do not occlude the arteries of the arm, preventing blood flow.

4. Place the cuff on the bare arm, following the instructions on the cuff for putting it over the artery (Figure 20.7 on page 109).

5. Begin by inflating the cuff until the radial pulse disappears. Then slowly release air from the cuff until the pulse reappears. At that point, check the gauge for the systolic blood pressure. With the palpation method, no diastolic reading is available.

6. Document your finding as the systolic blood pressure over "P" or "PALP" for palpation, as well as the time of the reading.

   Rationale: It is extremely important to document your findings in order to have a history of facts and events that occurred at the scene. Serial vital signs establish a pattern over time; therefore, the time at which vitals were assessed is important to note.

▶ PROBLEM SOLVING

▷ Be familiar with normal blood pressures so that you can immediately note whether your findings indicate a possible problem.

▷ It may be difficult to fit a blood pressure cuff on a very thin adult, who may need a child-sized cuff. Alternately, a very muscular or obese adult may need an extra-large cuff or thigh cuff.

▷ When the stethoscope is placed over clothing or under the cuff itself, the sounds heard may be mistaken for the blood pressure but actually be external noises from the articles touching the stethoscope. It is important to place the stethoscope on bare skin and not to tuck it underneath the cuff.

 GERIATRIC NOTE:

Because geriatric patients do not regulate their body temperatures as easily as younger patients, it is common for them to feel cold, even in warm homes. This causes geriatric patients to layer their clothing. Placing the blood pressure on bare skin is the most accurate means of obtaining the blood pressure. Therefore, even though it requires additional time to remove all the layers of clothing, whenever possible, care should be taken to do so.

SKIN

The skin is the largest organ in the body, but not as essential to survival as other organs such as the heart or brain. Because the skin is very vascular, blood will be drawn away from the skin in order to perfuse more vital organs during times of physical stress. As a result, the skin can provide valuable clues to blood loss as well as a variety of other conditions.

In assessing the skin, you should check color, temperature, condition, and, in children under 6 years, capillary refill time. You assess the skin when you collect baseline vitals and during your ongoing assessment.

The best place to assess skin color in adults is in the nail beds, inside the cheek, and inside the lower eyelid. In infants and children, the best places to look are the palms of the hands and the soles of the feet. Usually, the skin in any of these places is pink. Variations in color may suggest poor circulation or other problems. For example:

▷ Pale skin may be a sign of blood loss, shock, heart attack, fright, anemia, hypotension, or emotional distress.

▷ **Cyanosis** in skin points to inadequate oxygenation and perfusion, inadequate respirations, heart attack, or poisoning.

▷ Flushed skin suggests heat exposure, emotional excitement, an allergic reaction, hypotension, or **carbon monoxide poisoning.**

▷ **Jaundiced skin** results from liver disease.

▷ Mottled, or blotchy, skin is occasionally seen in cases of shock.

Both the temperature and condition of the skin can vary as well:

▷ Cool, clammy skin is a sign of shock or anxiety.

▷ Cold, moist skin means that the body is losing heat.

▷ Cold, dry skin results from an exposure to cold.

▷ Hot, dry skin or hot, moist skin indicates a high fever or heat exposure.

▷ "Goose bumps" accompanied by shivering, chattering teeth, blue lips, and pale skin can result from chills, cold exposure, pain, fear, or a communicable disease.

PROCEDURE: Assessing the Skin

1. Apply BSI precautions.

   Rationale: Gloves and eye protection are required at minimum, and a gown may be needed if large amounts of blood or fluid are present to prevent exposure to infectious diseases.

2. Evaluate the color of the patient's skin by observing the overall complexion plus the inside of the lower eyelids, the nail beds, or the inside of the cheek.

   Rationale: Note abnormalities in skin color.

3. Determine the skin temperature by feeling the forehead with the back of your hand. If the skin feels cool due to ambient temperatures, check a more central body temperature by placing your hand on the abdomen beneath the clothing (Figure 20.8).

4. Assess the condition of the skin for moisture. Note any moisture on the skin (Figure 20.9).

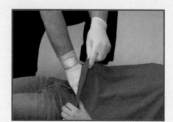
Figure 20.8

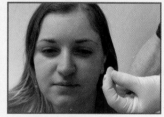
Figure 20.9

5. Document skin color, temperature, and condition on the prehospital care report.

   Rationale: It is extremely important to document your findings in order to have a history of facts and events that occurred at the scene. Serial vital signs establish a pattern over time; therefore, the time at which vitals were assessed is important to note.

PUPILS

The pupil is the black center of the eye and can be directly correlated with neurological function. Pupils should ordinarily be round and reactive to light.

PROCEDURE: Assessing the Pupils

1. Apply BSI precautions.

   Rationale: Gloves and eye protection are required at minimum, and a gown may be needed if large amounts of blood or fluid are present to prevent exposure to infectious diseases.

2. Note the size of the pupils before you shine any light into them.

   Rationale: It is important to note the size before shining light into the pupils because light will cause them to change size immediately.

3. Next cover one eye as you shine a penlight into the other eye.

   Rationale: This step is optional and is done to prevent light from one eye's assessment from dilating or constricting the pupil in the other eye.

4. The pupil should constrict when the light is shining into it and enlarge when you remove the light (Figure 20.10).

5. Repeat with the other eye.

   Rationale: Pupils that are dilated, constricted to pinpoint size, unequal in size or reactivity, or

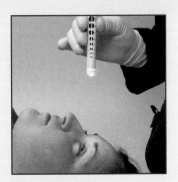

Figure 20.10

nonreactive may indicate a variety of conditions including drug influence, head injury, or eye injury.

6. Any deviations from normal should be reported and documented.

   Rationale: It is extremely important to document your findings in order to have a history of facts and events that occurred at the scene. Serial vital signs establish a pattern over time; therefore, the time at which vitals were assessed is important to note.

ONGOING ASSESSMENT

Vital signs should be reassessed every 5 minutes for critical patients and every 15 minutes for stable patients. All patients should have an initial or baseline set of vital signs taken, as well as at least one more set taken prior to arrival at the hospital or transfer of care to another agency or unit.

Be sure to note baseline vital signs and any changes in vital signs on the patient care report.

▶PROBLEM SOLVING

▶ It may be difficult to assess pupil size and constriction on a sunny day or in a brightly lit room. In these instances, it may be beneficial to conduct the pupillary assessment in the back of the ambulance or another sheltered area.

▶CASE STUDY

You are responding to assist a 59-year-old male with a history of being ill for the last week. On your arrival, you find the patient lying supine on his bed with his eyes closed. On approaching the patient, you attempt to determine his level of consciousness and note that he is unresponsive.

Upon arriving at the patient's side, you determine that the patient is breathing at a rate of 12 breaths per minute and that those breaths are shallow. You then attempt to palpate his radial and carotid pulses and find that they are weak. The patient is in critical condition and you make the decision to begin transporting him immediately. While in the back of the ambulance, your partner attempts to auscultate a blood pressure and states that he is unable to hear anything. He then attempts to palpate a blood pressure. Upon palpation, your partner states that the patient has a pressure of "90 over palp." Your patient's skin is cool to the touch and his pupils are slow to react but they do react.

As you continue transporting your patient, your partner reassesses his vital signs and reports that the patient no longer has a palpable radial pulse but still has a weak carotid pulse. His airway remains patent with an intact gag reflex and he is still breathing shallowly at a rate of 12. You put the patient in shock position and continue to transport him rapidly to the emergency department. ■

(continued)

1. Serial vital sign measurements for a patient complaining of chest pain should be taken every:

   a. 5 minutes

   b. 10 minutes

   c. 15 minutes

   d. Serial measurements are not necessary because the patient should already be at the emergency department.

2. Which of the following vital sign measurements may be omitted on pediatric patients and why?

   a. capillary refill, because it is not a good measure of perfusion in pediatric patients

   b. capillary refill, because it will be less than 2 seconds due to the small size of pediatric patients

   c. blood pressure, because the proper equipment is not always available

   d. breath sounds, because pediatric patients cry too much to measure accurately

3. Which of the following vital signs can be measured without any special equipment?

   a. pulse and papillary response

   b. pulse and skin color, temperature, and condition

   c. blood pressure and respirations

   d. pulse and respiratory quality

CHAPTER 21
Initial Assessment

OBJECTIVE

The student will successfully identify and treat any life-threatening problems that can cause compromise to the airway, breathing, or circulatory status of the patient.

INTRODUCTION

The **initial assessment,** formerly referred to as the primary assessment, is aimed at identifying any life-threatening problems. Abnormal findings in the initial assessment should be treated immediately, before proceeding with any further assessment. The EMT is required to quickly assess the situation and form an impression about the nature and severity of the call. Many important treatment and management decisions are determined from the initial assessment.

KEY TERMS

Baseline mental status

Chief complaint

General impression

Hemodynamically unstable

Initial assessment

Level of consciousness

Level of distress

Life threats

►EQUIPMENT

You will need the following equipment in order to complete the initial assessment:

► One or more rescuers
► Stethoscope

ASSESSMENT

The initial assessment begins with an assessment of the scene itself. Contact with the patient should not be made until scene hazards have been identified and rectified, number of patients determined, and additional help summoned as needed. Use this time, as well, to determine the nature of the illness if clues on scene expose this information.

PROCEDURE: Initial Assessment

1. Apply BSI precautions.

   Rationale: Gloves and eye protection are required at minimum, and a gown may be needed if large amounts of blood or fluid are present to prevent exposure to infectious diseases.

2. Conduct a scene size-up as you approach or come on scene. Determine that the scene is safe and free of hazards. Determine the nature of the illness such as an overdose, vomiting, or shortness of breath. Identify the number of patients and whether additional resources such as law enforcement personnel or firefighters will be necessary. If additional resources are needed, request those resources now.

   Rationale: Once you make contact with the patient, it will be difficult to disengage to determine the scene size-up.

3. If the patient appears unconscious and is on the ground or could have otherwise suffered trauma, direct manual stabilization of the cervical spine (Figure 21.1).

   Rationale: Full spinal immobilization may be necessary if you cannot rule out trauma.

4. Verbalize your **general impression** of the patient regarding her **level of distress** and other obvious findings such as positioning and surroundings. The general impression is your immediate sense or assessment of the severity of the situation (Figure 21.1). A general impression is made by combining the dispatch information, scene size-up, immediate patient findings, and even a little intuition. Some providers refer to the general

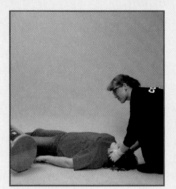
Figure 21.1

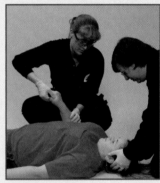
Figure 21.2

impression as "the view from the door" or a determination of "sick or not sick."

   Rationale: Verbalizing your general impression helps your team members respond with the same level of intensity as you.

5. Determine **level of consciousness** of the patient using the AVPU method. This initial assessment is used to determine whether the patient is ALERT, responsive to VERBAL stimuli, responsive to PAINFUL stimuli, or UNRESPONSIVE. An alert patient is aware of your presence, follows commands, and answers your questions. A patient responsive to verbal stimuli will seem unaware of your presence until you speak to her. If you have to shout at the patient to gain a response, altered mental status is likely. A patient responsive to painful stimuli only responds when pain is provoked, such as a pinch or sternum rub (Figure 21.2). Care should be taken not to injure the patient when trying to illicit a response. An

unresponsive patient does not respond to stimuli regardless of the intensity.

Rationale: Some systems may require that you obtain a Glasgow Coma Score. However, this may take longer to determine and is often difficult for EMTs to remember. Therefore, in the initial assessment, AVPU is all that is required at this time.

PEDIATRIC NOTE:

Children can also be evaluated on the AVPU scale. If they are alert, they will be aware of your presence and track your movement in the room. A verbal response from a child could be anything from grunting to actual words uttered in response to your verbal stimulation. Responsiveness to pain and unresponsiveness are determined for the child in the same manner as for adults, with stimuli dictated by local protocol.

GERIATRIC NOTE:

Compared to the younger adult population, a higher percentage of elderly patients have dementia. When any alteration of mental status is identified, it is helpful to attempt to ascertain from family or caregivers the **baseline mental status** of the patient. Baseline mental status is used to determine if the altered mental status is chronic or acute. When no history is available, always assume the abnormal findings are from an acute problem that may need your intervention such as a head injury, hypoglycemia, or stroke.

6. Ensure airway patency. If the airway is not open, open it using the head-tilt/chin-lift maneuver as long as no trauma is present. When trauma is suspected, open the airway using the jaw-thrust maneuver. Insert an airway adjunct to maintain patency. Consider suctioning or foreign body removal if indicated.

Rationale: Protection of the airway is the first element of patient care.

7. Determine the **chief complaint** or apparent **life threats.** If the patient can communicate, ask for her chief complaint. The chief complaint can often be determined by asking why the ambulance was called, what is bothering the patient today, or what is the matter.

Rationale: Identification of a chief complaint allows you to refine your assessment to the specific problem being experienced by the patient. In the event of an unconscious patient, form a general impression of the life threats that are readily visible such as unconsciousness, hemorrhage, or cyanosis.

8. Assess the rate and quality of breathing. Assess for adequate tidal volume by observing chest rise and fall. Ensure lung sounds are present and equal (Figure 21.3). Note any abnormal respiratory noises such as stridor, snoring, or gurgling. The chest should be examined for use of accessory muscles or retractions. Apply high-flow oxygen. For the apneic patient, begin rescue breathing with supplemental oxygen if possible.

Rationale: If the patient is not breathing, she will not survive. Inadequate respirations must be corrected immediately by the EMT.

9. Check central and peripheral pulses for rate, strength, and regularity (Figure 21.4). Assess skin color, temperature, and condition. Control external bleeding with direct pressure. Initiate shock management if indicated with Trendelenburg positioning or application of a pneumatic anti-shock garment (PASG). If circulation is absent, begin CPR.

Rationale: Poor perfusion is life threatening and must be corrected by the EMT during the initial assessment if at all possible.

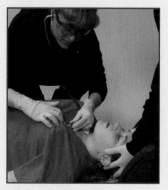

Figure 21.3

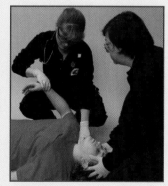

Figure 21.4

continued...

10. Determine priority of the patient and make a transport decision. Patients with threats to airway, breathing, or circulation should be prepared for transport immediately (Figure 21.5).

    Rationale: Stable patients or those with minor illnesses can be treated on scene and transported with less urgency. Examples of high-priority patients include those who are unresponsive, have difficulty breathing, show signs of shock, have uncontrolled bleeding or an altered mental status, and those who are **hemodynamically unstable.**

11. Document your findings.

    Rationale: It is extremely important to document your findings in order to have a history of facts and events that occurred at the scene.

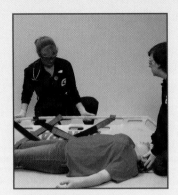

Figure 21.5

ONGOING ASSESSMENT

Should the condition of the patient worsen at any time, immediately return to the initial assessment and reassess airway, breathing, and circulation. It may be necessary to stop further assessment and treatment in order to initiate transport immediately if changes in the initial assessment occur.

▶PROBLEM SOLVING

▶ The most common error that occurs during the initial assessment is that EMTs fail to treat the life threats as they find them. Commonly, EMTs will only"make note of "a life-threatening finding, finish the assessment, and return to the problem. This approach costs the patient precious time and can often mean the difference between life and death. It is imperative that life threats be identified and treated immediately.

▶ The initial assessment should take less than 1 minute to complete if there are no treatments indicated. Much of the initial assessment is completed before you even touch the patient.

You are called to the scene of a motor vehicle collision with ejection. Upon arriving on scene, the fire department advises that there is only one patient, and she is lying in the grass. You proceed to the patient, making sure that you are out of the way of passing motorists and not in danger of being injured yourself. Your partner goes to the patient's head and provides manual cervical spine immobilization. At the same time, you talk to the patient to determine her level of responsiveness. The patient does not respond, so you try painful stimuli. The patient is still unresponsive. You and your partner agree that this is a critical patient and ask for backup. You also ask the fire department to get the immobilization equipment.

Then you have your partner open the patient's airway with a modified jaw-thrust maneuver. You assess the airway, which is patent, and respirations, which are normal at 20 times per minute. Next, you assess for a carotid and radial pulse. The patient has good, strong pulses at 100 per minute. Fire department personnel arrive with your equipment, and you inspect the neck, then measure and place a cervical collar. You then proceed with the rest of your assessment, finding no other major life threats. You log roll the patient and secure her to the backboard.

After transferring the patient to the ambulance, your backup arrives. You have them transport you and your partner to the emergency department (ED). En route, you complete a detailed assessment and physical examination while your partner places the patient on high-flow oxygen, completes the baseline vital signs, and alerts the ED. Upon arrival at the ED, the patient is becoming responsive. Your partner tries to calm her as you give your report to the ED staff. ■

(continued)

1. What does the *P* in AVPU stand for?
   a. pulses
   b. painful stimuli
   c. presentation
   d. purposeful movement

2. Which of the following injuries/presentations would be treated during the initial assessment?
   a. a femur fracture requiring traction splinting
   b. a laceration to the arm that is slowly bleeding
   c. a patient with a carotid pulse, but no radial pulse
   d. a patient who is breathing only 8 times per minute

3. Which of the following patients would be considered for a priority transport?
   a. a female who is 34 weeks pregnant complaining of abdominal pain
   b. a male patient involved in an accident complaining of a sore back
   c. a male patient who has abdominal pain
   d. a male patient who is short of breath and sweating

CHAPTER 22
Rapid Trauma Assessment

OBJECTIVE

The student will successfully identify major injuries that require immediate treatment by the EMT.

INTRODUCTION

The **rapid trauma assessment** allows the EMT to quickly assess major areas of the body for injuries that require immediate treatment. The rapid trauma assessment is completed after the initial assessment and only on major trauma patients. Patients with isolated or minor injuries would receive, in place of the rapid trauma assessment, a focused physical exam of only the injured body part. Minor injuries such as **abrasions** are noted, but should not be treated until additional help is available. Although information related to the cause of the incident and past medical history are helpful, much of the trauma patient assessment can be gathered from physical cues surrounding the patient and scene.

KEY TERMS

Abrasions

Burns

Contusions

Crepitation

Deformities

Lacerations

Paradoxical motion

Penetrations

Punctures

Rapid trauma assessment

Swelling

Tenderness

▶ EQUIPMENT

You will need the following equipment:

- ▶ Long spine board
- ▶ Cervical collar
- ▶ Stethoscope
- ▶ Penlight
- ▶ Scissors
- ▶ Bandaging supplies
- ▶ Splinting devices

ASSESSMENT

At this point in the assessment, the patient will have all threats to ABCs managed. The patient is likely to have oxygen and spinal immobilization devices in place. Moving expeditiously from head to toe, examine each body part for the following abnormalities: **deformities, contusions,** abrasions, **punctures** and **penetrations, burns, tenderness, lacerations,** or **swelling.** Additionally, the discovery of a life threat during the rapid trauma assessment should cause you to reconsider both the need for additional resources and transport priority.

PROCEDURE: Rapid Trauma Assessment

1. Apply BSI precautions.

   Rationale: Gloves and eye protection are required at a minimum, and a gown may be needed if large amounts of blood or fluid are present to prevent exposure to infectious diseases.

2. Reassess mechanism of injury. Be sure you understand the mechanism by which the patient sustained injury.

   Rationale: Acknowledgment of the mechanism of injury is important because you will be asked to explain it to the hospital staff.

3. The patient may already have a cervical collar (C-collar) in place. If not, you may place one now after assessing the neck and throat for injuries.

   Rationale: A C-collar is needed for any trauma patient suspected of having neck or back injuries to minimize the risk of paralysis.

4. Reconsider resources, such as the need for advanced life support (ALS) personnel, and your transport decision. If the patient's condition is worsening or unstable, call for ALS assistance and prepare the patient for immediate transport.

   Rationale: Trauma patients have the best chances for survival when they can be transported to a trauma center with surgical capabilities within 1 hour.

5. Reassess the level of consciousness of the patient using the AVPU method (see Chapter 21).

   Rationale: A decreasing level of consciousness indicates that the patient is worsening and should be transported immediately.

6. Begin at the head. Palpate and observe for any abnormality or injury, including **crepitation** of the skull and facial bones (Figure 22.1).

   Rationale: Beginning the assessment at the head provides a systematic approach that will help eliminate missed injuries.

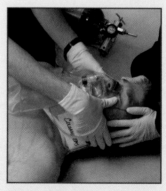

Figure 22.1

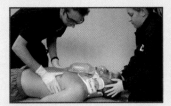
Figure 22.2

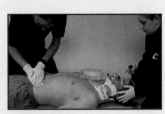
Figure 22.3

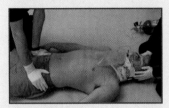
Figure 22.4

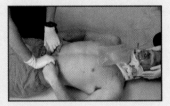
Figure 22.5

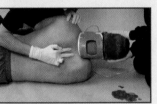
Figure 22.6

7. Check the neck for injuries, plus jugular venous distension, tracheal deviation, and crepitation of the cervical spinal bones. This should be done before a cervical collar is placed.

   Rationale: Careful assessment of the neck can prevent serious injuries that result in paralysis.

8. Assess the chest for injuries, including crepitation, **paradoxical motion,** and breath sounds (Figure 22.2).

   Rationale: Any injury to the chest can impede breathing or circulation and become life threatening.

9. Assess the abdomen for injuries including firmness and distension (Figure 22.3).

   Rationale: Injuries to the abdomen can result in significant blood loss and eventually shock.

10. Assess the pelvis for injuries by observation and gentle downword pressure or the pelvic bones. Do *NOT* rock the pelvis. Note any pain, tenderness, or lack of motion (Figure 22.4).

    Rationale: Rocking the pelvis can injure the spine.

11. Assess all four extremities for injuries, plus distal pulse, motor function, and sensation (Figure 22.5).

    Rationale: Absence of distal circulation, motor function, or sensation can result in loss of limb.

12. Roll the patient to his side and assess the posterior chest, buttocks, and legs for injuries (Figure 22.6).

    Rationale: The kidneys are solid organs located in the retroperitoneal space that can bleed significantly and cause shock if left undetected.

13. Treat injuries identified by the rapid trauma assessment.

    Rationale: Treatment often includes bandaging and splinting, which prevent further injuries or worsening of existing injuries.

14. Document your findings.

    Rationale: It is extremely important to document your findings in order to have a history of facts and events that occurred at the scene.

ONGOING ASSESSMENT

Should the condition of the patient worsen at any time, immediately return to the initial assessment and reassess airway, breathing, and circulation. It may be necessary to stop further assessment. Provide treatment and transport immediately.

▶ PROBLEM SOLVING

▶ The most common problem encountered with the rapid trauma assessment is disorganization, which leads to missed injuries. Conduct the assessment as described, without omitting any steps, and injuries will be identified in a systematic fashion leading to timely treatment and transport.

▶ Clothing should be removed when possible to allow for optimal inspection and palpation of the body.

▶ Rocking the pelvis to assess for stability is no longer acceptable. Gentle pressure lateral to medial and anterior to posterior is appropriate and will identify most pelvic injuries without compromising the spine.

▶ CASE STUDY

You are responding to the scene where a 29-year-old female bicyclist was struck by a car. A bystander advises you that the patient was riding on the side of the road when a car swerved over and struck her. The bystander estimates the speed of the car at about 60 miles per hour.

On your arrival, the patient is lying supine and motionless. You observe a helmet lying beside the patient. The patient has an obvious femur fracture on her left leg and an avulsion of her left hand. The patient is unresponsive and has been from the time of impact according to the bystander. You call your dispatcher and request an additional unit. Her airway is patent; her respirations are shallow but appear to be unlabored. After assessing the circulation, you conduct a rapid trauma assessment. The patient is then immobilized to a backboard with a C-collar and head immobilization device in place and transferred rapidly to the ambulance for transfer to the emergency department.

While en route to the hospital, a detailed physical exam is conducted. The patient's baseline vital signs are obtained. The blood pressure is 106/52, the heart rate is 94, strong and regular, and the patient is breathing at 18 times per minute. In addition to the previously identified fracture, your evaluation reveals the patient to have abrasions and contusions across her chest. Because of the shallow respirations, you elect to provide positive pressure ventilations. En route, you continue to reassess the patient for changes, as well as anything that you may have overlooked.

During the transport, you notify the trauma center about your patient. They advise you to continue your interventions and take the patient directly to the trauma room. After completing the detailed physical exam, you and your partner are able to apply a traction splint to the injured extremity. On completing the task, you are at the emergency department. You take the patient into the trauma room and give a thorough report to the trauma team. ■

1. The rapid trauma assessment would be appropriate for all of the following *except:*
   a. a 32-year-old patient who fell down four steps and has an altered mental status.
   b. a 15-year-old patient who slipped on the ice and was unresponsive initially.
   c. a 15-year-old patient who slipped on the ice and has an open ankle fracture.
   d. a 74-year-old patient who fell out of bed, has an apparent hip fracture, and is confused.

2. What is the primary objective of the rapid trauma assessment?
   a. manual cervical spine immobilization
   b. ensuring scene safety
   c. obtaining baseline vital signs
   d. inspecting for injuries

3. When should the bones of the neck be palpated and inspected?
   a. after the initial assessment
   b. before a cervical collar is put in place
   c. immediately upon contact with the patient
   d. after vital signs have been taken

CHAPTER 23
Detailed Physical Exam

KEY TERMS

Abrasions

Burns

Contusions

Crepitation

Deformities

Lacerations

Paradoxical motion

Penetrations

Punctures

Swelling

Tenderness

Thermoregulatory

OBJECTIVE

The student will successfully identify all injuries suffered by the patient.

INTRODUCTION

The detailed physical exam is performed most commonly on major trauma patients while en route to the hospital. All life threats must have already been detected and treated during the initial assessment or rapid trauma assessment before beginning the detailed physical exam. Nontransporting units may have time to complete a detailed physical exam on scene while awaiting arrival of the transporting unit. The purpose of the detailed physical exam is to identify all injuries suffered by the patient. It can, however, be omitted if you must dedicate personnel to the ABCs. Some injuries will require treatment by the EMT, whereas others will only be treated by the hospital staff but should be reported by the EMT in both a verbal and written report.

▶ EQUIPMENT

You will need the following equipment:

- ▶ Long spine board
- ▶ Cervical collar
- ▶ Stethoscope
- ▶ Penlight
- ▶ Scissors
- ▶ Bandaging supplies
- ▶ Splinting devices

ASSESSMENT

Many of the patient's injuries would have been identified during the rapid trauma assessment. However, because that exam is so brief, the detailed physical exam will reveal signs or symptoms that may have been missed or may have changed since the rapid trauma assessment. For example, bruising takes several minutes to develop, and may not be readily apparent during the initial assessment or rapid trauma assessment, but may become noticeable during the detailed physical exam.

During the detailed physical exam, the EMT systematically inspects and palpates each part of the body for abnormalities including **deformities, contusions, abrasions, punctures** and **penetrations, burns, tenderness, lacerations,** or **swelling.** At this point in the assessment, the patient will have all threats to ABCs managed. The patient is likely to have oxygen, spinal immobilization, and other treatments in place.

PROCEDURE: Detailed Physical Exam

1. Apply BSI precautions.
   Rationale: Gloves and eye protection are required at minimum, and a gown may be necessary if large amounts of blood or fluids are present to prevent exposure to infectious diseases.

2. Reassess mechanism of injury.
   Rationale: Additional information may become available as the call progresses and bystanders are interviewed. This additional information may be helpful during your assessment.

3. Repeat your initial assessment including general impression, mental status, airway, breathing, and circulation.
   Rationale: The initial assessment will reveal life threats as the patient's condition worsens. If a life threat is discovered, begin treatment and/or transport immediately.

4. Remove the patient's clothing, being sure to protect his privacy and prevent exposure to the elements.
   Rationale: The EMT must be able to see all injuries to effectively treat the patient.

 GERIATRIC NOTE:
Geriatric patients commonly have failing **thermoregulatory** systems and may not be able to stay warm after their clothes have been removed for an assessment. Be sure to cover the patient with blankets to prevent shivering and hypothermia.

5. Begin at the head. Palpate and observe for injuries including **crepitation** of the skull and facial

continued...

bones. Check the ears and nose for abnormalities plus bleeding or drainage of cerebrospinal fluid. Inspect the mouth for broken teeth, foreign objects, lacerations of the tongue, and unusual odors on the breath. Check the eyes for pupil size, reactivity, and blood in the anterior chamber of the eye, which indicates significant blunt force trauma (Figure 23.1).

Rationale: The assessment is begun at the head to ensure no injuries are missed by skipping around to different body regions.

6. Check the neck for injuries plus jugular vein distension, tracheal deviation, and crepitation of the cervical spinal bones (Figure 23.2).

Rationale: Note that a cervical collar will obscure any assessment of the neck region; therefore, ideally the neck is assessed before the collar is applied.

7. Assess the chest for any injuries plus crepitation, **paradoxical motion,** and the presence of breath sounds (Figure 23.3).

Rationale: Injuries to the chest can be life threatening.

8. Assess the abdomen for abnormalities plus firmness, tenderness, or distension (Figure 23.4).

Rationale: Injuries to the abdominal organs can cause significant internal hemorrhage and should be detected as soon as possible.

 PEDIATRIC NOTE:

Children have poorly developed abdominal muscles and are more prone to injuries to this area. Assess the abdomen often for signs of injury to hollow or solid organs.

9. Assess the pelvis for injuries by observation and gentle downward pressure on the pelvic bones. Do *not* rock the pelvis. Note any pain, tenderness, or lack of motion (Figure 23.5).

Rationale: Rocking the pelvis can injure the spine.

10. Assess all four extremities for injuries plus distal pulse, motor function, and sensation (Figures 23.6 and 23.7).

Rationale: Lack of movement or feeling can indicate a spinal injury.

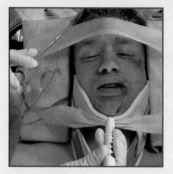
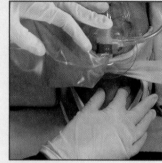

Figure 23.1

Figure 23.2

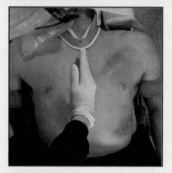
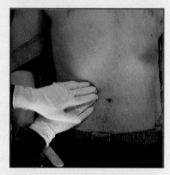

Figure 23.3

Figure 23.4

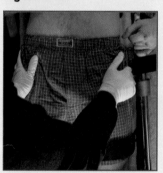
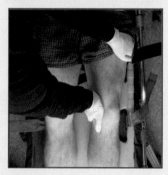

Figure 23.5

Figure 23.6

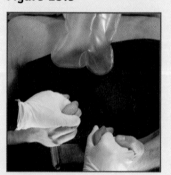

Figure 23.7

11. Roll the patient to his side and assess the posterior chest, buttocks, and legs for abnormalities.

    Rationale: The back and buttocks cannot be effectively assessed without rolling the patient and exposing this area.

12. Treat injuries identified in the detailed physical exam. If time permits, treat the injuries identified in the detailed physical exam. Treatment might include bandaging or splinting.

13. Document your findings.

    Rationale: It is exremely important to document your findings in order to have a history of facts and events that occurred at the scene.

ONGOING ASSESSMENT

If the patient's condition worsens at any time, immediately return to the initial assessment and reassess airway, breathing, and circulation. It may be necessary to stop further assessment and treatment and transport immediately. The detailed physical exam is usually completed en route to the hospital and can be repeated if the transport time is long.

▶ PROBLEM SOLVING

▶ The most common problem encountered with the detailed physical exam is disorganization, which leads to missed injuries. Conduct the assessment as described, without omitting any steps, and injuries will be identified in a systematic fashion leading to timely treatment and transport.

▶ Clothing should be removed when possible to allow for optimal inspection and palpation of the body.

▶ Rocking the pelvis to assess for stability is no longer acceptable. Gentle pressure lateral to medial and anterior to posterior is appropriate and will identify most pelvic injuries without compromising the spine.

▶ CASE STUDY

You have just responded to a motor vehicle collision in which a motorcycle hit a tree. The first responders tell you that the patient is awake, alert, and oriented. His vital signs are stable and he is complaining of pain in his chest, back, right leg, and his right shoulder. On your arrival, the patient is lying supine about 30 feet from his motorcycle with his helmet off. He was reportedly wearing his helmet at the time of the accident.

You ask the first responders to assist you in placing the patient on a backboard. On rolling him, you palpate and inspect his back and note no deformities or wounds, and he denies having any midspinal pain. The patient is then secured to the backboard and transferred on a stretcher to the ambulance.

Once in the ambulance, you reassess the patient's ABCs and find them to be unchanged. You begin your detailed physical exam. Starting at the head, you note no deficits. As you move down the body, you come across the neck and note the jugular veins to be normal, and the trachea to be midline. As you palpate the chest, the patient complains of pain in the right upper chest. On inspection, you note a large area of bruising but the chest is rising equally on inspiration. On palpation of the abdomen, the patient denies pain and inspection does not reveal anything remarkable. The pelvis is stable. As you move down the left leg, the patient denies pain, and he has good pulse, motor, and sensory response. Moving down the right leg, you find that the patient is complaining of intense pain just below his knee. On inspection, you note gross deformity of the right lower leg with lacerations and abrasions. Moving to the left arm, the patient denies pain and he has good pulse, motor, and sensory response. Moving down the right arm, you find that the patient is complaining of intense pain in his upper arm. On inspection, you note gross deformity of the right upper arm.

Throughout the transport, the patient's condition remains unchanged and you and your partner work to splint the right arm and right leg. ■

1. Which of the following is true about the detailed physical exam?
   a. It is required to be performed on every patient, regardless of time.
   b. It should be completed on scene to prevent further injuries.
   c. It can be omitted if you must dedicate personnel to the ABCs.
   d. It is the point at which you treat the life threats found in the initial and rapid trauma assessment.

2. What is the primary goal of the detailed physical assessment?
   a. to reassess interventions
   b. to identify and thoroughly inspect all injuries
   c. to initiate life saving interventions
   d. to obtain a SAMPLE history

3. You are in the middle of your detailed physical exam when your patient no longer responds appropriately. How would you proceed?
   a. Finish the exam and then recheck the patient.
   b. Have your partner stop the ambulance and help you.
   c. Call for backup and finish your exam.
   d. Stop the exam and repeat the initial assessment.

CHAPTER 24
Ongoing Assessment

KEY TERMS

Ongoing assessment

Perfusion

Serial vital signs

OBJECTIVE

The student will successfully reassess the patient, identifying any changes to the ABCs, vital signs, or physical presentation of the patient.

INTRODUCTION

The **ongoing assessment** provides an opportunity to reassess the patient's signs and symptoms and assess your interventions for effectiveness. The ongoing assessment is usually done after treatment is completed for the patient, but can also be done anytime there has been a change in the patient's condition. All patients should have an ongoing assessment completed prior to arrival at the receiving facility unless life-saving measures prevent such assessment.

▶ EQUIPMENT

You will need the following equipment:

▶ Blood pressure cuff
▶ Stethoscope
▶ Penlight
▶ One or more rescuers

ASSESSMENT

The ongoing assessment begins with reassessment of the findings from the initial assessment. Problems with the airway, breathing, or circulation should be treated without delay. Vital signs are reassessed and changes noted. It is during the ongoing assessment that **serial vital signs** are established. The focused physical exam should be repeated to determine if any further treatment is needed (see Chapter 23). You should be able to report to the hospital any changes in the patient's condition and whether or not your interventions helped the patient.

PROCEDURE: Ongoing Assessment

1. Apply BSI precautions.
   Rationale: Gloves and eye protection are required at minimum, and a gown may be necessary if large amounts of blood or fluid are present to prevent exposure to infectious diseases.

2. Reassess level of consciousness using the AVPU method (see Chapter 21) (Figure 24.1).
   Rationale: Changes in mental status can indicate an improvement or deterioration in the patient's neurological function and should be reported to the hospital.

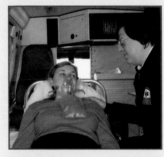

Figure 24.1

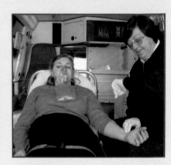

Figure 24.2

3. Reassess ABCs. Maintain an open airway and assist with breathing as needed by ventilating the patient or applying supplemental oxygen. Reassess the strength and quality of the pulse and the color, temperature, and condition of the skin. Be sure all bleeding has remained controlled (Figure 24.2).
   Rationale: Any change in airway, breathing, or circulatory status can be life threatening.

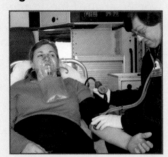

Figure 24.3

4. Re-establish patient priorities.
   Rationale: If the patient's condition has deteriorated, it may be necessary to change your priority or transport status. Critical patients should be transported immediately by safe and expeditious means.

5. Obtain vital signs, including respiratory rate, heart rate, and blood pressure (Figure 24.3).
   Rationale: This second set of vital signs, called *serial vital signs,* is used to establish a pattern in patient condition.

continued...

PEDIATRIC NOTE:

If properly sized equipment is not available, then blood pressures may not have been taken for small children. **Perfusion** can be assessed and reassessed using distal pulses, skin color, and capillary refill instead.

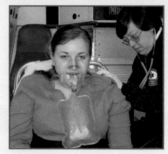
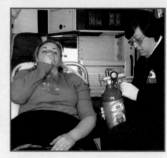

Figure 24.4   **Figure 24.5**

6. Repeat the focused physical exam of the affected body system or area. The focused physical exam includes inspection and palpation of the isolated area of complaint such as abdomen or chest. Or, if a detailed physical exam was done, repeat this exam (Figure 24.4).

   Rationale: The physical exams are repeated in order to identify any changes in patient condition that may need to be addressed by either the EMT or hospital staff.

7. Check interventions to be sure your treatments are helping the patient and are still

appropriate to the patient situation (Figure 24.5).

   Rationale: Patient needs change, and a treatment may become harmful if not observed carefully, such as an oxygen tank running out of oxygen or a splint occluding distal circulation.

8. Document your findings.

   Rationale: It is extremely important to document your findings in order to have a history of facts in events that occurred at the scene.

ONGOING ASSESSMENT

The ongoing assessment should be repeated every 5 minutes for critical patients and every 15 minutes for stable patients. Every patient should have at least two sets of vital signs assessed before arrival at the hospital. Should the condition of the patient worsen at any time, immediately return to the initial assessment and reassess airway, breathing, and circulation. It may be necessary to stop further assessment and treatment and transport immediately.

▶PROBLEM SOLVING

▶ Be sure to re-evaluate your treatments. Many things could happen that make an intervention harmful to your patient such as an oxygen tank running out or a splint applied so tightly that it impedes circulation.

▶ Do not be afraid to upgrade your response to the hospital if your patient's condition worsens.

▶ Contact medical control if you have a significant change in the patient's condition. The receiving facility will need time to prepare the proper resources for the patient.

▶CASE STUDY

Your squad responds to a call about a 4-year-old male with a history of fever, noisy breathing, and drooling. His mother states that the fever began this morning and spiked this afternoon. The noisy breathing was alarming to the child's parents and, as a result, 911 was called. The mother states that the child has not taken anything by mouth since he became ill.

Your assessment reveals the child's pulse to be 144; respirations of 32, even, and shallow; BP is 100/66; and his pulse oximetry reading is 90 percent on room air. He appears alert, awake, and to be having significant trouble breathing. He appears to prefer an upright or forward leaning position. Lung sounds are clear and equal across the chest. The child does have inspiratory stridor.

As you approach the patient, you note that he is seated in a tripod position with accessory muscle use. The patient is transferred to the ambulance and transport is initiated. While en route to the hospital, the child continues to experience respiratory difficulty. The child was given blow-by oxygen and a detailed physical exam was conducted. You check the patient's vital signs again and find them unchanged.

As transport continues, the patient becomes more anxious and appears to be experiencing greater difficulty in breathing. The child tolerates the oxygen well and will allow you to give it to him by nonrebreather mask. Throughout the remainder of the transport, you continue to evaluate his ABCs and watch for any other changes.

As you approach the pediatric emergency care center, you call to report on the patient. Upon arrival, you transfer the patient care to the staff and give them a thorough report. ■

1. Which of the following best describes the use of the ongoing assessment?
    a. It may not be completed prior to arrival at the hospital.
    b. It should be completed on all patients, even if you omit something else.
    c. It is a reassessment of all previous assessments and interventions.
    d. It only looks at previous interventions and does not allow for change.

2. A patient is complaining of ankle pain after tripping down the stairs. How frequently should the ongoing assessment be performed?
    a. every 5 minutes
    b. every 10 minutes
    c. every 15 minutes
    d. Ongoing assessment is not necessary because the patient only has an isolated injury.

3. The ongoing assessment includes all of the following *except*:
    a. the ABCs
    b. the focused physical examination
    c. the detailed physical examination
    d. the hospital notification of patient changes

CHAPTER 25

Assessment of the Responsive Medical Patient

OBJECTIVE

The student will successfully assess a responsive medical patient, identifying and treating signs and symptoms of illness through the use of proper history gathering and physical examination.

INTRODUCTION

In contrast to the trauma patient assessment, which relies heavily on the physical exam to identify life-threatening injuries, the medical patient assessment requires thorough history taking. The **past medical history** and history of present illness are easily obtained from the conscious medical patient. Treatable signs or symptoms should be managed by the EMT. Often, however, no prehospital treatment is indicated and a thorough assessment and transport to a hospital are the only tasks required of the EMT.

KEY TERMS

Chief complaint

Field impression

Focused history

General impression

Level of distress

Life threats

Nature of the illness

Past medical history

▶EQUIPMENT

You will need the following equipment:

- ▷ Blood pressure cuff
- ▷ Stethoscope
- ▷ Pen light
- ▷ Scissors
- ▷ One or more rescuers

ASSESSMENT

The responsive medical patient assessment begins with an assessment of the scene itself. Contact with the patient should not be made until scene hazards have been identified and rectified, number of patients determined, and additional help summoned as needed. Use this time, as well, to determine the **nature of the illness** if clues on scene expose information such as empty pill bottles, suggesting an overdose, or oxygen equipment at the home of a chronic respiratory patient.

PROCEDURE: Assessment of the Responsive Medical Patient

1. Apply BSI precautions.
   Rationale: Gloves and eye protection are required at a minimum, and a gown may be needed if large amounts of blood or fluid are present to prevent exposure to infectious diseases.

2. Conduct a scene size-up as you approach or come on scene. Determine that the scene is safe and free of hazards. Determine the nature of the illness such as an overdose, vomiting, or shortness of breath. Identify the number of patients and whether additional resources such as law enforcement personnel or firefighters will be necessary. If additional resources are needed, request those resources now.
   Rationale: Once you make contact with the patient, it will be difficult to disengage to determine the scene size-up.

3. If the patient appears unconscious and is on the ground or could have otherwise suffered trauma, direct manual stabilization of the cervical spine.
   Rationale: Full spinal immobilization may be necessary if you cannot rule out trauma.

4. Verbalize your **general impression** of the patient regarding her **level of distress** and other obvious

findings such as positioning and surroundings (see also Chapter 21).
   Rationale: Verbalizing your general impression helps your team members respond with the same level of intensity as you.

5. Determine level of consciousness of the patient using the AVPU method. This initial assessment is used to determine whether the patient is ALERT, responsive to VERBAL stimuli, responsive to PAINFUL stimuli, or UNRESPONSIVE (see Chapter 21 for details about the AVPU method).
   Rationale: A *baseline* assessment of mental status is needed to determine if the patient is capable of answering other questions. Unresponsive patients receive a different assessment process (see Chapter 26).

6. Determine the **chief complaint** or apparent **life threats.** If the patient can communicate verbally, ask for the chief complaint. Otherwise, visualize the nature of the illness (Figure 25.1).
   Rationale: The chief complaint will guide both the order and urgency of the assessment.

7. Ensure airway patency. If the airway is not open, use the head-tilt/chin-lift maneuver as long as no

trauma is present. Insert an airway adjunct to maintain patency if needed.

Rationale: No further assessment should be done if the airway is not controlled.

8. Assess the rate and quality of breathing. Assess for adequate tidal volume by observing chest rise and fall. Ensure lung sounds are present and equal. Apply high-flow oxygen here. Repositioning the patient may assist with keeping the airway open and improving breathing (Figure 25.2) (see also Chapter 21).

Rationale: Breathing must be adequate before any other assessment is completed. Inadequate respirations must be corrected immediately by the EMT.

9. Check central and peripheral pulses for rate, strength, and regularity. Assess skin color, temperature, and condition. Control external bleeding with direct pressure. Initiate shock management with Trendelenburg positioning, if applicable, or application of a pneumatic anti-shock garment (PASG). Major bleeding can be found by inspection after the patient has been exposed or by palpation and inspection for blood on the gloves of the rescuer (see also Chapter 21).

Rationale: Bleeding is considered a life threat and would need to be controlled before any further assessment can be completed.

 GERIATRIC NOTE:

Peripheral pulses may be difficult to palpate in the geriatric patient due to peripheral vaso-constriction and arteriosclerosis. It may be necessary to palpate central pulses, such as the carotid, to determine a pulse rate in the geriatric patient.

10. Determine priority of the patient and make a transport decision.

Rationale: Patients with threats to airway, breathing, or circulation should be prepared for transport immediately. Stable patients, or those with minor illnesses, can be treated on scene and transported with less urgency.

The above steps, from determination of responsiveness to transport decision, make up the initial assessment and resuscitation.

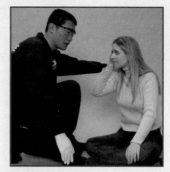
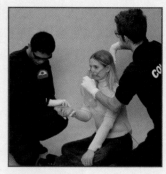

Figure 25.1   **Figure 25.2**

11. Begin transport of the critical patient.

Rationale: If the patient is critical, no further on-scene assessment will improve the patient's condition. All further assessment findings can be completed en route to the proper receiving facility.

12. Perform the **focused history** by gathering information about the history of the present illness using the OPQRST method, in which you inquire about *O*nset, *P*rovocation, *Q*uality, *R*adiation, *S*everity, and *T*ime. Ask now about related signs and symptoms and other questions related to the chief complaint.

Rationale: OPQRST works very well for patients describing some type of pain or discomfort.

13. Obtain a SAMPLE history, which includes Signs and symptoms, Allergies, Medications, Pertinent post medical history, Last oral intake, and Events leading up to the incident. The history may be obtained from the patient if she is still conscious, or from a family member, bystander, or witness if needed. Patients may also carry this information in their purse or wallet, glove box, cupboard, etc. (Figure 25.3).

Rationale: The history is often the most valuable element in the assessment of the medical patient

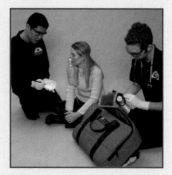

Figure 25.3

continued...

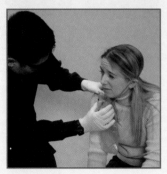

Figure 25.4

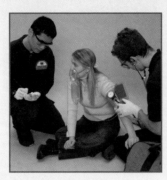

Figure 25.5

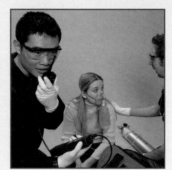

Figure 25.6

to determine the presenting problem and how best to help the patient.

 PEDIATRIC NOTE:

Children may not know their medical history. It is appropriate to ask parents, relatives, or caregivers for past medical history.

14. Complete a focused physical exam of the affected body system or area. A focused physical exam includes inspection and palpation of the isolated area of complaint such as the head, abdomen, or chest (Figure 25.4).

    Rationale: A head-to-toe exam is not needed if the chief complaint is isolated to one specific body area.

15. Obtain vital signs, including respiratory rate, heart rate, and blood pressure. This task may be delegated to a partner (Figure 25.5).

    Rationale: Vital signs will help complete the assessment picture for the EMT to determine the cause of the patient's problem and what treatment might be needed.

16. Complete any diagnostic tests needed such as cardiac monitoring, pulse oximetry, or blood sugar testing.

    Rationale: In some systems, EMTs have protocols to conduct diagnostic tests.

 GERIATRIC NOTE:

Geriatric patients often have factors of comorbidity or past medical problems that can affect or be affected by their current medical problem. Diagnostic tests can help to determine what effect, if any, those previous problems are exerting on the current situation. For example, the chief complaint may be a headache, but if the patient has a history of diabetes, it would also be appropriate to check her blood sugar to ensure that it is within normal limits.

17. Determine and state a **field impression** of the patient.

    Rationale: Your field impression will often determine which protocol or algorithm should be used to treat your patient.

18. Determine the appropriate treatment plan for your patient and call medical control for orders if necessary (Figure 25.6).

    Rationale: In many systems, EMTs require online medical control for treatment orders.

19. Re-evaluate your transport decision.

    Rationale: If the patient's condition has worsened, you may decide to upgrade your response to the hospital. Additionally, be sure you are transporting to the most appropriate receiving facility for the illness suffered by your patient.

PEDIATRIC NOTE:

Ensure that the receiving facility to which you intend to take your patient is appropriate for a child. Some facilities do not have equipment that is sized for pediatric patients. Therefore, a pediatric emergency room may be a better choice for your patient.

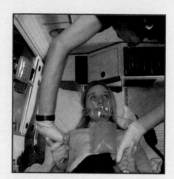

Figure 25.7

20. Complete an ongoing assessment, which includes repeating the initial assessment, vital signs, and focused history and physical exam as well as evaluating response to treatments (Figure 25.7).

    Rationale: You may need to modify your treatment as the patient's condition changes.

21. Document your findings.

    Rationale: It is extremely important to document your findings in order to have a history of facts and events that occurred at the scene.

ONGOING ASSESSMENT

Assessment should be repeated every 5 minutes for critical patients and every 15 minutes for stable patients. Every patient should have at least two sets of vital signs assessed before arrival at the hospital. Should the condition of the patient worsen at any time, immediately return to the initial assessment and reassess airway, breathing, and circulation. It may be necessary to stop further assessment and treatment and transport immediately.

▶PROBLEM SOLVING

▶ The most common problem with the medical patient assessment is poor history taking leading to missed symptoms. Ask open-ended questions that allow patients to describe their complaints in their words. Then, ask follow-up questions for clarification.

▶ Because the history is so important in the medical patient assessment, good communication with your patient is a must. Create an environment conducive to conversation. When a language barrier exists, find an interpreter or alternate means of communication such as signing, pointing, or writing.

▶CASE STUDY

You are responding to the home of a 39-year-old female who is reportedly having trouble breathing. On your arrival, the patient is seated upright in a tripod position complaining of difficulty breathing. The patient appears to be breathing shallowly and has labored respirations.

The patient is responsive and appears to be anxious. She has an open and patent airway. The patient's radial and carotid pulses are equal at a rate of 118. The patient's skin is warm and moist. On further assessment, you note that the patient's lung sounds are diminished with inspiratory and expiratory wheezes on the left side of her chest.

The patient states she has a history of asthma, but has not had an attack since she was a teenager. She continues to tell you that she has no other medical problems aside from being sick for the last week or so. She denies taking medications and says she has no allergies to medications either.

While en route to the hospital, the patient's vital signs were obtained and were as follows: Pulse is 132 weak and regular; respirations are 28, labored and shallow; and BP is 100/56. As the patient deteriorates you administer an Epi-pen and continue to transport her to the emergency department. ■

1. What does the *P* in OPQRST stand for?
   a. number of patients
   b. past medical history
   c. How bad is the pain?
   d. What makes it worse?

2. The responsive medical patient assessment consists of:
   a. the initial assessment and a focused history.
   b. a detailed physical exam and baseline vitals.
   c. an initial and rapid medical assessment.
   d. more physical assessment and less history.

3. After determining the level of consciousness of the responsive medical patient, the patient should only be interviewed for additional history information if he is:
   a. unresponsive.
   b. alert and oriented.
   c. responsive to painful stimuli.
   d. responsive to verbal stimuli.

CHAPTER 26

Assessment of the Unresponsive Medical Patient

KEY TERMS

High-priority conditions

Index of suspicion

Presenting problem

Trendelenburg positioning

Unresponsiveness

Vegetative state

OBJECTIVE

The student will successfully assess an unresponsive medical patient, identifying the probable cause for unresponsiveness through proper physical examination and interview of bystanders or caregivers when possible.

INTRODUCTION

The patient assessment unlocks the keys to the patient's illness or **presenting problem.** The unresponsive patient presents a challenge to the EMT because the EMT cannot interview, or ask questions of, the patient. The communication barrier presented by an unresponsive patient causes the EMT to rely on physical findings and an **index of suspicion** for what might be causing the unconsciousness. **Unresponsiveness** can be a life-threatening condition, but it can also be a **vegetative state** that is normal for the patient. Through proper use of the physical exam and questioning of bystanders and caregivers, clues to the patient's needs can be discovered and proper patient care delivered.

EQUIPMENT

You will need the following equipment:

- Blood pressure cuff
- Stethoscope
- Penlight
- Scissors

ASSESSMENT

The medical patient assessment begins with an assessment of the scene itself. Contact with the patient should not be made until scene hazards have been identified and rectified, number of patients determined, and additional help summoned as needed. Use this time, as well, to determine the nature of the illness if clues on scene reveal this information, such as an odor in the air that could indicate a toxic inhalation situation or drug paraphernalia that could indicate an overdose. Assessment of the unresponsive medical patient may resemble that of rapid trauma assessment depending on the condition of the patient.

The unresponsive patient falls into a category for treatment and transport referred to as *high priority*. **High-priority conditions** require immediate transport because they could be life threatening. Other high-priority patients, in addition to unresponsive patients, include poor general impression, responsive but not following commands, difficulty breathing, shock, complicated childbirth, chest pain with systolic blood pressure less than 100, uncontrolled bleeding, and severe pain.

PROCEDURE: Assessment of the Unresponsive Medical Patient

1. Apply BSI precautions.
   Rationale: Gloves and eye protection are required at minimum, but a gown may be needed if large amounts of blood or fluid are present to prevent exposure to infectious diseases.

2. Perform a scene size-up as you approach or come on the scene. Determine that the scene is safe and free of hazards. Determine the nature of the illness such as respiratory failure, shock, or gastrointestinal bleeding. Identify the number of patients and if additional resources such as law enforcement personnel or firefighters will be necessary. If additional resources are needed, request those resources now (Figure 26.1).
   Rationale: Once you make contact with the patient, it will be difficult to disengage to determine the scene size-up.

PEDIATRIC NOTE:

For children, note where the patient was found upon your arrival, such as the crib or bed, but also specifically ask where the patient was found by the family members. Children are easily moved from their original locations because they can be picked up and carried about by an adult.

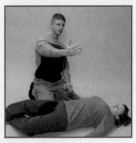

Figure 26.1

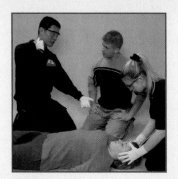

Figure 26.2

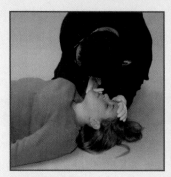

Figure 26.3

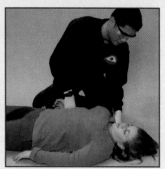

Figure 26.4

3. If the unconscious patient is on the ground or could have otherwise suffered trauma, direct manual stabilization of the cervical spine (Figure 26.2).

   Rationale: Full spinal immobilization may be necessary if you cannot rule out trauma.

4. Verbalize your general impression of the patient regarding her level of distress, which will be severe or serious for the unconscious patient, and other obvious findings such as positioning and surroundings.

   Rationale: Verbalizing your general impression helps your team members respond with the same level of intensity as you.

5. Determine level of consciousness of the patient using the AVPU scale. This initial assessment is used to determine whether the patient is ALERT, responsive to VERBAL stimuli, responsive to PAINFUL stimuli, or UNRESPONSIVE (Figure 26.3).

   Rationale: Even if the patient appears unconscious, he or she may respond to loud verbal or painful stimuli. Only a true measure of level of responsiveness will assist in determining a treatment plan.

6. Determine the chief complaint or apparent cause for unresponsiveness. For the unconscious patient, form a general impression from the life threats that are readily visible such as unconsciousness, hemorrhage, or cyanosis.

   Rationale: The chief complaint or presenting problem will determine the order and type of assessment conducted.

7. Ensure airway patency. If the airway is not open, open it using the head-tilt/chin-lift maneuver as

long as no trauma is present. Insert an airway adjunct or suction to maintain patency as needed (Figure 26.4).

Rationale: No further assessment should be conducted until the airway is managed.

PEDIATRIC NOTE:

Be sure not to hyperextend the neck of pediatric patients because this will actually occlude their airway. The airways of children are very flexible and susceptible to damage when hyperextended.

8. Assess the rate and quality of breathing. Assess for adequate tidal volume by observing chest rise and fall. Ensure lung sounds are present and equal. Apply high-flow oxygen (Figure 26.5).

   Rationale: Unconscious patients often have inadequate rate and tidal volume. Assisting ventilations with a bag-valve-mask unit may be required. Repositioning the patient may assist with keeping the airway open and improving breathing.

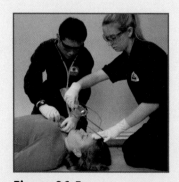

Figure 26.5

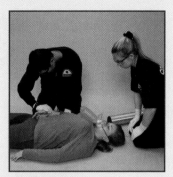

Figure 26.6

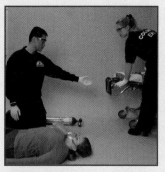

Figure 26.7

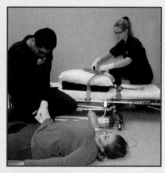

Figure 26.8

9. Check central and peripheral pulses for rate, strength, and regularity. Assess skin color, temperature, and condition. Control external bleeding with direct pressure. Initiate shock management if indicated with **Trendelenburg positioning** or application of a pneumatic anti-shock garment (PASG). Major bleeding can be found by inspection after the patient has been exposed or by palpation and inspection for blood on the gloves of the rescuer (Figure 26.6).

   Rationale: Any insult to the circulatory system could potentially be life threatening and indicate a need for immediate transport.

10. Determine priority of the patient and make a transport decision (Figure 26.7).

    Rationale: Patients with threats to airway, breathing, or circulation should be prepared for transport immediately. Usually, an unconscious patient will require rapid transport. However, if the unconscious state is chronic, and normal for this patient, routine transport may be appropriate. Stable patients or those with minor illnesses can be treated on scene and transported with less urgency.

    The above steps, from determination of responsiveness to transport decision, make up the initial assessment and resuscitation.

11. Perform a rapid assessment of the entire body (Figure 26.8). Examine each of the following body regions:

    A. Head for vomit or other abnormalities
    B. Neck for jugular vein distension or medical identification devices
    C. Chest for presence and equality of breath sounds
    D. Abdomen for distension, firmness, or rigidity
    E. Pelvis for incontinence of urine or feces

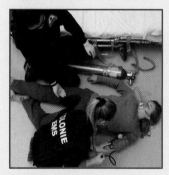

Figure 26.9

    F. Extremities for PMS and medical identification devices
    G. Posterior for bleeding or incontinence

    Rationale: You are checking each body region for any signs that would indicate the cause of unconsciousness such as a bruise that might signify a fall, bleeding that might indicate a gynecological emergency, or a distended abdomen that might indicate an abdominal emergency.

12. Take vital signs including respirations, pulse, skin signs, pupils, and blood pressure (Figure 26.9).

    Rationale: Vital signs will help establish a baseline for the patient's condition and further determine priority for patient treatment and transport.

13. Consider a request for advanced life support (ALS) personnel.

    Rationale: If an ALS assist is unavailable, you will have to decide whether the patient should be transported to a more specialized—and perhaps more distant—medical facility given her particular signs and symptoms. For example, if the patient appears to have suffered a stroke, the most appropriate receiving facility for that patient would be one with an operating computed tomography (CT) scanner.

continued...

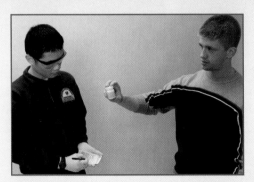

Figure 26.10

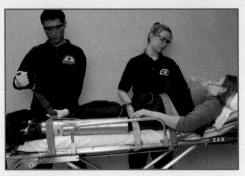

Figure 26.11

14. Interview family and bystanders to obtain as much of the SAMPLE history as possible (Figure 26.10).

   Rationale: The unresponsive patient will not be able to relay past medical history that may be pertinent to her care, such as a history of seizures. The SAMPLE history includes Signs and symptoms, Allergies, Medications, Pertinent past medical history, Last oral intake, and Events leading up to the incident.

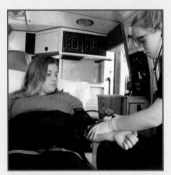

Figure 26.12

15. Using the physical exam and history information gathered, determine the patient's presenting problem and formulate a treatment plan.

   Rationale: Most systems provide algorithms or protocols for treatment once the presenting problem has been determined.

16. Perform necessary interventions and transport to an appropriate receiving facility (Figure 26.11).

   Rationale: Life-saving treatment should be performed on scene, but other interventions can be performed en route. For critical patients, arrival at the appropriate receiving facility is more important than minor care provided on scene.

17. Complete an ongoing assessment, which includes repeating the initial assessment, vital signs, and focused history and physical exam as well as evaluating response to treatments (Figure 26.12).

   Rationale: Your treatment may need to be adjusted depending on changes in the patient's condition.

 GERIATRIC NOTE:

Any changes in the condition of the geriatric patient should be attended to quickly because geriatric patients do not compensate as well as other patients due to their degenerating body systems and complicating medical conditions.

18. Document your findings.

   Rationale: It is extremely important to document your findings in order to have a history of facts and events that occured at the scene.

Retake vital signs every 5 minutes in an unstable patient and every 15 minutes in a stable patient. You should have a least two—and preferably three—sets of vitals by the time you reach the hospital.

If the patient's condition worsens at any time, immediately return to the initial assessment and re-evaluate the ABCs. Adjust your treatment and transport priorities as needed.

▶PROBLEM SOLVING

▷ When the patient is unresponsive, the history may be difficult to obtain. Be sure to use the clues on scene to put together as much of the story as possible. Remember that you are the eyes and ears for the emergency department staff. They will rely on you to observe and report any elements of the scene or situation that could be helpful when treating the patient.

▷ Unresponsiveness leads to airway and breathing problems because such a patient is unable to maintain her own airway. The EMT may be very busy managing airway and breathing and unable to obtain every element of the history.

▶CASE STUDY

You are responding to the home of a 30-year-old male who is reportedly having trouble breathing. A bystander advises you that the patient was cutting some bushes when a swarm of yellow jackets attacked him. The patient has numerous areas of swelling about his chest, face, and arms.

On your arrival, the patient is lying supine and motionless. The patient appears to be breathing very shallowly. He is unresponsive and has been for the last 10 minutes according to the bystander. His airway is open and you hear stridor; his respirations are shallow and labored. The patient's radial and carotid pulses are at a rate of 126 but unequal. The carotid pulse is substantially stronger than the radial. The patient's skin has hives and is very red. On further assessment, you note that the patient's lung sounds are diminished and equal with inspiratory and expiratory wheezes.

While en route to the hospital, the patient's vital signs were obtained and were as follows: Pulse is 132 weak and regular; respirations are 28, labored and shallow; and BP is 100/56. As the patient deteriorates you administer the epinephrine auto-injector and continue to transport him to the emergency department. ■

(continued)

1. The unresponsive medical patient assessment most closely resembles:
   a. the responsive medical patient assessment.
   b. the rapid trauma assessment.
   c. the focused history.
   d. none of the above

2. Clues to the nature of the illness in an unresponsive medical patient can be obtained through each of the following except:
   a. bystanders.
   b. the scene.
   c. medications.
   d. detailed history.

3. What is the most important aspect of caring for the unresponsive medical patient?
   a. maintaining the ABCs
   b. completing a detailed physical exam
   c. questioning family
   d. completing an ongoing assessment

CHAPTER 27

Assessment of the Trauma Patient with No Significant Mechanism of Injury

OBJECTIVE

The student will successfully demonstrate assessment of the trauma patient with minor injuries from an incident with no significant mechanism of injury.

INTRODUCTION

Assessment of the trauma patient is focused on cervical spinal protection, identification and treatment of life-threatening injuries, and rapid transport to an appropriate receiving facility. **Life threats,** or insults to the mental status, airway, breathing, or circulation, should be treated as soon as they are found. However, not all trauma patients have life-threatening injuries. Many will have only minor injuries for which a thorough assessment and proper treatment can be performed while still on scene. Information related to the cause of the incident or **mechanism of injury (MOI)** and past medical history are likely to be available from the patient, and can complete the picture formed from your trauma patient assessment.

▶ EQUIPMENT

You will need the following equipment:

▷ Long spine board

▷ Cervical collar (set)

▷ Head blocks or towel rolls

▷ 2- or 3-inch tape

▷ Backboard straps

▷ Blood pressure cuff

▷ Stethoscope

▷ Penlight

▷ Scissors

▷ Bandaging supplies (e.g., occlusive dressing)

▷ Portable suction unit and rigid Yankauer tip

▷ OPAs and/or NPAs

▷ Oxygen and appropriate tubing

▷ BVM, reservoir, and tubing

▷ Nonrebreather mask

ASSESSMENT

The trauma patient assessment begins with an assessment of the scene itself. Because the trauma patient with no significant mechanism of injury is almost always conscious, he can describe the mechanism of injury and his chief complaint. All trauma patients will still receive an initial assessment because, occasionally, even a minor MOI can cause serious injuries that should be identified as early as possible. But after the initial assessment is completed, the focused history and physical exam will be the appropriate assessment format. Once an area of complaint is identified, such as wrist pain from a skateboard fall, a focused trauma assessment of that specific injury will follow, with minor treatment provided on scene to minimize pain or further injury.

PROCEDURE: Assessment of the Trauma Patient with No Significant Mechanism of Injury

1. Apply BSI precautions.

   Rationale: Gloves and eye protection are required at a minimum, and a gown may be needed if large amounts of blood or fluid are present to minimize exposure to infectious diseases.

2. Perform a scene size-up as you approach or come on scene. Determine that the scene is safe and free of hazards. Use clues found on scene to determine the mechanism of injury such as a fall or vehicle collision. Identify the number of patients and whether additional resources are needed, such as highway patrol officers for traffic control. If additional resources are needed, request those now.

   Rationale: Once you make contact with the patient, it will be difficult to disengage to determine the scene size-up, and necessary resources could then be delayed.

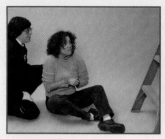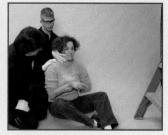

Figure 27.1   **Figure 27.2**

3. Approach the patient from her front or side, introduce yourself, and instruct the patient not to move (Figure 27.1).

   Rationale: You should assume that all trauma patients have the potential for a spinal injury. Approaching from the front or side minimizes the possibility that the patient will turn her head to view you, possibly exacerbating a spinal injury.

 PEDIATRIC NOTE:

   If no parent is on scene when you arrive, immediately send a bystander to get the parent or guardian. In many cases, you will need parental consent to treat and transport the child.

4. Until the cause of the patient's trauma and her chief complaint have been determined, direct manual stabilization of the cervical spine (Figure 27.2).

   Rationale: If it turns out that there is no complaint of neck or back pain, and your protocol allows, you may be able to release spinal stabilization later in the assessment.

5. Verbalize your general impression of the patient regarding her level of distress and other obvious findings such as positioning and surroundings.

   Rationale: Verbalizing your general impression helps your team members respond with the same level of intensity as you.

6. Determine level of consciousness of the patient using the AVPU method. This initial assessment is used to determine whether the patient is ALERT, responsive to VERBAL stimuli, responsive to PAINFUL stimuli, or RESPONSIVE.

   Rationale: A baseline assessment of mental status is needed to determine if the patient is capable of answering other questions. Note that the trauma patient with no significant mechanism of injury is likely to be unresponsive.

7. Ensure airway patency. If the airway is not open, open it using the jaw-thrust maneuver. Insert an airway adjunct or suction to maintain patency if needed.

   Rationale: The assessment process should not be continued if the airway is not controlled. However, management of the airway is not likely to be needed in this type of trauma patient.

8. Determine the chief complaint or apparent life threats. Because the patient is likely to be able to communicate, ask about her chief complaint. Otherwise, visualize the mechanism of injury and use your **index of suspicion** to estimate the probable injuries suffered.

   Rationale: The chief complaint will guide both the order and urgency of the assessment.

9. Assess the rate and quality of breathing. Assess for adequate tidal volume by observing chest rise and fall. Ensure lung sounds are present and equal. Apply high-flow oxygen. Repositioning the patient may assist with keeping the airway open and improving breathing.

   Rationale: Breathing must be adequate before any other assessment is completed. Even minor trauma patients may require supplemental oxygen.

 GERIATRIC NOTE:

   Pain can cause patients to **hypoventilate,** which can be problematic for the elderly patient. Supplemental oxygen is likely to be indicated for the geriatric trauma patient, even if the injuries are minor.

10. Check central and peripheral pulses for rate, strength, and regularity. Assess skin color, temperature, and condition. Control external bleeding with direct pressure. Initiate shock management if indicated with Trendelenburg positioning or application of pneumatic anti-shock garment (PASG). Major bleeding can be found by inspection after the patient has been exposed or by palpation and inspection for blood on the gloves of the rescuer (Figure 27.3).

    Rationale: Bleeding is considered a life threat and needs to be controlled before any further assessment is completed.

continued...

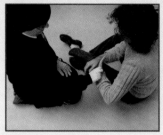
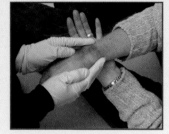

Figure 27.3   **Figure 27.4**

 PEDIATRIC NOTE:

Carotid and radial pulses can be difficult to find on small children. The recommended place to check pulses on a small child is the brachial artery.

11. Determine priority of the patient and make a transport decision.

    Rationale: Patients with threats to airway, breathing, or circulation should be prepared for transport immediately. However, the trauma patient with no significant mechanism of injury is likely to be stable and can be treated on scene and transported with less urgency.

    The above steps, from determination of responsiveness to transport decision, make up the initial assessment and resuscitation.

12. Perform a focused trauma assessment of the injured body part identified by the patient's chief complaint. You will evaluate the injury using inspection and palpation. Look and feel for any abnormalities such as bruising, deformity, pain, swelling, or bleeding (Figure 27.4).

    Rationale: The assessment of the injured area will dictate what treatment is appropriate, such as splinting or bandaging.

13. Obtain baseline vital signs, including respirations, pulse, skin signs, pupils, and blood pressure. This task may be delegated to a partner (Figure 27.5).

    Rationale: Vital signs will help complete the assessment picture for the EMT and further confirm that the mechanism of injury was not significant and the injury quite minor.

14. Obtain a past medical (SAMPLE) history: Signs and symptoms, Allergies, Medications, Pertinent past medical history, Last oral intake, and Events leading up to the incident. The history should be obtained from the patient first, but a family member, bystander, or witness may also be questioned if necessary.

    Rationale: Although the history of the minor trauma patient is not as important as is the history of major trauma patient, the information may help complete the picture for the patient's presentation. For example, if the patient seems unusually upset about a minor injury, and you then discover the patient has an anxiety disorder, it may help you understand the patient's fears and help to calm her.

 GERIATRIC NOTE:

Remember that elderly patients often have significant medical histories that may have caused the traumatic incident to occur. For example, the patient may have been experiencing chest pain before he crashed his vehicle or may have stood up too quickly, causing him to get dizzy and fall to the floor. Be sure to thoroughly evaluate the medical history of geriatric trauma patients.

15. Treat the injuries found with bandaging or splinting as needed (Figure 27.6).

    Rationale: The minor trauma patient has time for you to splint or bandage injuries before transport. In most cases, the treatment serves to not only minimize further injury, but decrease the patient's pain, making her experience with EMS more pleasant.

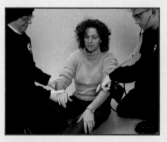
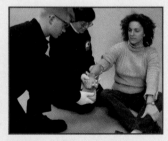

Figure 27.5   **Figure 27.6**

16. Prepare patient for transport (Figure 27.7).

   Rationale: Most patients who sustain any type of traumatic injury will need to be transported to the hospital for further evaluation, which may include X-rays or sutures.

17. Document findings.

   Rationale: It is extremely important to document your findings in order to have a history of facts and events that occurred at the scene.

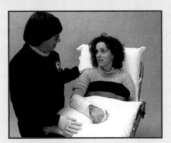

Figure 27.7

ONGOING ASSESSMENT

Assessment should be repeated every 5 minutes for critical patients and every 15 minutes for stable patients. Every patient should have at least two sets of vital signs assessed before arrival at the hospital.

Should the condition of the patient worsen at any time, immediately return to the initial assessment and reassess airway, breathing, and circulation. It may be necessary to stop further assessment and treatment and transport immediately.

▶PROBLEM SOLVING

▷ A common mistake made in the assessment of a minor trauma patient is failure to protect the cervical spine immediately upon making contact with the patient. Often, the EMT engages the patient in conversation about the incident and the patient's injuries, during which time the patient might be moving about and talking animatedly, before any manual spinal precautions are taken. All trauma patients should have the benefit of manual spinal immobilization immediately upon arrival of the EMTs. When it is later discovered that no possibility of neck or back injury exists, manual stabilization can be discontinued.

▷ Many EMTs fail to properly assess mechanism of injury for trauma incidents. When a patient appears injured, the EMT often goes directly to the patient, becomes involved in his care, and never goes back to evaluate the potential for injuries based on the **kinematics** of the incident. This is why it is important to assess the scene before engaging with the patient or, in the worst case scenario, to at least go back to assess the damage once the patient is packaged for transport and a partner has assumed care for the victim.

►CASE STUDY

You respond to the scene of a bicycle accident and find a 19-year-old male complaining of pain in his left elbow and side after falling from his bicycle. During your assessment of the scene, you note the patient to be standing directly in front of his bike with no obvious injuries and no significant damage to the bike. The patient states that he was riding along the road when a car came by and made him run off of the road. He said that as he swerved to avoid the curb, he fell off his bike into the tree.

The patient appears alert and is oriented to person, place, time, and events of the incident. The patient denies striking his head and says he has recollection of all events leading up to and including the incident. His airway is patent, his respirations are even and unlabored, and his vital signs are a blood pressure of 128/74, heart rate of 88, and the patient is breathing 24 times per minute. Your evaluation reveals the patient to have a bruise on the lateral aspect of his elbow and some point tenderness of the thoracic wall. Pulse, motor function, and sensation are intact in all four extremities and there is no variation between the extremities. No instability or crepitus is noted on the patient's chest and the patient denies difficulty in breathing, point tenderness along his spine, or abdominal pain.

The patient, after being evaluated by you determines that he does not want to be transported to the emergency department and refuses transport. He signs a refusal form and is left standing next to his bike. ■

1. Your patient tripped and fell while walking. She is complaining of right wrist pain after trying to stop the fall. What would be the best way to approach this patient?

   a. from the front, applying manual spinal immobilization until no longer needed

   b. from the front, talking to the patient to rule out the need for immobilization

   c. from the front, without manual spinal immobilization because of the MOI

   d. from the rear, applying manual spinal immobilization before the patient moves

2. The goal for treating the trauma patient with no significant mechanism of injury is to:

   a. determine any injuries and release the patient.

   b. treat the patient as needed and release the patient.

   c. do a thorough assessment and treat as needed.

   d. transport all patients for a more thorough evaluation.

3. Of the following, which would you do first in the assessment of the trauma patient with no significant mechanism of injury?

   a. Call for an additional unit to get a second opinion.

   b. Ensure that the patient is breathing adequately.

   c. Perform a focused trauma assessment to determine the extent of the injury.

   d. Assess for cervical spinal injury so you can release spinal immobilization.

CHAPTER 28

Assessment of the Trauma Patient with a Significant Mechanism of Injury

KEY TERMS

Altered mental status

Index of suspicion

Inspection

Mechanism of injury (MOI)

Palpation

OBJECTIVE

The student will successfully demonstrate assessment of the trauma patient who has been involved in an incident with a significant mechanism of injury.

INTRODUCTION

Assessment of the trauma patient is focused on cervical spinal protection, identification and treatment of life-threatening injuries, and rapid transport to an appropriate receiving facility. Patients with significant mechanism of injuries are likely to have life-threatening injuries. Life threats, or insults to the mental status, airway, breathing, or circulation must be treated as soon as they are found. In contrast, minor injuries such as abrasions should be noted, but should not be treated until additional help is available and the patient is en route to a trauma center. Although information related to the cause of the incident or **mechanism of injury (MOI)** and past medical history is helpful, this information may not be available if the patient is unconscious. Therefore, much of the trauma patient assessment will be gathered from physical cues surrounding the patient and scene.

▶EQUIPMENT

You will need the following equipment:

- ▶ Long spine board
- ▶ Cervical collar (set)
- ▶ Head blocks or towel rolls
- ▶ 2- or 3-inch tape
- ▶ Backboard straps
- ▶ Blood pressure cuff
- ▶ Stethoscope
- ▶ Penlight
- ▶ Scissors
- ▶ Bandaging supplies (i.e., occlusive dressing)
- ▶ Portable suction unit and rigid Yankauer tip
- ▶ OPAs and/or NPAs
- ▶ Oxygen and appropriate tubing
- ▶ BVM, reservoir, and tubing
- ▶ Nonrebreather mask

ASSESSMENT

The trauma patient assessment begins with an assessment of the scene itself. Contact with the patient should not be made until scene hazards have been identified and rectified, the number of patients determined, and additional help summoned as needed. Once you make contact with the patient, it will be difficult to disengage to determine the scene size-up. The consequences could be dangerous to you, your crew, and your patients.

This assessment is based on a trauma patient with a significant mechanism of injury. Significant mechanisms of injury include ejection from a vehicle; death in the same passenger compartment; falls of more than 15 feet or three times the patient's height; rollover of a vehicle; high-speed vehicle collision; vehicle-pedestrian collision; motorcycle crash; unresponsiveness or **altered mental status;** and penetrations of the head, chest, or abdomen, for example, stab and gunshot wounds. Additional significant mechanisms of injury for children include falls from more than 10 feet, bicycle crashes, and medium-speed vehicle collisions.

When assessing a patient who has experienced any of the above MOIs, know that his mechanism of injury is significant, and his potential for injury great. Therefore, the focus will be on rapid assessment and preparation for transport. A detailed assessment will be performed en route to the hospital if time permits.

PROCEDURE: Assessment of the Trauma Patient with a Significant Mechanism of Injury

1. Apply BSI precautions.

   Rationale: Gloves and eye protection are required at a minimum, and a gown may be needed if large amounts of blood or fluid are present to minimize exposure to infectious diseases.

2. Perform a scene size-up as you approach or come on scene. Determine that the scene is safe and free of hazards (Figure 28.1). Use clues found on scene to determine the mechanism of injury such as a fall or vehicle collision. Identify the number of patients and whether additional resources are needed, such as highway patrol officers for traffic control. If additional resources are needed, request those now.

   Rationale: Once you make contact with the patient, it will be difficult to disengage to determine the scene size-up, and necessary resources could then be delayed.

3. Approach the patient from his front side, introduce yourself, and instruct the patient not to move. Even if the patient appears unconscious, he or she may still be able to hear you.

   Rationale: You should assume that all trauma patients have the potential for a spinal injury. Approaching from the front minimizes the possibility that the patient will turn his head to view you, possibly exacerbating a spinal injury.

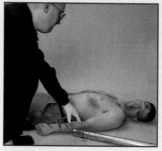

Figure 28.1

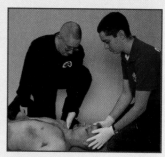

Figure 28.2

5. Verbalize your general impression of the patient regarding his level of distress and other obvious findings such as positioning and surroundings.

   Rationale: Verbalizing your general impression helps your team members respond with the same level of intensity as you.

6. Determine level of consciousness of the patient using the AVPU method. This initial assessment is used to determine whether the patient is ALERT, responsive to VERBAL stimuli, responsive to PAINFUL stimuli, or UNRESPONSIVE.

   Rationale: A baseline assessment of mental status is needed to determine if the patient is capable of answering other questions. Altered mental status is an indication for priority transport.

 PEDIATRIC NOTE:

A child is likely to be frightened by his injuries. If a family member is on scene, allow him or her to remain near the child for comfort, as long as the family member is not interfering with your ability to care for the child.

 GERIATRIC NOTE:

Although some elderly patients do suffer from dementia, most do not. When an altered mental status is illicited from a trauma patient, it should be assumed that this is *NOT* normal for the patient and, instead, a sign of serious injury suffered from the traumatic incident.

4. Direct manual stabilization of the cervical spine (Figure 28.2).

   Rationale: You should always assume that trauma patients with a significant mechanism of injury have potential spinal injuries. Nearly all major trauma patients should be placed on a long spine board.

7. Ensure airway patency. If the airway is not open, open it using the jaw-thrust maneuver (Figure 28.3).

8. Determine the chief complaint or apparent life threats. Because the patient may not be able to communicate, visualize the mechanism of injury

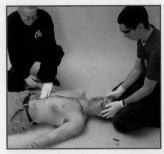

Figure 28.3

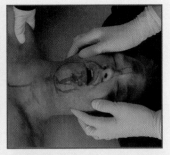

Figure 28.4

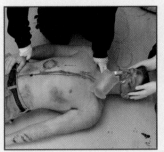

Figure 28.7

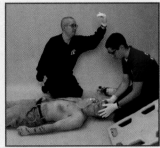

Figure 28.8

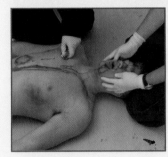

Figure 28.5

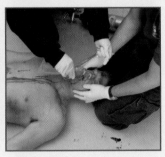

Figure 28.6

and use your **index of suspicion** to estimate the probable injuries suffered (Figure 28.4).

Rationale: The chief complaint or presenting problem will guide both the order and urgency of the assessment.

9. Insert an airway adjunct or suction to maintain patency if needed.

Rationale: The assessment process should not be continued if the airway is not controlled.

10. Assess the rate and quality of breathing. Assess for adequate tidal volume by observing chest rise and fall. Ensure lung sounds are present and equal. Apply high-flow oxygen (Figures 28.5 and 28.6).

11. Repositioning the patient may assist with keeping the airway open and improving breathing.

Rationale: Breathing must be adequate before any other assessment is completed.

12. Check central and peripheral pulses for rate, strength, and regularity. Assess skin color, temperature, and condition. Control external bleeding with direct pressure. Initiate shock management if indicated with Trendelenburg positioning or application of a pneumatic anti-shock garment (PASG). Major bleeding can be found by **inspection** after the patient has been

exposed or by **palpation** and inspection for blood on the gloves of the rescuer (Figure 28.7).

Rationale: Bleeding is considered a life threat and needs to be controlled before any further assessment is completed.

> **PEDIATRIC NOTE:**
>
> Children may be very sensitive or embarrassed to be exposed. Capillary refill is a relatively reliable indicator of perfusion status for children. Determine capillary refill in the distal extremities to assess circulation.

13. Determine priority of the patient and make a transport decision (Figure 28.8).

Rationale: Patients with threats to airway, breathing, or circulation should be prepared for transport immediately.

The above steps, from determination of responsiveness to transport decision, make up the initial assessment and resuscitation.

14. Reconsider the mechanism of injury.

Rationale: Often, additional information will become available while you are on scene that may enhance or even change your first impression of the mechanism and therefore what potential injuries the patient has suffered as a result of the mechanism. For example, it may first appear that the patient has fallen from a ladder. However, a bystander could come forward informing you that the patient actually fell from the second story roof, and just knocked the ladder down during the fall. This new information could significantly change your interpretation of the potential injuries suffered by the patient.

continued...

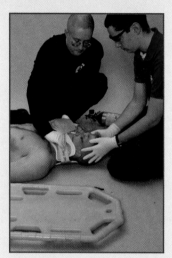

Figure 28.9

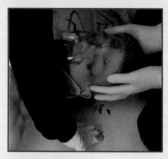

Figure 28.10

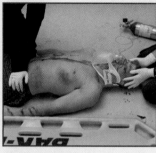

Figure 28.11

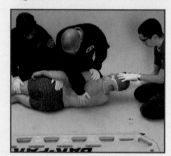

Figure 28.12

15. Continue spinal stabilization. If you wish, you may apply a cervical collar now after assessing the bones and soft tissue that will be covered by the collar (Figure 28.9).

Rationale: Because spinal immobilization is likely to be indicated, application of a cervical collar will help keep the patient from moving.

 GERIATRIC NOTE:

Many geriatric patients suffer from some anatomical changes in their spines. If the patient's normal anatomy does not allow application of a cervical collar to maintain neutral alignment, then manual stabilization should be continued until other equipment can be improvised such as towel rolls or blankets.

16. Consider a request for advanced life support (ALS).

Rationale: Should ALS not already be on scene, they should be notified to start coming to the scene at this time to prevent delays in patient care or transport.

17. Reconsider your transport decision.

Rationale: Changes in the patient presentation or information gathered could increase your index of suspicion for serious injury. You may decide to transport the patient without further delay, or to change your receiving facility destination to one that is more appropriate for a trauma patient, such as a trauma center.

18. Reassess mental status using the AVPU method (see step 6).

Rationale: A patient with deteriorating mental status is a high-priority patient who should be transported without delay to the proper receiving facility, such as a trauma center.

19. Conduct a rapid trauma assessment by inspecting and palpating for any abnormalities such as bleeding, bruising, swelling, deformities, or pain in all major body areas including the head, neck, chest, abdomen, pelvis, extremities, and posterior (Figures 28.10, 28.11, and 28.12).

Rationale: A quick check of all major body areas should reveal any injuries that are a threat to life or limb and require either immediate treatment or transport. A rapid trauma assessment is usually only conducted on major trauma patients after the initial assessment.

20. Provide any lifesaving treatment needed for major injuries found during the rapid trauma assessment, such as hemorrhage control or application of an occlusive dressing to a sucking chest wound.

Rationale: Life threats should be treated as soon as they are identified.

21. Obtain baseline vital signs, including respirations, pulse, skin signs, pupils, and blood pressure. This task may be delegated to a partner (Figure 28.13).

Rationale: Vital signs will help complete the assessment picture for the EMT and help to estimate the internal damage done by the traumatic incident that may not be visible on the outside of the body.

22. Obtain a past medical (SAMPLE) history including Signs and symptoms, Allergies, Medications, Pertinent past medical history, Last oral intake, and Events leading up to the incident. The history should be obtained from the patient if conscious, but a family member, bystander, or witness may also be questioned if necessary.

Rationale: While the history is not as important to the trauma patient as it is to the treatment of a medical patient, the information may help complete the picture for the patient's presentation. For example, if it is discovered that the patient is diabetic, the unconsciousness you see may be a result of the trauma, or hypoglycemia, and would warrant a blood glucose check that may otherwise not be indicated for another trauma patient.

23. Begin transport of the patient now if transport was not initiated earlier.

Rationale: Transport should have been initiated at whatever point in the assessment life-threatening injuries were identified and treated. There is no such thing as field stabilization of the major trauma patient, and no time should be wasted on scene. Transport should begin as soon as the life threats have been managed and the patient packaged for transport.

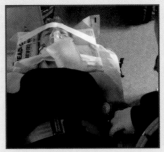
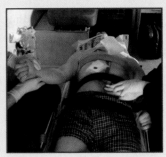

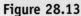

Figure 28.13   **Figure 28.14**

24. Conduct a detailed physical exam if time permits. Use your penlight to check pupillary response; the ears and nose for blood or drainage; the mouth for loose teeth or other debris; the neck veins for jugular venous distension; the chest, abdomen, and pelvis for development of any other bruising, bleeding, swelling, deformities, crepitus, or pain; and the extremities for injuries as well as pulses, motor function, and sensation (Figure 28.14).

Rationale: The detailed physical exam is used to help the EMT check every body area carefully to discover any other injuries that were either missed earlier or have developed since the rapid trauma assessment was completed. For example, bruising does not occur instantly. The abdomen may have initially looked normal, but now exhibits a bruise consistent with improper seat belt use. This bruise should then increase your index of suspicion for internal abdominal bleeding from compression of abdominal organs caused by the improperly applied seat belt.

25. Document findings.

Rationale: It is extremely important to document your findings in order to have a history of facts and events that occurred at the scene.

Assessment should be repeated every 5 minutes for critical patients and every 15 minutes for stable patients. Every patient should have at least two sets of vital signs assessed before arrival at the hospital. Should the condition of the patient worsen at any time, immediately return to the initial assessment and reassess airway, breathing, and circulation. It may be necessary to stop further assessment and treatment and transport the patient immediately.

The ongoing assessment also allows you to check interventions. Ensure that the oxygen flow is still adequate for the patient, that bandages have continued to control bleeding, and that splints have not become too tight as swelling has continued. If any interventions need adjustment, do so now.

▶PROBLEM SOLVING

▶ Many EMTs fail to properly manage cervical stabilization of the trauma patient. Manual stabilization should be applied immediately upon contact with the patient.

▶ Some EMTs will discount a significant mechanism of injury because the patient is alert and talking upon arrival of EMS. The mechanism of injury is supposed to trigger an index of suspicion about the potential severity of injuries suffered by the patient. The EMT, not the patient, should determine the urgency of the response and likelihood of serious injuries that need to be evaluated and treated.

▶CASE STUDY

You are responding to the scene where a 39-year-old male pedestrian was struck by a car. A bystander advises you that the patient was standing on the sidewalk when a car appeared to go out of control and struck him. The speed of impact was estimated to be between 40 and 50 miles per hour.

On your arrival, the patient is lying supine and motionless. The patient has an obvious tibia/fibula fracture on his left leg and a humerus fracture on the left arm. The patient is unresponsive and has been from the time of impact according to the bystander. His airway is patent; his respirations are shallow and appear to be labored. The patient is immobilized to a backboard with a C-collar and cervical immobilizer device (CIDs) in place, transferred rapidly to the ambulance, and then transported to the emergency department. While en route to the hospital, the patient's vital signs were obtained: blood pressure of 138/72, respirations of 20, and a heart rate of 100. In addition to the previously identified fractures, your evaluation reveals the patient to have crepitus and deformity of the left side of his chest. The patient is ventilated with the bag-valve-mask unit and the chest fractures are stabilized with 2-inch tape.

As you approach the trauma center, a report is called in, no orders are received, and upon arrival, care is turned over to the emergency staff. ■

1. Which of the following mechanisms of injury alone does *Not* qualify a patient for immediate transport?

   a. automobile versus pedestrian accident

   b. fall from 13 feet

   c. ejection from the vehicle

   d. death of the driver

2. You find a man lying on the ground beside a ladder that extends to the roof of the second floor. Your patient is moving all extremities well and is trying to sit up. What should be your initial action?

   a. Move the ladder so that it is no longer a threat to your safety.

   b. Approach the patient from the rear so that you do not startle him.

   c. Approach from the front and apply manual in-line stabilization.

   d. Approach from the side and help the patient to his feet so you can talk.

3. Life threats found during the initial assessment should be treated:

   a. when the patient is en route to the hospital to expedite transport.

   b. after completing the initial and rapid trauma assessment to find them all.

   c. as soon as they are found and prior to completing any other assessment.

   d. after completing each assessment, based on the severity of the life threat.

SECTION 2
PATIENT ASSESSMENT

1. Components of the initial assessment include:
   A. assess mental status, airway, breathing, and circulation.
   B. form a general impression.
   C. determine priority for transport.
   D. all of the above

2. A helpful mnemonic while assessing the trauma patient is DCAP-BTLS. In this mnemonic, the "L" represents:
   A. lumps.
   B. lacerations.
   C. large open wounds.
   D. lacrimation.

3. Which of the following is NOT a high priority transport situation?
   A. unresponsiveness
   B. uncontrolled bleeding or severe pain
   C. compound ankle fracture
   D. chest pain, diastolic blood pressure less than 100

4. A focused physical exam differs from a rapid trauma assessment in that the rapid trauma assessment:
   A. is performed more quickly, and in a more focused area than the focused physical exam.
   B. does not include eyes, ears, nose, and mouth, where the focused physical exam always does.
   C. is a complete, head-to-toe rapid exam.
   D. is performed while en route to the hospital.

5. BSI personal protective equipment can include:
   A. masks and gowns.
   B. eye protection.
   C. disposable gloves.
   D. all of the above

6. Assessment of perfusion in the pediatric patient may include assessment of:
   A. distal pulses.
   B. capillary refill.
   C. skin color.
   D. all of the above

7. The "A" in the mnemonic "AVPU" stands for:
   A. Aware.
   B. Alert.
   C. Altered.
   D. none of the above

8. In assessing the pelvis of a trauma patient, you should:
    A. avoid any type of pressure.
    B. rock the pelvis to assess stability.
    C. apply gentle lateral-to-medial and anterior-to-posterior pressure.
    D. none of the above

9. You suspect your patient has a spinal injury. Manual stabilization should occur:
    A. after completing the initial assessment.
    B. upon first contact.
    C. after competing the focused history and physical exam.
    D. at any time you have additional personnel.

10. The first set of vital signs are called?
    A. starting vital signs
    B. baseline vital signs
    C. serial vital signs
    D. parallel vital signs

11. All of the following are principles of proper body mechanics EXCEPT:
    A. position feet on a firm surface, shoulder width apart.
    B. keep the patient's weight away from your body.
    C. keep your back straight.
    D. use legs, not back to lift.

12. Components of the ongoing assessment include:
    A. repeat vital signs.
    B. recheck interventions.
    C. repeat initial assessment.
    D. all of the above

13. Once you complete the focused physical exam to assess injuries, you will:
    A. immediately transport the patient.
    B. splint all injuries.
    C. begin a detailed physical exam.
    D. assess baseline vitals.

14. Vital signs should be reassessed:
    A. every minute in an unstable patient and every 5 minutes in a stable patient.
    B. every 5 minutes in an unstable patient and every 10 minutes in a stable patient.
    C. every 5 minutes in an unstable patient and every 15 minutes in a stable patient.
    D. every 10 minutes in an unstable patient and every 20 minutes in a stable patient.

15. While assessing the neck of a trauma patient, you should check for:
    A. deformity.
    B. jugular vein distension.
    C. crepitation.
    D. all of the above

16. Which of the following is NOT a significant mechanism of injury for an adult?
    A. death in the same passenger compartment
    B. falls of under 15 feet or 3 times the patient's height
    C. unresponsiveness or altered mental status
    D. penetrations of the head, chest, or abdomen

17. The patient you are transporting has been diagnosed with tuberculosis. You should use a:
    A. surgical mask.
    B. HEPA or N–95 mask.
    C. SCBA.
    D. none of the above

18. Assessment of the trauma patient's chest should include all of the following EXCEPT:
    A. crepitation.
    B. paradoxical motion.
    C. distal pulse, motor, and sensory.
    D. breath sounds.

19. Medical patient assessment differs from trauma patient assessment in that:
    A. the medical patient relies heavily on history whereas the trauma patient relies heavily on physical exam.
    B. the trauma patient relies heavily on history whereas the medical patient relies heavily on physical exam.
    C. both the medical and trauma patients rely heavily on history.
    D. both the medical and trauma patients rely heavily on physical exam.

20. The initial assessment is designed to:
    A. identify non-life-threatening problems and treat immediately.
    B. identify non-life-threatening problems and treat after completed assessment.
    C. identify life-threatening problems and treat immediately.
    D. identify life-threatening problems and treat after completed assessment.

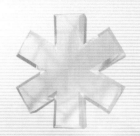

SECTION 3
MEDICAL EMERGENCIES

Many of the skills in this section cover administration of medications. As an EMT you will be responsible for the patient's self-administration of some medications, and in other cases you may be administering certain medications.

Medications are given to induce specific physiologic effects on the body. They also can alleviate many patient's symptoms and complaints, but medications can also cause harm if used inappropriately.

In all cases of medical emergency, it is essential that the EMT perform a detailed history and physical examination. In most EMS systems, detailed medical control policies and procedures must be followed to ensure that the patient is not placed in any danger.

CHAPTER 29
Administration of Activated Charcoal

KEY TERMS

Absorption

Activated charcoal

Alkali

Antidote

Aspirate

Constipation

Cyanide

Organic solvents

OBJECTIVE

The student will successfully administer activated charcoal to patients for whom it is indicated.

INTRODUCTION

Activated charcoal is one of the medications carried by EMT-Basics aboard an ambulance. It comes as a powder made from charred wood and is premixed with water for use in the field.

Activated charcoal is used primarily to treat patients who have swallowed a poison or who have taken an overdose orally. The medication should be administered according to medical direction and/or local policies or protocols.

Activated charcoal is not an **antidote**—a substance that neutralizes a poison or its effects. Instead, it works through **absorption,** the process in which one substance becomes attached to the surface of another. Activated charcoal has been manufactured to have many cracks and crevices, thereby increasing the surface area to which poisons might bind.

In many cases, absorption of poisons by activated charcoal reduces the amount of poison available for the body to absorb. However, activated charcoal will not absorb all poisons. It is difficult, if not impossible, to memorize a list of these poisons. Instead, you should consult with medical control on whether activated charcoal will be effective against a particular poison. Often medical control will contact a poison control center or refer to a computerized poison control index.

Keep in mind several groups of patients in which activated charcoal is generally contraindicated:

▶ Patients who cannot swallow obviously cannot take activated charcoal.

▶ Patients with an altered mental status might choke when swallowing the slurry and **aspirate** the substance into their lungs.

▶ Patients who have ingested acids or **alkalis** should not swallow activated charcoal. The caustic materials may have damaged the mouth, throat, and esophagus. Swallowing the slurry might cause further injury.

- Patients who have been poisoned by **cyanide, organic solvents,** iron, ethanol, and methanol should not be given activated charcoal because, again, swallowing the slurry might cause further injury.

The most common side effects from activated charcoal include:

- vomiting and/or nausea
- abdominal cramping
- **constipation**
- black stools

►EQUIPMENT

You will need the following equipment:

- BSI equipment
- Activated charcoal
- Covered container with lid
- Straw
- Suction unit

ASSESSMENT

Find out the name or type of toxic substance ingested and identify any possible contraindications for use of activated charcoal. Also determine when the substance was taken. Activated charcoal is most effective if given within 29 minutes of the poisoning or overdose. Communicate this information to medical control for approval to administer the slurry.

PROCEDURE: Administration of Activated Charcoal

1. Consult with medical control about the use of activated charcoal.

   Rationale: In many EMS systems activated charcoal may only be given under the direction of a base station hospital. If you have the authority to give activated charcoal under standing protocols, then do so. If you are unsure if the patient meets the protocol, consult medical control.

2. Apply BSI precautions.

   Rationale: Gloves and eye protection are required at a minimum, and a gown may be needed if large amounts of blood or fluid are present to prevent exposure to infectious diseases.

3. Keep in mind the six "rights" of patients when administering medications. Ensure that you have the:

   - right patient
   - right drug
   - right amount/dose
   - right route of administration
   - right time
   - right documentation

   Rationale: Following the six rights ensures that proper safety procedures are used for the administration of any medication.

4. Determine the correct dosage, which is usually *1 gram* of activated charcoal per kilogram of

   continued...

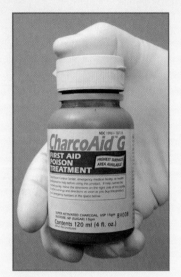

Figure 29.1

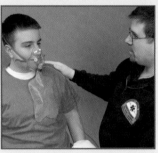

Figure 29.2

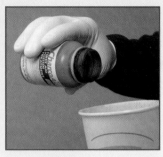

Figure 29.3

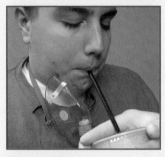

Figure 29.4

body weight. In general, the usual adult dose is 25–100 *grams*. (Figure 29.1).

 PEDIATRIC NOTE:
The usual pediatric dose is 12–25 *grams*.

Rationale: Drug dosage is based on kilograms. Remember that 1 kg is equal to 2.2 pounds. The drug dosage is 1 gram per kilogram.

5. Explain the procedure to the patient (Figure 29.2).

Rationale: For this procedure to work properly, it requires the assistance of the patient. Without the assistance of the patient, the procedure is less effective, which may affect the absorption of the medication. The patient is likely to be more cooperative if he understands the procedure. Explain the procedure in a way that the patient can understand what is required of him.

6. Shake the container thoroughly.

7. Place the mixture into a covered, non-see-through container with a straw (Figure 29.3).

Rationale: Activated charcoal is very dark black. It does not look good to drink. Placing the activated charcoal in a covered, non-see-through container keeps the patient from seeing what he is drinking. The straw also allows him to have minimal visual contact with the slurry. In some

cases, you do not have to put the charcoal into a different container.

8. Explain the procedure. Tell the patient that slurry is gritty and does not taste good, but will help him or her recover from the poisoning.

Rationale: Explaining to the patient that the mixture is gritty and does not taste good will prepare the patient for the experience. Not explaining the process can cause patients to refuse to drink the charcoal.

9. Ask patient to take the medication. The slurry may have to be shaken or stirred if it has settled (Figure 29.4).

Rationale: When the charcoal sits and has not been stirred, it has a tendency to reseparate and needs to be mixed occasionally so that its consistency is loose enough to be sucked through a straw.

10. If the patient vomits or spits up the medication, consider a second dose. Be sure to consult with medical direction before administering activated charcoal a second time. Keep suction available at all times to reduce the risks of aspiration.

Rationale: Obviously if the medication has not made it to the stomach or has not been there for a period of time, it has not had the ability to absorb the poison like it's supposed to. A second attempt might be necessary. This should only be done under medical direction.

11. Document this procedure. Be sure to include the time the drug was administered, the dosage, the patient's reaction to the drug, and serial vital signs.

Rationale: It is extremely important to document your findings in order to have a history of facts and events at the scene.

ONGOING ASSESSMENT

Constantly monitor the patient's mental status for changes due to absorption of toxic substances. Be prepared to manage the airway if the patient begins to vomit. Reassess vital signs every 5 minutes for critical patients and every 15 minutes for stable patients. If the patient vomits, save the vomitus for analysis in the emergency department.

▶PROBLEM SOLVING

▶ Once you have given the patient the activated charcoal it is *NOT* advisable to let the patient have milk, ice cream, or sherbet. These can reduce the effectiveness of the charcoal.

▶ Never force a patient to swallow activated charcoal.

▶ Notify medical control and provide ongoing assessment and care.

▶ The administration of charcoal can make the patient vomit. Have suction ready if the patient vomits to reduce the chances of aspiration. Also consider the patient's position; if he must lay down, keep him on his side.

▶ A patient may refuse to take it based on the slurry's muddy appearance.

▶CASE STUDY

You are responding to the home of a 34-year-old female who has reportedly taken 50 Tylenol tablets in a suicide attempt. On arrival at the patient's house, you find the patient to be awake, alert, and crying. As you begin assessing the patient, she tells you that she wanted to kill herself when she took the pills, but now realizes that she does not want to die. The patient states that she took the pills approximately 15 minutes ago. You complete the initial assessment, detailed assessment, and obtain the SAMPLE history while your partner obtains the patient's vital signs. He advises you that the patient has a blood pressure of 108/74, a heart rate of 106, and a respiratory rate of 22. You retrieve the bottle of medication from the bathroom sink, and confirm with the patient that it is the correct bottle and that she did not take anything else. You contact medical control concerning the administration of activated charcoal. They advise you to administer it as soon as possible.

Because the patient not experiencing any other complaints, you and your partner elect to carry the patient downstairs in the stair chair. After securing the patient to the cot and starting transport to the emergency department, you administer the activated charcoal. You shake it well to mix it, and then have the patient drink it through a straw. She is able to keep it down without getting nauseated. You contact medical control again with an update on the patient's status as well as serial vital signs. The hospital advises you to continue transport with no further orders. The patient is transported without any changes, and care is transferred to the emergency staff. ■

(continued)

1. Activated charcoal should be administered only after:
   a. contacting poison control.
   b. determining the ingested substance.
   c. contacting medical control.
   d. inducing vomiting with ipecac.

2. Activated charcoal is contraindicated for all of the following *except*:
   a. a patient who overdosed on Tylenol 30 minutes ago.
   b. a patient with an altered mental status from the overdose.
   c. a patient who has ingested bleach and other cleaning solutions.
   d. a patient who ingested alcohol with an overdose of multiple medications.

3. Prior to administering activated charcoal, the most important question to ask is which of the following?
   a. Is this the right dose for the patient?
   b. Does the patient have any allergies?
   c. Is this the right route for administration?
   d. Is this the right time to administer it?

CHAPTER 30
Administration of Glucose

KEY TERMS
Diabetes

Glucose monitoring

Hypoglycemia

Oral glucose

OBJECTIVE
The student will successfully administer glucose to a patient for whom it is indicated.

INTRODUCTION

Oral glucose is a form of glucose. Oral glucose is indicated for patients with a history of **diabetes** with an altered mental status, but who still have the ability to swallow on their own. Glucose can reverse a diabetic patient's potentially life-threatening **hypoglycemia** or low blood sugar condition. Oral glucose should be administered quickly, without compromising the patient's airway. Time to administration can sometimes make a critical difference in the outcome for the patient with diabetes.

Oral glucose usually comes in a tube and can be administered with the assistance of a tongue depressor. The tip of the tongue depressor is placed between the patient's cheek and gum or under the patient's tongue. The typical dose is one tube. Oral glucose has no major side effects when administered properly.

►EQUIPMENT

You will need the following equipment:

- ► BSI equipment
- ► Oral glucose tube (e.g., Glutose)
- ► Tongue depressor
- ► Suction available

ASSESSMENT

Determine the patient's mental status. Oral glucose should not be administered to a patient who is unresponsive or unable to swallow. Perform an initial and focused history and physical exam. Determine if the patient has a history of diabetes. If the patient does have such a history, determine the following:

- ► Determine if the patient takes insulin and/or oral hypoglycemic medications, and inquire about when the medication was last taken.
- ► Determine the last time the patient ate and inquire what he ate.
- ► Inquire whether the patient has recently overexerted himself.
- ► Inquire whether the patient vomited recently. If so, ask if it was after the last meal.
- ► Inquire if the altered mental status was rapid or slow in onset.
- ► Determine if the patient is alert enough to swallow and if the gag reflex is present.

PROCEDURE: Administration of Glucose

1. Consult with medical control about the use of oral glucose (Figure 30.1).

   Rationale: In many EMS systems, oral glucose may only be given under the direction of a base station hospital. If you have the authority to give glucose understanding protocols, then do so. If you are unsure if the patient meets the protocol, consult medical control.

2. Apply BSI precautions.

   Rationale: Gloves and eye protection are required at a minimum, and a gown may be needed if large amounts of blood or fluid are present to prevent exposure to infectious diseases.

3. Keep in mind the six "rights" of patients when administering medications. Ensure that you have the:
   - ► **right patient**
   - ► **right drug**
   - ► **right amount/dose**

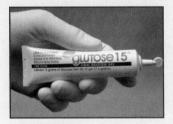

Figure 30.1

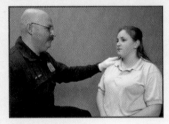

Figure 30.2

   - ► **right route of administration**
   - ► **right time**
   - ► **right documentation**

   Rationale: Following the six rights ensures that proper safety procedures are used for the administration of any medication.

4. Explain the procedure to the patient (Figure 30.2).

   Rationale: For this procedure to work properly, it requires the assistance of the patient. Without the assistance of the patient, the procedure is less effective, which may affect the absorption of the medication. The patient is likely to be more cooperative if she understands the procedure. Explain the procedure in a way that the patient can understand what is required of her.

5. Open the tube, making sure to keep it clean.

    Rationale: Keeping the tube clean reduces the risk of contamination to the patient.

6. Apply glucose to the tongue depressor by squeezing the tube (Figure 30.3).

    Rationale: Squeezing the glucose onto the tongue depressor allows you to control the amount of glucose to be administrated to the patient.

7. If the patient is wearing an oxygen mask, remove it. Explain to the patient that the oxygen will be replaced as soon as the procedure is done.

    Rationale: Access to the mouth is necessary to administer oral glucose.

8. Insert tongue depressor with glucose into the patient's mouth. Apply it between the cheek and

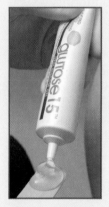

Figure 30.3

the gum (Figure 30.4). In some cases, the patient can self-administer the glucose by directly squeezing the glucose under their tongue. Ask the patient not to swallow the paste.

Rationale: You will find that using the tongue depressor is an easy way to administer and control the administration of oral glucose. Swallowing the paste will not allow absorption of the medication in a timely fashion.

9. Remove tongue depressor.

10. Confirm that the patient can swallow.

11. Reapply glucose to tongue depressor and continue the administration until all glucose from the tube has been used (Figure 30.5).

    Rationale: There is no specific dose for oral glucose; the entire tube should be used.

12. Immediately discontinue administration if the patient loses the ability to swallow or becomes unresponsive.

13. Readminister oxygen to the patient.

14. Consult with medical control as soon as possible.

15. Document this procedure.

    Rationale: It is extremely important to document your findings in order to have a history of facts and events that occurred at the scene.

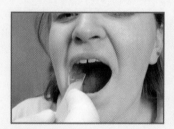

Figure 30.4

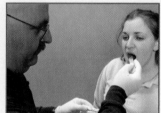

Figure 30.5

ONGOING ASSESSMENT

Constantly monitor for mental status changes. Monitor the patient's airway. Reassess vital signs every 5 minutes for an unstable patient and every 15 minutes for a stable patient. It can take up to 20 minutes before you start seeing any improvement in level of consciousness.

▶PROBLEM SOLVING

▷ In some cases, the patient may have a glucose monitor that someone can give you when you arrive so that you can take readings. In some EMS systems, EMT-Basics have the ability to do **glucose monitoring.** A value of less than 80 in a patient with an altered mental status is considered symptomatic and indicates the prompt administration of glucose. A glucose monitor should *NOT* be used unless approved by your EMS system.

▶ In most cases the administration of oral glucose should be limited to the patient who has a history of diabetes. Follow your local medical control policies and procedures for other possibilities of administration.

▶ If the patient does not have the ability to swallow, do *NOT* attempt to administer oral glucose. Any attempt could compromise the airway or cause the patient to aspirate.

▶ If advanced life support personnel are available, call them for possible IV dextrose administration.

▶CASE STUDY

You respond to the house of a 19-year-old male who states he is not feeling well. On your arrival, the patient states that he has not been feeling well for the last few days and today he has been unable to walk right and has felt dizzy. The patient's mother advises you that he is a diabetic and has been experiencing flu-like symptoms for the past week. He is currently taking Glucophage to control his diabetes, and he does not have any allergies.

Your assessment reveals a patient with no obvious injuries, a blood pressure of 128/64 and a heart rate of 88, who is breathing 12 times per minute. According to the patient's mother, he has not been acting appropriately and has been more and more confused during the last two days. You are allowed to do glucose monitoring, so you do a finger stick and note the patient's blood sugar level to be 54 mg/dL.

You administer oral glucose to the patient with a tongue depressor on the inside of his mouth. Because the oral glucose will take a few minutes to work, you and your partner load the patient onto the cot and begin transport to the local emergency department (ED). While en route, you repeat the vital signs and complete an ongoing assessment. The patient states he is feeling less dizzy and that he feels revitalized. The ED is notified and does not reply with any new instruction. You complete the transport without any other changes in the patient's condition. On arrival at the ED, care is turned over to the emergency staff.■

1. Oral glucose can be administered to which of the following patients?

   a. a 28-year-old with a history of diabetes who is unresponsive

   b. a 70-year-old confused diabetic with a blood glucose level of 165 mg/dL

   c. a 65-year-old nondiabetic with weakness and slurred speech

   d. a 54-year-old responsive diabetic who is not acting appropriately

2. Oral glucose should be applied under the tongue or between the cheek and gums:

   a. it prevents triggering the gag reflex.

   b. it allows for rapid absorption of the sugar.

   c. so it will not be aspirated by unresponsive patients.

   d. so patients do not have to swallow it without a drink.

3. Prior to administering oral glucose, you need to confirm all of the following except:

   a. that the patient is not allergic to any medications.

   b. that the patient has a history of diabetes.

   c. that the patient has a blood glucose level of < 80 mg/dL.

   d. that the patient does not have any difficulty swallowing.

CHAPTER 31
Administration of Metered-Dose Inhaler

KEY TERMS

Bronchioles

Bronchodilators

Chronic pulmonary disease

Metered-dose inhaler

(MDI)

OBJECTIVE

The student will successfully administer a metered-dose inhaler to a patient for whom it is indicated.

INTRODUCTION

A **metered-dose inhaler (MDI)** administers a prescribed dose of medication every time the inhaler is activated, usually to a patient with a history of **chronic pulmonary disease.** The most common medications administered by this route are **bronchodilators,** which are drugs that dilate, or enlarge, the smaller air passages, making breathing easier.

Most bronchodilators begin to work immediately and their effect can last for hours. The most common bronchodilators include albuterol (Proventil, Ventolin), metaproterenol (Metaprel, Alupent), and isoetharine (Bronchosol, Bronkometer). The device through which these drugs are administered consists of a metal canister and a plastic container with an attached mouthpiece. The metal container holds the medication and fits inside the plastic container. When depressed, the device delivers a metered, or exactly measured, dose of medication.

The patient must coordinate his or her inhalation with activation of the device so that the drug will deposit itself on the **bronchioles.** Because the coordination can be difficult at times, some metered-dose inhalers come with a chamber, or "spacer," that attaches to the plastic container. The chamber holds the medication until the patient inhales it.

Remember that patients will become agitated when they are short of breath. They also may not know how to use their inhaler properly. Although it is best for the patient to self-administer the medication, you may be requested to coach or assist. In such cases, medical control will authorize you to assist them. In some systems, EMT-Basics may actually carry MDIs on the ambulance and may have standing orders and/or protocols spelling out when and how MDIs may be used in the field.

The dose of the MDI is set. Each time the MDI is depressed, it delivers a precise dose of the medication. Regardless of the situation, consult with local protocols or medical control on the appropriate dose as well as guidelines on multiple usage. Finally, know (or find out about) the drug's indications, contraindications, and possible adverse side effects.

▶ EQUIPMENT

You will need the following equipment:

▶ BSI equipment

▶ Metered-dose inhaler

▶ Spacer

ASSESSMENT

Check the expiration date on the metered-dose inhaler and make sure that the device works. For the medication to be properly dosed, the inhaler should be at room temperature or warmer. Find out if the patient used the inhaler prior to your arrival. If so, ask how many times and over what time period.

In general, use of a metered-dose inhaler is indicated when:

▶ a patient exhibits shortness of breath and/or signs and symptoms of difficulty in breathing.

▶ the MDI has been prescribed to the patient by a physician.

▶ local protocols or medical control has approved the use of the device.

Use of a metered-dose inhaler is contraindicated when:

▶ the patient is unable to use the device, for example, when he or she is unresponsive.

▶ the patient has already taken the maximum number of doses prior to the arrival of EMT-Basics.

▶ permission has not been given by local protocols or medical control.

PROCEDURE: Administration of Metered-Dose Inhaler

1. Consult with medical control about the use of a metered-dose inhaler (Figure 31.1).

   Rationale: In many EMS systems a metered-dose inhaler may only be given under the direction of a base station hospital. If you have the authority to use an MDI under standing protocols, then do so. If you are unsure if the patient meets the protocol, consult medical control.

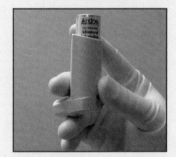

Figure 31.1

2. Apply BSI precautions.

   Rationale: Gloves and eye protection are required at a minimum, and a gown may be needed if large amounts of blood or fluid are present to prevent exposure to infectious diseases.

3. Keep in mind the six "rights" of patients when administering medications. Ensure that you have the:

   ▶ right patient
   ▶ right drug
   ▶ right amount/dose
   ▶ right route of administration
   ▶ right time
   ▶ right documentation

   Rationale: Following the six rights ensures that proper safety procedures are used for the administration of any medication.

continued...

4. Explain the procedure to the patient (Figure 31.2).

   Rationale: For this procedure to work properly, it requires the assistance of the patient. Without the assistance of the patient, the procedure is less effective, which may affect the absorption of the medication. The patient is likely to be more cooperative if he understands the procedure. Explain the procedure in a way that the patient can understand what is required of him.

5. Shake the MDI canister vigorously for at least 30 seconds.

   Rationale: The shaking of the canister mixes the medication and the propellant to a specific metered dose. If you do not shake it, the wrong dose might be administered.

6. If the patient is wearing an oxygen mask, remove it. Explain to the patient that the oxygen will be replaced as soon as the procedure is done.

   Rationale: Access to the mouth is necessary to administer an MDI dose.

7. Instruct the patient to hold the inhaler upright in his hand. If the patient cannot do so, then you should hold the inhaler. Place your thumb on the bottom of the canister and your index finger on the top (Figure 31.3).

   Rationale: Holding the container in a upright position allows for the best medication administration. If the patient has used a MDI before, and he is willing to self-administer the medication, then have him do it. The patient is sometimes better at doing this procedure than you.

8. Tell the patient to take a deep breath and to exhale fully.

   Rationale: Explain to the patient that this is the type of breath you will be asking him to do when the medication is administered.

9. Have the patient place his lips around the mouthpiece, making a tight seal (Figure 31.4).

   Rationale: A tight seal around the mouthpiece is essential for the medication to get to the lower airways. Without a tight seal, an improper dose may be delivered.

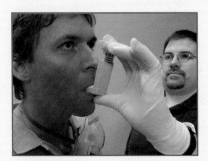

Figure 31.4

10. Direct the patient to take a deep, slow breath over a 5-second period. Simultaneously, either you or the patient should depress the canister. Make sure the patient has started inhalation before the canister is depressed (Figure 31.5).

    Rationale: The medication must be delivered during the inspiration phase of breathing. A deep and slow breath ensures that the medication gets to the lower airways and is absorbed. Poor timing or swallowing during breathing reduces the absorption.

11. Remove the inhaler, and request that the patient hold his breath for at least 10 seconds (Figure 31.6).

    Rationale: For the medication to absorb through the bronchioles, the medication must remain there for a short period of time. Asking the patient to hold his breath ensures the medication is absorbed. *Note:* This is a difficult task to ask of a patient suffering from shortness of breath.

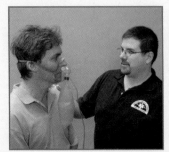

Figure 31.2

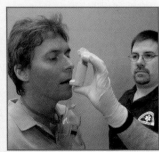

Figure 31.3

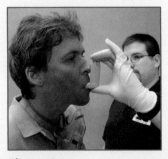

Figure 31.5

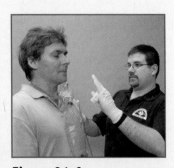

Figure 31.6

12. Coach the patient to exhale slowly with pursed lips.

Rationale: Exhaling slowly with pursed lips allows for greater airway pressures, which assist with medication absorption.

13. Readminister oxygen to the patient.

14. Document this procedure.

Rationale: It is extremely important to document your findings in order to have a history of facts and events that occurred at the scene.

ONGOING ASSESSMENT

Reassess vital signs and other earlier physical findings. Constantly monitor the patient for drug effects, including adverse reactions. Document any changes. Reestablish contact with medical control if the patient does not respond. Consider a second dose.

▶ PROBLEM SOLVING

▶ Timing is everything when delivering medication by a metered-dose inhaler. Inhalation and depression of the canister must be coordinated for the drug to be effective.

▶ In some cases, a spacer device may be added between the medication and the patient's mouthpiece (Figure 31.7). This reduces the difficulty some patients have in timing the inhalation with the administration of the drug. Follow manufacturer's recommendations when using a spacer.

▶ Consult with medical control prior to assisting, or giving, any additional doses. Wait at least 2 minutes before reusing the inhaler. In the interim, reassess the patient.

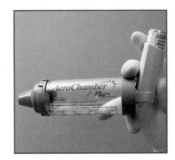

Figure 31.7

▶ If the canister is not at room temperature or warmer, consider holding it in your hands to warm it.

▶ CASE STUDY

You and your partner have just finished lunch at the station when you are called to respond to a "difficulty breathing" call. You are greeted at the door by a very anxious elderly woman who directs you to her 18-year-old granddaughter who is sitting on the couch and is clearly in respiratory distress. While your partner obtains vital signs, you begin your initial assessment and obtain a medical history. You find out that the 18-year-old female is an asthmatic and was recently prescribed a Metaprel metered-dose inhaler. Her present asthma attack started about 1 hour ago. She states she tried using her prescribed inhaler once about a half hour ago, but is not familiar with using an MDI and says that it just left a "funny taste" in her mouth. Her vital signs are as follows: pulse, 104; respirations, 36; blood pressure, 136/88; skin that is warm and dry. She is coughing frequently and is unable to complete long sentences.

The patient is not allergic to any medications and has never been hospitalized or intubated before. After consulting medical control, you receive an order to administer up to two doses of Metaprel from the patient's MDI. As you vigorously shake the medication canister for 30 seconds, you confirm the six rights in administering medications (Right patient, Right drug, Right amount/dose, Right route, Right time, and

Right documentation). You explain the procedure while you attach the plastic spacer to improve medication delivery. Through active coaching of the patient, you are able to instruct her to take a deep breath and fully exhale. You assist her in placing the mouthpiece in her mouth, and as she begins taking a slow deep breath you discharge the MDI.

The inhaler is removed from the patient's mouth, and you ask the patient to hold her breath as long as she can before slowly exhaling. Your partner provides supplemental oxygen, as you reassess your patient and evaluate whether a second dose is necessary. You provide oxygen to the patient while your partner prepares for transport. After the patient is loaded into the ambulance, you complete an ongoing assessment to determine the need for an additional dose of the MDI. The patient is still short of breath and you auscultate the chest and hear wheezing throughout. You recheck vital signs and administer a second dose of the MDI.

You notify the emergency department (ED) with an update on the patient and advise them that you have already administered the two doses of the MDI. They advise you to continue monitoring the patient and continue transport. Upon arrival at the ED, the patient is feeling much better. She is transferred to a bed for evaluation, and a report is given to the nurse. ■

1. An MDI should be administered to which of the following patients?
   a. a 17-year-old male who is wheezing and has an altered mental status
   b. an 80-year-old patient who is confused and cannot follow directions
   c. a 54-year-old patient who has chest pain and shortness of breath
   d. a 46-year-old female who is wheezing on inspiration only

2. To correctly administer an MDI, you must:
   a. have the patient inhale deeply after depressing the chamber.
   b. shake the MDI vigorously for 30 seconds prior to use.
   c. make sure the MDI is below room temperature.
   d. make sure the MDI is upside down to dispense the propellant.

3. An MDI is a:
   a. metered-dose inhaler.
   b. multi-dose inhaler.
   c. many dose inhaler.
   d. metered delivery inhaler.

CHAPTER 32

Administration of Nitroglycerin

KEY TERMS

Angina

Hypotension

Myocardial infarction

Nitroglycerin

Systolic blood pressure

Vasodilator

OBJECTIVES

The student will successfully administer nitroglycerin to a patient for whom it is indicated.

INTRODUCTION

Nitroglycerin, or "nitro," is a potent **vasodilator.** It helps dilate the coronary arteries that supply the heart muscle with blood, thereby relieving the chest pain associated with **angina** and acute **myocardial infarction.**

In many cases, the patient has been advised by his physician to take nitro whenever he experiences chest pain. EMT-Basics commonly arrive on scene to find that a cardiac patient has already taken nitro. In other cases, the patient may have the medication, but not yet thought of using it. Assisting the patient with the nitro may reduce myocardial damage.

To assist a patient with nitroglycerin, all of the following indications must be met:

▶ The patient complains of chest pain.

▶ The patient has a history of cardiac problems.

▶ The patient's physician has prescribed nitro.

▶ The patient has the medication with him.

▶ The patient's **systolic blood pressure** is greater than 100 systolic.

▶ Medical control, a standing medical order, or local protocol allows you to assist the patient with nitro.

Contraindications for the use of nitro include the following:

▶ The patient's systolic blood pressure is less than 100 (some systems use 90) systolic.

▶ The patient has already taken the maximum prescribed dosage.

▶ The patient is unable to open his mouth.

▶ The patient has taken sexually oriented vasodilation medication, for example, Viagra, within the last 6 hours.

▶ The patient has a head injury.

▶ The patient is an infant, child, or falls below an age limit set by local protocols.

Nitroglycerin is normally absorbed within 1 to 2 minutes, with a duration of between 20 and 30 minutes. Possible side effects include:

▶ **hypotension**

▶ headache

▶ changes in pulse rate

The normal dose of nitroglycerin is 0.4 mg (one tablet or one spray) under the tongue. This dose can be repeated in 3 to 5 minutes after the patient has been reassessed and the systolid blood pressure remains above 100 mmHg. In most EMS systems, the total dose of nitroglycerin should not be greater than three tablets. This includes any tablets taken before your arrival on scene.

▶EQUIPMENT

You will need the following equipment:

▶ Blood pressure cuff

▶ Patient's nitroglycerin tablets or nitroglycerin spray

▶ Stethoscope

ASSESSMENT

Complete an initial assessment. Administer high-concentration oxygen by nonrebreather mask and perform the focused history and physical exam prior to administering nitroglycerin to the patient. Make sure the patient meets all indications for the use of nitro and exhibits none of the contraindications. Ask the patient if he had taken nitroglycerin before your arrival. In some EMS systems, if the patient has taken a specific number of nitroglycerin tablets prior to your arrival, then nitroglycerin is contraindicated.

Be sure to take a full set of vital signs, including blood pressure, prior to administration. A patient's blood pressure in many EMS systems must be greater than 100 mmHg systolic before nitroglycerin can be administered. Ask the male patient if he has taken a sexually oriented medication within the last 6 hours. Medications like Viagra are contraindications for nitroglycerin administration if taken within the last 6 hours.

Check the expiration date of the nitroglycerin tablets. Remember that nitroglycerin tablets are light and heat sensitive. If the nitro is in tablet form, ask the patient when the container was first opened because air reduces the potency of nitroglycerin.

PROCEDURE: Administration of Nitroglycerin

1. Consult with medical direction about the use of nitroglycerin.

   Rationale: In many EMS systems, nitroglycerin may only be given under the direction of a base station hospital. If you have the authority to give nitroglycerin under standing protocols, then do so. If you are unsure if the patient meets the protocol, consult medical control.

2. Apply BSI precautions.

   Rationale: Gloves and eye protection are required at a minimum, and a gown may be needed if large amounts of blood or fluid are present to prevent exposure to infectious diseases.
   Warning: Nitroglycerin can be absorbed into your skin or through the membranes of your eyes.

3. Keep in mind the six "rights" of patients when administering medications. Ensure that you have the:

   ▷ right patient

   ▷ right drug

   ▷ right amount/dose

   ▷ right route of administration

   ▷ right time

   ▷ right documentation

   Rationale: Following the six rights ensures that proper safety procedures are used for the administration of any medication.

4. Explain the procedure to the patient (Figure 32.1).

   Rationale: For this procedure to work properly, it requires the assistance of the patient. Without the assistance of the patient, the procedure is less effective, which may affect the absorption of the medication. The patient is likely to be more cooperative if he understands the procedure. Explain the procedure in a way that the patient can understand what is required of him.

5. Place patient in a comfortable position, preferably one that will allow you to move the patient into a supine position if necessary.

   Rationale: The administration of nitroglycerin can immediately lower blood pressure. Having the patient in a position that allows you to place him in the shock position is important.

   If the patient's nitroglycerin comes in tablet form, go to step 6A; if it comes in spray form, go to step 6B.

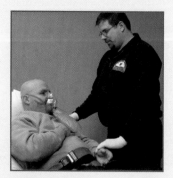

Figure 32.1

6A. If the patient's nitroglycerin comes in tablet form, take these steps:

   a. If the patient is wearing an oxygen mask, remove it. Explain to the patient that the oxygen will be replaced as soon as the procedure is done.

   Rationale: Access to the mouth is necessary to administer nitroglycerin.

   b. Ask the patient to open his mouth and lift his tongue. Place the tablet under the patient's tongue (Figure 32.2).

   c. Tell the patient not to swallow the pill. The nitroglycerin should dissolve under the tongue, where the medication will be quickly absorbed. Explain to the patient that the tablet will taste bitter, but again remind him to keep the pill under the tongue until it is completely dissolved.

Rationale: The tablet will be absorbed within the shortest amount of time and with the greatest absorption by the under-the-tongue method. If swallowed, nitroglycerin may not be absorbed.

6B. If the patient's nitroglycerin comes in the form of a spray, take these steps.

   a. Do *NOT* shake the canister.

   Rationale: Shaking the nitroglycerin canister displaces the propellant and the medication. This changes the metered dose.

   b. If the patient is wearing an oxygen mask, remove it. Explain to the patient that the oxygen will be replaced as soon as the procedure is done.

   Rationale: Access to the mouth is necessary to administer nitroglycerin.

   c. Ask the patient to open his mouth and lift his tongue.

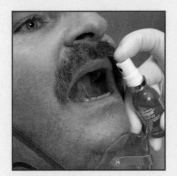

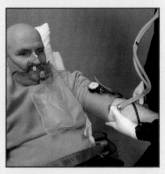

Figure 32.3 **Figure 32.4**

   d. Spray the medication under the tongue according to directions on the label (Figure 32.3).

   Rationale: Although the medication can be absorbed if sprayed on the tongue, it is better to spray it under the tongue.

   e. Ask patient to wait at least 10 seconds before swallowing. Readminister oxygen as needed.

Rationale: Asking the patient not to swallow allows for the medication to be absorbed.

7. Retake the patient's blood pressure within 2 minutes (Figure 32.4).

Rationale: Nitroglycerin is a very potent vasodilator and can lower the patient's blood pressure.

8. Because nitroglycerin is a potent vasodilator, if the patient becomes hypotensive and/or shows signs of shock, immediately place the patient in the shock position.

Rationale: Placing the patient in the shock position can immediately reverse the hypotension side effects associated with nitroglycerin.

9. If chest pain persists more than 5 minutes, consult with medical control and/or refer to standing medical orders or local protocols. In some EMS systems, multiple doses of nitroglycerin can be administered.

Rationale: In some cases, multiple does of nitroglycerin may be needed to reverse chest pain.

10. Document this procedure.

Rationale: It is extremely important to document your findings in order to have a history of facts and events that occurred at the scene.

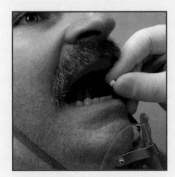

Figure 32.2

Retake vital signs every 5 minutes for critical patients and every 15 minutes for stable patients. Ask the patient about the effect of the medication on pain relief. Constantly monitor for changes.

▶PROBLEM SOLVING

▶ The most significant problem associated with the administration of nitroglycerin is the possibility of causing a hypotensive event. Usually you can relieve this condition by placing the patient in a supine position and raising the legs slightly.

▶ First-time users of nitroglycerin or patients who have ingested alcohol or who are taking hypertensive drugs can compound the side effects of hypotensive events.

▶ About 50 percent of patients taking nitroglycerin complain of associated headaches.

▶ If a patient does not have his prescription for nitroglycerin, then provide immediate transport or request for advanced cardiac life support backup.

▶CASE STUDY

You are called to a scene where a 63-year-old male is complaining of chest pain. Upon arrival, you and your partner determine the scene is safe and take appropriate BSI precautions. You make contact with the patient and begin your assessment. Through your interview, you learn the patient has chest pain radiating to his left arm and on the left side of his jaw. The patient rates his pain as a 7 on a scale of 1 to 10 and states he has a history of coronary artery disease and a myocardial infarction 2 years ago. The patient also tells you that he is on an aspirin regimen and has a prescription for nitroglycerin. He states he took one nitroglycerin tablet 15 minutes ago, with some relief. Your partner places the patient on high-flow oxygen using a nonrebreather mask at 15 liters per a minute. You assess vital signs and find that the patient's blood pressure is 162/114 and heart rate is 110, weak and regular. His respirations are 24 and seem to be shallow and labored. Patient is cool, pale, and diaphoretic. His pupils are equal and reactive.

Your local protocols allow you to administer nitroglycerin when a patient complaining of chest pain has a history of cardiac problems, a systolic blood pressure over 100, a physician prescription for nitroglycerin, and has the medication present. Because your patient has met all indications for nitroglycerin administration, you ask the patient if he has taken any Viagra within the last 6 hours and rule out all other contraindications for nitroglycerin administration. You position the patient comfortably and administer one 0.4-mg tablet of nitroglycerin sublingually, with instructions for the patient to let the tablet dissolve completely under his tongue.

While waiting for the nitroglycerine to work, you and your partner prepare the cot for transport. After 2 minutes you recheck his blood pressure, which is now 148/98. You load the patient onto the cot and into the ambulance. En route, after 5 minutes, you ask about his chest pain, and he reports he still has chest pain at a 4 on a scale of 1 to 10. Per your protocols, you reassess the patient and administer a second dose of 0.4 mg of nitroglycerin. Two minutes after administering the second nitroglycerin dose, you recheck the patient's blood pressure and find it is now 134/90. You notify the emergency department (ED) of the patient's condition, and after arriving at the ED, transfer the patient to the emergency staff with no further changes. ■

1. Nitroglycerin should be administered at which point in the assessment?
   a. as soon as you determine that the patient is complaining of chest pain
   b. after completing both the focused history and detailed exam
   c. only after ALS backup is on scene in case of hypotension
   d. after you obtain baseline vital signs with a systolic pressure >100 mmHg

2. Nitroglycerine should be administered:
   a. under the tongue to prevent the patient from aspirating.
   b. under the tongue to avoid the patient drinking water to help swallow it.
   c. under the tongue to increase the rate of absorption.
   d. between the cheek and the gums to avoid swallowing the pill.

3. Which of the following patients would qualify for nitroglycerin administration?
   a. a 70-year-old patient complaining of chest pain throughout the day
   b. a 64-year-old male complaining of chest pain after falling and striking a table
   c. a 56-year-old patient that has no cardiac history, but has his father's nitro
   d. an 18-year-old patient complaining of chest pain after running 2 miles

CHAPTER 33
Administration of Epinephrine Auto-Injector

KEY TERMS

Bronchioles

Edema

Epinephrine auto-injector

Hypoperfusion

Hypotension

Severe allergic reaction

OBJECTIVE

The student will successfully administer an epinephrine auto-injector to a patient for whom it is indicated.

INTRODUCTION

Injectable drugs are not commonly used at the EMT-Basic level. However, an **epinephrine auto-injector**—a truly lifesaving device—is an exception. This medication is physician prescribed, which is one reason an EMT-Basic can assist in its administration. An epinephrine auto-injector is a disposable prepackaged delivery system that allows the patient to self-administer a single dose of medication into the thigh muscles via a spring-loaded injection needle and syringe.

Epinephrine is prescribed for patients who are suspected to have a **severe allergic reaction.** In the patient with a severe reaction, it will constrict blood vessels and dilate the **bronchioles.** The actions will assist with the patient suffering from **hypotension** and/or shortness of breath. With the approval of medical control, you may administer or help the patient administer the medication. The recommended location for delivery is usually on the outside of the lateral thigh midway between the waist and knee. When the auto-injector is placed on the thigh and pushed, a spring-loaded mechanism drives a needle into the thigh and automatically injects the medication.

 PEDIATRIC NOTE:

Adults and children usually have different auto-injectors, each of which delivers a single dose of epinephrine. The adult injector delivers 0.3 mg, and in pediatrics it is 0.15 mg. It is usually not customary to use more than one dose.

▶ EQUIPMENT

You will need the following equipment:

- ▶ BSI supplies
- ▶ Patient's epinephrine auto-injector
- ▶ Sharps box or portable biohazard container
- ▶ Oxygen equipment

ASSESSMENT

Assess the patient for signs of severe allergic reaction, these may include:

- ▶ altered level of consciousness
- ▶ skin signs
- ▶ rash
- ▶ hives
- ▶ **edema**
- ▶ shortness of breath
- ▶ signs of **hypoperfusion** (shock)
- ▶ pale, cool, moist skin
- ▶ rapid pulse
- ▶ thirst
- ▶ low blood pressure

In addition, check the expiration date of the medication. Confirm that the patient is not allergic to this medication.

PROCEDURE: Administration of Epinephrine Auto-Injector

1. Consult with medical control about the use of an epinephrine auto-injector (Figure 33.1).

   Rationale: In many EMS systems, epinephrine may only be given under the direction of a base station hospital. If you have the authority to give epinephrine under standing protocols, then do so. If you are unsure if the patient meets the protocol, consult medical control.

2. Apply BSI precautions.

   Rationale: Gloves and eye protection are required at a minimum, and a gown may be needed if large amounts of blood or fluid are present to prevent exposure to infectious diseases.

3. Keep in mind the six "rights" of patients when administering medications. Ensure that you have the:

   - ▶ right patient
   - ▶ right drug
   - ▶ right amount/dose
   - ▶ right route of administration

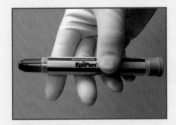

Figure 33.1

continued...

▶ **right time**

▶ **right documentation**

Rationale: Following the six rights ensures that proper safety procedures are used for the administration of any medication.

4. Explain the procedure to the patient.

Rationale: For this procedure to work properly, it requires the assistance of the patient. Without the assistance of the patient, the procedure is less effective, which may affect the absorption of the medication. The patient is likely to be more cooperative if he understands the procedure. Explain the procedure in a way that the patient can understand what is required of him.

5. Remove the safety cap from the auto-injector.

6. Expose the thigh area (Figure 33.2).

Rationale: Removal of clothing is suggested. Pulling clothes up to expose the area can impede circulation and cause reduction in absorption.

7. Place the auto-injector device on the lateral thigh midway between the knee and the waist (Figure 33.3).

Rationale: This area has a large amount of muscle mass that allows for good absorption of epinephrine.

8. Tell the patient he may feel a stick from the needle.

Rationale: Not advising the patient could cause a sudden move that could result in injury or make the device malfunction.

9. In a smooth, direct 90-degree angle, push the injector firmly until you hear the device inject the needle (Figure 33.4).

Rationale: This angle reduces pain and allows for the most direct route of administration of the epinephrine.

10. Hold the injector in place until the medication is injected or for at least 10 seconds.

Rationale: Removing the injector too early will not allow the epinephrine to be administered.

11. Remove the auto-injector.

12. Dispose of the injector in a sharps box or biohazard container.

Rationale: To reduce any chance of needle stick, carefully remove the device and place in a sharps container.

13. Reassess the patient for improvement (Figure 33.5).

14. Document this procedure.

Rationale: It is extremely important to document your findings in order to have a history of facts and events that occurred at the scene.

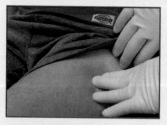

Figure 33.2

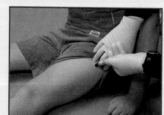

Figure 33.3

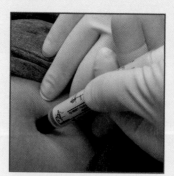

Figure 33.4

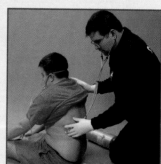

Figure 33.5

ONGOING ASSESSMENT

Reassess the vital signs and patient condition to see if the medication has helped. Consider the need for a second dose if the patient's condition deteriorates and if approved by medical direction. Assess:

- chief complaint
- blood pressure
- pulse
- respirations
- skin signs
- other earlier positive physical findings

Constantly monitor the patient for drug effects, including adverse reactions. Pay special attention to the patient's ABCs.

▶ PROBLEM SOLVING

- The spring-loaded device requires firm pressure against the thigh to make it work. Make sure you are pressing hard enough.
- If at any time you or anyone becomes stuck by a needle, consult local protocols and implement needle-stick procedures immediately.
- Immediately consult with medical control if the patient experiences any adverse effects from the medication.

▶ CASE STUDY

You and your partner respond to the local city park for a report of an unknown medical problem. Once at the park, you put on appropriate BSI and confirm scene safety as you proceed to the patient's location. Upon arrival, you find a 36-year-old male sitting at a picnic table with his family, complaining of shortness of breath. You observe the patient has facial edema, hives, and his skin is cool and clammy. His radial pulse is rapid and very weak. Your partner notices what looks to be an insect bite or sting on the patient's left forearm. The patient confirms that he is allergic to bees, but does not recall being stung. As you continue to obtain further information, the patient's wife remembers that their doctor recently prescribed something for bee stings. She hands you the patient's epinephrine auto-injector, saying, "Our doctor gave us this, but I don't remember what we are supposed to do with it."

Your partner places the patient on high-flow oxygen using a nonrebreather mask at 15 liters per a minute. As you prepare to administer the epinephrine auto-injector, you review the six "rights" in administering medications (Right patient, Right drug, Right amount/dose, Right route, Right time, and Right documentation) and advise the patient of the procedure. You expose the patient's thigh, remove the safety cap from the epinephrine auto-injector, and, holding it at a 90-degree angle, place it flush against the lateral thigh midway between the knee and the waist. After telling the patient he may feel the stick from the needle, you firmly push the epinephrine auto-injector until you hear the device inject the needle. You hold the epinephrine auto-injector in place for 10 seconds, and observe that the medication was injected. After disposing of the epinephrine auto-injector in a sharps container, you and your partner conduct an ongoing assessment of the patient, including vital signs, and then prepare for transport.

En route, you continue to monitor the patient for signs that the allergic reaction is returning. You notify the emergency department (ED) and do not receive any orders; you continue to transport. You arrive at the ED with the patient feeling much better. You transfer care to the emergency nurse and prepare for the next call. ■

(continued)

1. Which of the following is *not* part of the assessment prior to administering epinephrine?

   a. Assess for signs of an allergic reaction.

   b. Check to confirm the six rights.

   c. Confirm that the patient is not allergic to epinephrine.

   d. Complete the focused history and exam.

2. The epinephrine auto-injector should be administered to which of the following patients?

   a. an 18-year-old male having a severe asthma attack

   b. a 26-year-old patient who has edema around a bee sting

   c. a 32-year-old male who is hypotensive after ingesting peanuts

   d. a 50-year-old patient who is unresponsive from a bee sting and has his daughter's epinephrine auto-injector

3. Which of the following patients received the correct dose of epinephrine?

   a. a 15-year-old received 0.3 mg

   b. an 18-year-old received 0.15 mg

   c. a 24-year-old received 0.15 mg

   d. a 28-year old received 0.3 mg

CHAPTER 34
Administration of Nebulized Medication

OBJECTIVE

The student will successfully administer nebulized medication to a patient for whom it is indicated.

KEY TERMS

Handheld nebulizer

Nebulizer chamber

T-tube

INTRODUCTION

A nebulizer is a device that is used to aerosolize medications into a mist for delivery directly to the lungs. Medication is then absorbed from the lower airways and the lungs into the bloodstream. This is one of the fastest non-invasive ways to deliver medications. Knowledge of the medication being administered is essential. Knowing the indications, contraindications, and adverse reactions and doses are important.

The nebulizer device needs to be connected to a medical air compressor or, as in most EMS systems, to oxygen. A nebulizer requires the patient to be alert enough to assist in the delivery process. If the patient is not alert, then a nebulized medication may not work.

A **handheld nebulizer** has a chamber where the medication is placed and it is connected to either a mask or a mouthpiece. In most EMS systems, the mouthpiece is the delivery method of choice.

▶ EQUIPMENT

You will need the following equipment:

▶ BSI equipment

▶ Medication

▶ Handheld nebulizer

▶ Connection tube

▶ **Nebulizer chamber**

▶ **T-tube**

▶ 6-inch flex tube

▶ Mouthpiece

▶ Oxygen supply tank

ASSESSMENT

Determine that the patient has the ability to use the handheld nebulizer. Determine which drug is to be administered, such as albuterol or atrovent. Confirm that the patient is not allergic to this medication. Consult with medical control or follow local policies and procedures for administration.

PROCEDURE: Administration of Nebulized Medication

1. Consult with medical control about the use of the handheld nebulizer (Figure 34.1).

   Rationale: In many EMS systems, a nebulizer may only be given under the direction of a base station hospital. If you have the authority to use a nebulizer under standing protocols, then do so. If you are unsure if the patient meets the protocol, consult medical control.

2. Apply BSI precautions.

   Rationale: Gloves and eye protection are required at a minimum, and a gown may be needed if large amounts of blood or fluid are present to prevent exposure to infectious diseases.

3. Keep in mind the six "rights" of patients when administering medications. Ensure that you have the:

   ▶ right patient

   ▶ right drug

   ▶ right amount/dose

   ▶ right route of administration

   ▶ right time

   ▶ right documentation

   Rationale: Following the six rights ensures that proper safety procedures are used for the administration of any medication.

4. Explain the procedure to the patient (Figure 34.2).

   Rationale: For this procedure to work properly, it requires the assistance of the patient. Without the assistance of the patient, the procedure is less effective, which may affect the absorption of the medication. The patient is likely to be more cooperative if she understands the procedure. Explain the procedure in a way that the patient can understand what is required of her.

5. Unscrew the lid of the nebulizer chamber.

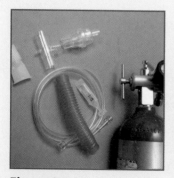

Figure 34.1

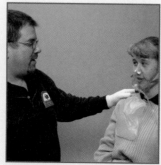

Figure 34.2

6. Add medication as directed (Figure 34.3).

7. Reattach the lid.

8. Fasten the T-tube to the nebulizer chamber (Figure 34.4).

9. Connect the mouthpiece to one end of the T-tube and the flex tube to the other end (Figure 34.5).

10. Attach tubing from the nebulizer to the oxygen source. Adjust oxygen to 6 liters per minute. You should be able to see a mist coming out of both the flex tube and the mouthpiece (Figure 34.6).

11. Ask the patient to sit as upright as possible.

12. You may hold the nebulizer or ask the patient to hold the nebulizer in her hand and to place the mouthpiece firmly in her mouth. Lips should be sealed tightly around mouthpiece. Ask her to breathe deep and slowly through her mouth (Figure 34.6). At times it may be necessary to shake the chamber slightly to remove medication attached to the wall of the chamber.

13. Continue this treatment until the full amount of the medication is gone.

14. Reassess the patient.

15. Document this procedure.

    Rationale: It is extremely important to document your findings in order to have a history of facts and events that occurred at the scene.

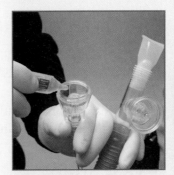
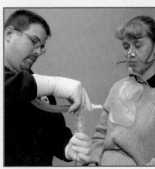

Figure 34.3   **Figure 34.4**

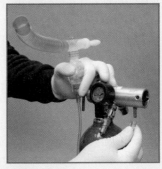

Figure 34.5

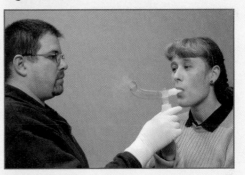

Figure 34.6

ONGOING ASSESSMENT

Assess:

▶ chief complaint

▶ blood pressure

▶ pulse

▶ respirations

▶ skin signs

▶ other earlier positive physical findings

Constantly monitor the patient for drug effects, including adverse reactions.

▶PROBLEM SOLVING

▶ For this delivery system to work well, the patient must be alert and have a fair respiratory tidal volume. Contact medical control for potential options if you have concerns.

▶ Immediately consult with medical control if the patient experiences any adverse effects from the medication.

▶CASE STUDY

A 68-year-old female calls EMS after experiencing shortness of breath for 35 minutes. When the EMTs arrive on scene they ensure scene safety and BSI. Upon entering the house, they find the patient in the kitchen in a tripod position, trying to catch her breath. She has rapid, shallow respirations and is only able to speak in two- to three-word sentences. The patient's husband is on the scene and provides the pertinent medical history on his wife.

He tells the EMTs that she has a 40-year history of smoking one pack a day and was diagnosed with chronic obstructive pulmonary disease 5 years ago. The patient uses home oxygen as needed. Before the current episode of shortness of breath, the patient had just returned from walking her poodle around the block. During the initial assessment, the EMTs find a blood pressure of 146/82, heart rate of 125, skin that is ashen and moist, respirations at 36 to 40 per minute with wheezes, and accessory muscle use.

The EMTs confirm that the patient is not allergic to albuterol. On-line medical control is consulted and the order is given for 2.5 mg of nebulized albuterol (0.5 cc of 0.5% solution diluted in 2.5 cc of normal saline). As the EMTs prepare to administer the nebulized medication, they explain the procedure to the patient and confirm the six "rights" in administering medications (Right patient, Right drug, Right amount/dose, Right route, and Right documentation).

After adding the medication to the nebulizer chamber and making the appropriate connections, they adjust their portable oxygen source to 6 liters per minute. Upon seeing the mist come out of the mouthpiece and flex tubing, they place the nebulizer in the patient's hands and coach the patient in taking slow, deep breaths while maintaining a tight seal on the mouthpiece. The patient is kept sitting as close to upright as possible while transportation is initiated. Once the medication is finished, the EMTs reassess the patient and document the procedure. The emergency department is called with a report and gives an order to provide a second treatment if necessary. The patient remains relaxed and is breathing well so you elect not to give the second treatment. While transferring care to the emergency staff, you advise them that the patient only received one dose of the albuterol.■

1. Which of the following patients would receive nebulized albuterol?
   a. a patient with difficulty breathing and very shallow respirations
   b. a patient who was wheezing then became unresponsive
   c. a patient who has chest pain and shortness of breath
   d. a patient who has been wheezing and short of breath all day

2. Nebulizer therapy should be administered at which of the following flow rates?
   a. <6 lpm to provide good nebulization
   b. 6–8 lpm for proper nebulization
   c. 10–15 lpm to ensure adequate oxygenation
   d. none of the above

3. When administering the nebulizer, it is important to:
   a. coach the patient to ensure adequate delivery.
   b. listen to lung sounds throughout to make sure the medication is working.
   c. make sure the patient is unresponsive.
   d. use two types of nebulizers.

Automated External Defibrillation

OBJECTIVE

The student will successfully demonstrate the ability to perform defibrillation using an automated external defibrillator.

INTRODUCTION

The single most important link in the "Chain of Survival" for the cardiac arrest patient is the successful use of the defibrillator. Studies show that time to **defibrillation** may be even more important than cardiopulmonary resuscitation (CPR).

An **automated external defibrillator (AED)** is a device that delivers an electronic shock, through the chest wall, to a heart that is fibrillating or is in **ventricular tachycardia (VT).** The device has the ability to recognize **ventricular fibrillation (VF)** or VT as a shockable rhythm without the need for interpretation by the user. The device can also interpret rhythms that are not VF or VT as nonshockable rhythms. Because these devices interpret the rhythm, they do not require the expertise of rhythm recognition as does a manual defibrillator. This makes AEDs simpler to operate and increases the possibilities of who can use them. Studies have shown that AEDs can deliver a shock quicker in most cases than can **manual defibrillation.**

There are two categories of AEDs. Semiautomatic AEDs (semi-AEDs) are devices that interpret the rhythms and give the operator the command to deliver the shock. Automatic AEDs (auto-AEDs) are simpler to use. They also interpret the rhythm, but they deliver the shock without the assistance of the operator. Currently, auto-AEDs and semi-AEDs come in two types. These two types use a different form of energy delivery: **Monophasic** and **biphasic energy levels.** The difference is not noticeable to the operator.

Patients are defibrillated by means of pads that are placed on the chest. These pads also serve to monitor the patient's rhythm. For the pads to be effective they must be properly placed and stick firmly to the chest wall.

The AED is manufactured with sensors that can detect movement, improperly applied and/or loose leads, and rhythms that can be misleading. The device is manufactured so that it does not shock a patient who should not be shocked. The AED is programmed at the factory to meet the current standard of care for cardiac arrest patients.

The AED is contraindicated in patients with cardiac arrest of trauma origin, and, depending on your EMS system, AEDs may be contraindicated in infants and children (less than 8 years or 55 lb).

Most AEDs come equipped with a quality improvement module that allows for recording of all activity that is associated with the AED. A voice recorder may also be supplied. This recorded information is then available at the end of the procedure for medical direction review.

You should become very familiar with the AED equipment, because many AED models are on the market. The time to become familiar with the equipment is *NOT* when it is needed. Because of the many available types and models of defibrillators, the procedure discussed here will be generic to all AEDs. Check with the manufacturer for details about a specific AED.

▶ EQUIPMENT

You will need the following equipment:

- ▶ BSI equipment
- ▶ AED
- ▶ Defibrillation pads
- ▶ BVM, with reservoir attachment
- ▶ Oxygen cylinder
- ▶ Suction and catheter
- ▶ Razor

ASSESSMENT

The patient will be unresponsive and will not have respirations or a pulse. If CPR was being administered prior to your arrival, have the core providers stop and assess for pulse. Check for mechanism of injury or trauma. Check the patient's age. Bare the patient's chest and check for a **pacemaker** and **nitroglycerin patch** or patches. If possible, check for a **Do Not Resuscitate (DNR) order.**

Check the environment for safety and consider removing the patient if:

- ▶ the environment is unstable.
- ▶ significant water is present in the environment.
- ▶ the patient is on a metal surface.
- ▶ an explosive environment is a concern.

NO movement of the patient, ventilations, or chest compressions should be performed during the analysis phase. CPR should be performed whenever possible.

PROCEDURE: Automated External Defibrillation

1. Apply BSI precautions.

   Rationale: Gloves and eye protection are required at a minimum, and a gown may be needed if large amounts of blood or fluid are present to prevent exposure to infectious diseases.

2. Place the patient in the supine position on a dry, **nonmetallic surface.**

   Rationale: This needs to be done as quickly as possible. Energy from the AED could transfer to you without it moving. Also consider moving a

   continued...

patient who is in a tight space so that you have enough space on which to work.

3. One EMT confirms that no pulse is present and performs CPR.

   Rationale: If only one EMT is present, application of the AED has priority.

4. Bare the patient's chest, including removing a bra if present, and make sure the patient's chest is dry (Figure 35.1).

   Rationale: Any fluid on the chest could interfere with pad placement and could reduce the energy transfer.

5. Use a razor to remove any hair from the area on the patient's chest with which the pads will come into contact.

   Rationale: Any hair on the chest will interfere with pad placement and will reduce energy transfer.

6. Turn on power to the AED.

7. Place the pads on the patient's chest. The sternum paddle or pad is placed on the anterior right side of the chest, just inferior to the clavicle at the **midclavicular line.** The apex pad is placed on the anterior left side of the chest, at the fourth or fifth **intercostal space,** at the **anterior-axillary line** (Figure 35.2).

   Rationale: Improper pad placement could interfere with AED use.

8. If required, and the AED comes equipped with a voice recorder, give a verbal report.

9. Stop CPR, and state verbally to "stand clear."

   Rationale: For the AED to evaluate the patient's rhythm, no movement, including CPR, can be done while the AED is analyzing the rhythm. If movement or CPR is done, the AED might not function properly.

10. If using a semi-AED, press the analyze button. This is done automatically by on auto-AED, which usually has a voice prompt that will alert you of the situation (Figure 35.3).

11. At this point the AED will assess the rhythm, and either go into shockable or nonshockable mode.

    If a shockable rhythm is identified, go to step 12. If nonshockable, go immediately to step 16.

12. If using a semi-AED, visually check the area and state loudly and clearly "Stand clear." Some EMS systems require you to say the following: "I'm clear, you're clear, everyone clear." Once everyone is clear, press the shock button (Figure 35.4). The shock is delivered automatically with the auto-AED, which usually has a voice prompt that will alert you of the situation.

    Rationale: Safety must be a prime concern during defibrillation. Your priority is to make sure that no one gets shocked accidentally.

13. Press the analyze button again. In auto-AEDs and in some semi-AEDs, this happens automatically. The auto-AED usually has a voice prompt that will alert you of the situation.

14. If the AED gives an alert that another shock is required, repeat steps 12 and 13 two more times. Otherwise, go on to step 15.

15. Check with your local protocols for the total number of shocks that can be delivered. In some cases, steps 12 and 13 are done in series of three with 1 minute of CPR done in between.

16. If at any time a no-shock-indicated response is received from the AED, check for a pulse. If there is still no pulse, do 1 minute of CPR.

    Rationale: If you get a pulse, *STOP* CPR, check for respirations, and after 1 minute check for blood pressure.

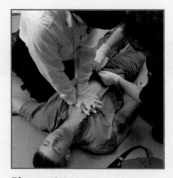

Figure 35.1

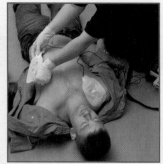

Figure 35.2

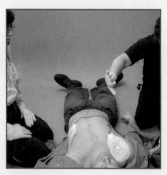

Figure 35.3

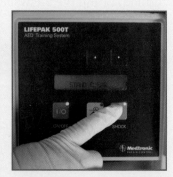

Figure 35.4

17. Press the analyze button (Figure 35.5).

18. If the rhythm changes and the AED alerts you that a shock is needed, resume steps 12 and 13, resume CPR for 1 minute, and analyze a third time. If no shock is indicated, resume CPR and transport.

19. Document findings.

    Rationale: It is extremely important to document your findings in order to have a history of facts and events that occurred at the scene.

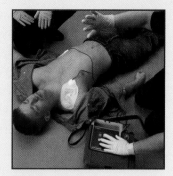

Figure 35.5

ONGOING ASSESSMENT

If you receive a no-shock-indicated response from the AED and a pulse is present, check for breathing. If breathing is fast enough and the volume is sufficient, check for a blood pressure and prepare to transport. If ventilations are not sufficient, continue ventilations and prepare for transport. If the rhythm changes, most AEDs will prompt you to press the analyze button.

▶ PROBLEM SOLVING

▶ Time to defibrillation can make the difference between a successful resuscitation and not. Make sure that you are familiar with the equipment and are trained appropriately before attempting to use the AED.

▶ Safety for the patient and for the EMS provider is essential during defibrillation. To reduce the risk of injury to the patient or the EMS provider, the following must be considered:

　▶ Place the patient in an environment that gives you plenty of space in which to work. Move the patient if necessary to create that space.

　▶ Make sure the environment that the patient is in is dry. Move the patient if necessary.

　▶ Make sure the environment the patient is resting on is not metal. Move the patient if necessary.

　▶ Make sure there are no explosive agents in the environment. If necessary, remove the patient from an unsafe area.

　▶ Make sure that nobody, including yourself, is in direct contact with the patient during defibrillation. Visual and verbal warnings reduce this risk.

　▶ If the patient's chest is wet, make sure that it is dry prior to defibrillation.

　▶ If the patient is wearing a bra or has metal jewelry on, consider removing such items before defibrillation to prevent burning of the chest wall.

　▶ If the patient has a considerable amount of hair in the areas where the paddles or pads are placed, consider quickly shaving prior to defibrillation to prevent burning of the chest wall.

　▶ The AED will not function properly in the analyze mode if ventilations, chest compressions, or patient movement is occurring.

　▶ If the pads are not firmly placed on the patient, the AED will not analyze properly. In some cases, the AED will voice prompt that there is a problem with the electrodes.

- A large amount of breast tissue (adipose) may interfere with paddle or pad placement on the left side of the chest. Make sure the pad is on the chest wall and *NOT* on the breast tissue. Reduced energy delivered to the heart could occur, possibly interfering with conversion of the rhythm.

- If the patient has a pacemaker, do *NOT* place pad directly over the pacemaker. Movement to one side is the only option.

- If the patient is wearing a nitroglycerine patch, remove it before defibrillation.

- If the patient is hypothermic, consider transport after three unsuccessful shocks.

- If you turn on the AED and nothing happens, consider a problem with the batteries. Immediately switch to new batteries and continue.

- Consult the owner's manual of your defibrillator to become familiar with the product.

PEDIATRIC NOTE:

On the basis of the published evidence to date, the Pediatric Advanced Life Support Task Force of the International Liaison Committee on Resuscitation has made the following recommendation (October 2002):

Automated external defibrillators (AEDs) may be used for children 1 to 8 years of age who have no signs of circulation. Ideally the device should deliver a pediatric dose. The arrhythmia detection algorithm used in the device should demonstrate high specificity for pediatric shockable rhythms, i.e., it will not recommend delivery of a shock for nonshockable rhythms (Class IIb).

In addition:

- Currently there is insufficient evidence to support a recommendation for or against the use of AEDs in children <1 year of age.

- For a lone rescuer responding to a child without signs of circulation, the task force continues to recommend provision of 1 minute of CPR before any other action, such as activating the emergency medical services system or attaching the AED.

- Defibrillation is recommended for documented ventricular fibrillation (VF)/pulseless ventricular tachycardia (VT) (Class I).

▶CASE STUDY

You are working on Medic 10 when you are dispatched to help a "man not feeling well" at a youth soccer field on a drizzly October afternoon. You and your partner arrive to find a crowd of onlookers surrounding an older male, probably in his 50s, lying supine on the bleachers. A bystander is performing CPR on the patient. His wife stands by sobbing.

After ensuring appropriate BSI and scene safety, your partner checks for respirations and a carotid pulse, confirming that the man is in full arrest. You find out from bystanders that he collapsed just minutes after his wife called 911 to report that her husband was not feeling well. You and your partner quickly assess the scene and make the determination that you will need to move the man off of the metal bleachers. Using your plastic backboard, you relocate the man to a nearby dry area under a portable canopy.

Your partner and a bystander resume CPR using a bag-valve-mask unit attached to supplemental oxygen, while you prepare the automated external defibrillator. Once you are set up, they stop CPR and your partner confirms there is no pulse. Making sure the chest is dry and free of hair under the pads, you place the AED defibrillator pads in position on the chest. The AED is turned on, and you direct people to "stand clear" as you press the analyze button. The machine responds with "SHOCK ADVISED." Advising everyone to again "stand clear," you visually confirm and reconfirm that you, your partner, and everyone else is clear of the patient before you press the "SHOCK" button. The patient responds with the usual extremity jerk. You repeat the AED analysis, are advised to shock, and deliver a second shock. Upon pressing the analyze button the third time, however, the AED indicates "NO SHOCK ADVISED." Your partner assesses the patient and finds a weak carotid pulse, but no respirations.

You begin "bagging" the patient and frequently reassess the patient while you and your partner initiate transportation to the nearest hospital facility. You notify the emergency department (ED) about your patient, and continue to closely monitor him throughout transport. Upon arriving at the ED, you transfer care to the emergency physician and nurse. ■

(continued)

1. Which of the following patients qualifies for defibrillation with a regular, semi-automated AED?
   a. a 6-year-old patient who has been in a drowning accident
   b. a 50-pound patient who collapsed at home
   c. a 16-year-old patient who has experienced a motor-vehicle collision (MVC)
   d. a 55-year-old patient who had complained of chest pain

2. Which of the following will *not* disrupt rhythm analysis?
   a. moving while en route to the hospital
   b. continuing ventilatory support
   c. completing the focused history
   d. providing chest compressions

3. Which patient does not need to be moved prior to defibrillation?
   a. a patient lying back in a recliner
   b. a patient who is on the floor of a boat
   c. a patient who is lying on metal bleachers
   d. a patient who collapsed on the driveway while shoveling snow

CHAPTER 36
Applying Soft Restraints

OBJECTIVE

The student will successfully apply soft restraints to patients for whom they are indicated.

INTRODUCTION

Occasionally, patients will need to be physically restrained during ambulance transport. These patients are usually severely agitated, combative, and violent for a multitude of reasons. Keep in mind that medical emergencies can cause a patient to become unruly (e.g., **hypoglycemia, hypoxia,** head injury, overdose). Ambulance transport is indicated because these patients do require medical care, whether they realize it or not.

When the determination has been made that the patient is a danger to himself or others, reasonable force and restraints are used. **Reasonable force** is the minimum amount of force needed to control the patient. The goal is to restrain the patient, not to hurt him. Physical restraint is always the last option; EMT-Basics should always attempt verbal persuasion first. *NEVER* attempt to restrain a patient alone. **Positional asphyxia** has been reported in the literature when patients have been "hog-tied" or restrained in a manner that impairs breathing. Patients should be restrained in a face-up or **lateral position,** not face down. Follow local protocols when restraining uncooperative patients. In many areas, law enforcement or medical control must authorize restraint and treatment of patients against their will.

KEY TERMS

Hypoglycemia

Hypoxia

Lateral position

Positional asphyxia

Reasonable force

Soft restraints

▶EQUIPMENT

You will need the following:

▶ BSI equipment for all involved in the restraining process

▶ **Soft restraints** (or wide tape and sheets)

▶ Sufficient personnel; one person per extremity at a minimum

▶ Surgical mask or oxygen mask

ASSESSMENT

Always consider physiological causes of a patient's behavior. Make sure the patient is not carrying a weapon. You can perform a "pat-down" during the patient assessment. Attempt to determine what triggered the patient's unruly behavior. Quickly perform a scene assessment. Make sure that the scene is safe.

Law enforcement should be required to intervene if the patient is extremely combative or yielding a weapon. Always have an exit planned and stay at least an arm's distance from the patient. All of these factors should be incorporated into your assessment.

PROCEDURE: Applying Soft Restraints

1. Apply BSI precautions.

   Rationale: It is not uncommon for patients to spit at EMTs during restraining. Gloves and eye protection are required at a minimum, and a gown may be needed if large amounts of blood or fluid are present to prevent exposure to infectious diseases.

2. Plan your actions ahead of time.

   Rationale: Preplanning is important. Make sure all individuals involved in the restraining procedure know their jobs. Discussion with the patient is controversial. In some cases, it could make attempts to restrain the patient more difficult.

3. At least four people are required to restrain a patient. Each person should be preassigned a limb to restrain. Rescuers should act all at once to overwhelm the patient (Figure 36.1).

   Rationale: Safety for both the patient and the individuals involved in the restraining process is a priority.

4. Attempt to grab clothing or large joints. Avoid placing pressure on the neck or chest (Figure 36.2).

   Rationale: Grabbing joints reduces the patient's ability to move. Again for the safety of the patient, be careful about which area you grab. Keep an eye on all other patient areas during the restraining process.

5. Avoid getting close to the patient's mouth, because some patients may try to bite rescuers.

6. An EMT-Basic should be assigned to reassure the patient throughout the procedure (Figure 36.3).

   Rationale: Reassuring the patient that she will be not injured can reduce the patient's anxiety.

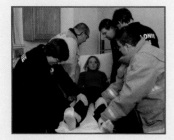

Figure 36.1

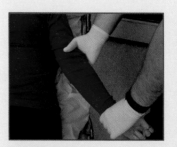

Figure 36.2

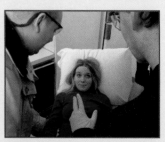

Figure 36.3

7. Secure all four limbs with soft restraints approved by local protocols.

8. The patient should be secured on the ambulance gurney in a supine or lateral position (Figure 36.4).

   Rationale: Patients should not be restrained in a prone position because it can make breathing difficult.

9. If the patient is spitting at rescuers, a surgical mask or oxygen mask (connected to oxygen) can be placed over the patient's face. If the patient's face is covered, monitor the airway carefully.

10. Continually monitor distal circulation in restrained extremities (Figure 36.5).

    Rationale: Because of the excitement of the restraining process, restraints may initially be placed too tightly. Trauma to an extremity or under the restraints could cause swelling. Monitoring distal perfusion can reduce the risk of complications from tight restraints.

11. Once restrained, do not leave the patient at any time.

12. Consider having extra personnel in the ambulance's patient compartment during transport.

13. Monitor ABCs during transport (Figure 36.6).

    Rationale: Patients may have drugs or alcohol in their system. Constant monitoring for decreased level of consciousness and reduced respiratory functions is important.

14. Do not remove restraints unless sufficient personnel are available to control the patient (usually at the hospital).

15. Document why and how the patient was restrained as well as distal assessments.

    Rationale: It is extremely important to document your findings in order to have a history of facts and events that occurred at the scene.

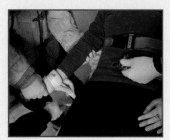

Figure 36.4

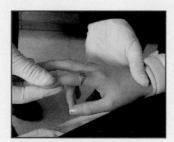

Figure 36.5

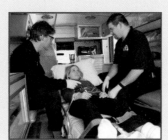

Figure 36.6

ONGOING ASSESSMENT

Constantly reassess distal circulation in restrained extremities during transport. ABCs should always be monitored in the restrained patient. Patients who calm down may actually be deteriorating, so be vigilant. Attempt to take vital signs every 15 minutes if patient is stable.

▶PROBLEM SOLVING

▶ During a scuffle is not the time to learn how to apply restraints. Be familiar with the soft restraints that are carried in ambulances.

▶ Soft restraints are commercially available but can be improvised with cravats (triangular bandages), roller bandages, or sheets and wide tape.

▶ If the patient continues to struggle violently, requiring multiple people for restraint, consider advanced life support resources for chemical restraint.

▶ Do not place your hands near the patient's mouth; you might get bitten.

►CASE STUDY

You have responded to a local bar to aid a patient who is reportedly intoxicated and has demonstrated episodes of violent outbreaks. On arrival, you find a very muscular patient who has been subdued by the local police department. As you approach, you note that the patient is being restrained face down with wrist and ankle cuffs.

On your arrival at the patient's side, the police officer in charge tells you that they asked the patient to leave the premises and he immediately became violent and attacked them. The officer states that they have had a difficult time restraining the patient and he suggests that you transport him to the emergency department just as he is restrained.

You determine that the patient should be restrained on your cot and that you would like the police officers to assist you in restraining him on the cot and in removing the wrist and ankle cuffs. After moving the patient to the cot, you and your partner apply soft restraints to all four of the patient's extremities. After applying the soft restraints and securing them to the cot, you have the police department remove the wrist and ankle cuffs. The patient is then transported to the hospital for evaluation. ■

1. An patient may be unruly as a result of:
   a. head injury.
   b. overdose.
   c. hypoglycemia.
   d. all of the above

2. What is the minimum number of people needed to restrain a patient?
   a. 2
   b. 4
   c. 6
   d. 8

3. _____ may result if the patient is restrained face down and develops respiratory distress or arrest.
   a. Positional breathing
   b. Restrained patient arrest
   c. Positional asphyxia
   d. Positional aspiration

CHAPTER 37
Assisting with Childbirth

KEY TERMS

Amniotic sac

Childbirth

Contractions

Crowning

Fontanelles

Oxytocin

Placenta

Trimesters

Umbilical cord

OBJECTIVE

The student will successfully assist the patient with childbirth.

INTRODUCTION

Childbirth is an exciting and rewarding experience. During your career, you may be called upon to assist the delivery process. Remember that pregnancy normally lasts nine months and is divided into three **trimesters.** Labor also is divided into three stages. The first stage begins when **contractions** start and the cervix becomes fully dilated. The second stage ends when the infant is delivered. Finally, the third stage ends with the delivery of the **placenta.**

When contractions begin, they usually last for 30 seconds to 1 minute and occur at 2- to 3-minute intervals. Contractions less than 2 minutes apart are a sign of imminent delivery. Mothers who have delivered previously can usually tell you of imminent birth. These women are commonly straining and have an urge to go to the bathroom. A transport decision will have to be made whether to stay and deliver or to begin rapid transport. The procedure outlined in this chapter is for a normal full-term delivery.

Remember, childbirth is a rewarding experience. It has occurred naturally for thousands years without the aid of EMT-Basics. Your role is to assist as needed. Otherwise, let nature take its course.

▶EQUIPMENT

You will need the following equipment:

▷ BSI equipment
▷ Obstetric kit, which contains the following:

1. Sterile gloves
2. Plastic bag (to store placenta)
3. Umbilical cord clamps or ties
4. Umbilical cord scissors
5. Towels or sheets (to keep delivery area as sterile as possible)
6. Bulb syringe (to suction baby)
7. Sanitary pads (to help control bleeding)
8. Gauze sponges or towels (to dry baby)
9. Baby blanket and hat

If you are lacking some of these items, you can improvise using clean sheets, shoelaces, plastic bags, rubber gloves, and other such items.

ASSESSMENT

To begin your evaluation of the mother, ask the following questions:

▷ What is the due date?
▷ What prenatal care have you received?
▷ Have you had any complications in your pregnancy?
▷ Is this your first pregnancy?
▷ Describe your contractions—how long and how far apart are they?
▷ Have you had any vaginal discharge. If so, what color and how much? Has your water broken?
▷ Do you have the urge to urinate or defecate?
▷ Do you have the urge to push?

The physical examination and questions are personal and private in nature. Be respectful and accommodate the patient's privacy.

You should also take a SAMPLE history and baseline vital signs. Be vigilant for hypertension. Look for signs of **crowning,** that is, the baby's presenting part (usually the head), through the vaginal opening. Contractions can be felt by placing a hand on the patient's abdomen. If contractions are less than 2 minutes apart, prepare for imminent delivery.

PROCEDURE: Assisting with Childbirth

1. Apply BSI precautions.
   Rationale: Significant amounts of body fluids will be present during delivery. Take extreme precautions. Gloves, eye protection, and a gown are required to prevent exposure to infectious disease.

continued...

2. Visualize the vaginal area. Take note of any blood or "bloody show." Remove clothing that obstructs the vaginal opening (Figure 37.1).

3. If possible, clean vaginal area with antiseptic Towlettes™. Wipe in an anterior to posterior motion.

   Rationale: Keeping the area cleaned can reduce the chances that the mother will get an infection.

4. Using sheets, drape delivery area leaving the vaginal opening exposed (Figure 37.2).

5. As the baby's head presents, support the head and apply slight counterpressure. Spread your fingers across the head, avoiding the **fontanelles** (Figure 37.3).

   Rationale: Counterpressure prevents rapid birth, which may cause trauma to the vaginal area. Avoid putting pressure on the infant's face.

6. Make sure the membrane **(amniotic sac)** surrounding the baby has ruptured. If not, gently puncture the sac with your fingers, removing it from the baby's face.

   Rationale: In most cases, the amniotic sac ruptures. If it does not, the infant will be unable to breathe, so rupturing the sac is essential. Use your fingers to rupture the sac and then push it away from the infant's head.

7. Check to make sure the **umbilical cord** is not wrapped around the infant's neck (Figure 37.4).

   Rationale: If the umbilical cord is wrapped around the infant's neck, strangulation could occur.

8. If the umbilical cord is wrapped around the baby's neck, gently remove it. If you cannot free the cord from around the neck, clamp the cord in two places and cut between the clamps.

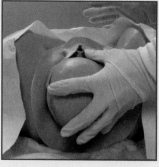

Figure 37.3

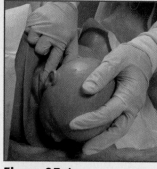

Figure 37.4

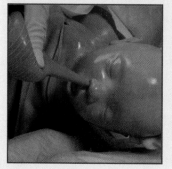

Figure 37.5

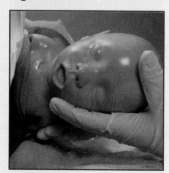

Figure 37.6

9. Once the head has been delivered, quickly suction the baby's mouth then each nostril, cradling the head during the suctioning (Figure 37.5).

   Rationale: Suction should be done as soon as possible. If the infant tries to breathe before the mouth and/or nose are suctioned, aspiration could occur.

10. After the head is delivered, the anterior shoulder comes next. As the anterior shoulder delivers, apply gentle downward pressure.

    Rationale: The slight downward pressure allows for delivery of the posterior shoulder.

11. After the anterior shoulder, the posterior shoulder will deliver. As the posterior shoulder delivers, apply gentle upward pressure (Figure 37.6).

12. Support the trunk and feet as the rest of the infant delivers (Figure 37.7).

    Rationale: Be careful to hold onto the baby. Babies are very slippery!

13. After delivery, dry off the infant and continue to monitor the airway, suctioning as needed. Wrap the infant in blankets to conserve warmth (Figure 37.8).

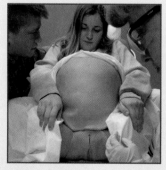

Figure 37.1

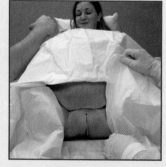

Figure 37.2

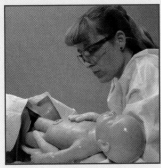

Figure 37.7

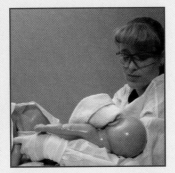

Figure 37.8

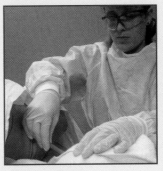

Figure 37.9

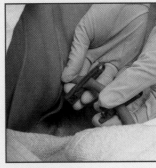

Figure 37.10

Rationale: Infants get very cold very quickly. Drying off the infant reduces heat loss. The airway may need to be constantly suctioned. If the infant does not immediately start to breathe, you must provide ventilations and reassess after 30 seconds. If the infant is not breathing, immediately start respirations.

14. Keep the infant at the same level as the vagina until the umbilical cord stops pulsating (Figure 37.9).

   Rationale: Elevating the infant above the mother's vagina could cause a change in perfusion of the child. Do *NOT* elevate the child until the cord stops pulsating.

15. Once the cord has stopped pulsating, you will need to cut it. Place an umbilical clamp 10 inches from the infant. Place the second clamp about 7 inches from the infant and cut the cord between the two clamps (Figure 37.10).

   Rationale: Cutting the cord removes the infant from being dependent on the mother. After the cord has been clamped, the infant can be moved. Monitor the ends of the cord periodically for any excessive bleeding.

16. Note the time of birth.

17. The mother may want to immediately nurse the baby. This will help control any postpartum bleeding.

   Rationale: The mother produces a hormone during nursing that causes the uterus to contract, reducing bleeding.

18. Placental delivery usually begins several minutes after delivery of the baby. Do not pull or tug on the umbilical cord! The placenta will be expelled on its own.

19. Save the placenta, because the receiving physician will want to examine it.

20. Place one or two sanitary napkins over the vaginal area.

   Rationale: This can reduce some bleeding. It is normal for the mother to have slight tearing in the area between the vaginal opening and the anus.

21. Monitor the mother and infant constantly during transport to the hospital.

22. Document findings.

   Rationale: It is extremely important to document your findings in order to have a history of facts and events that occurred at the scene.

ONGOING ASSESSMENT

Infant:

▷ Immediately assess infant after birth and 5 minutes later.

▷ Monitor breathing, heart rate, crying, movement, and skin color.

▷ Maintain warmth.

▷ If the infant is not breathing after 30 seconds of stimulation, resuscitation will be necessary. The EMT-Basic should focus on these measures:

   1. drying, warming, positioning, suction, and tactile stimulation

   2. oxygen

3. bag-mask ventilation

4. chest compressions, if no pulse or if pulse less than 60

Mother:

▷ Placenta usually delivers several minutes after childbirth.

▷ Keep all afterbirth tissue. The receiving physician will examine it for abnormality.

▷ The mother may continue to bleed vaginally, but usually no more than 500 cc.

▷ If excessive bleeding occurs, sanitary pads may be placed over (not into) the vagina to help control bleeding.

▷ Massaging the uterus through the abdomen stimulates uterine contractions, which stop bleeding.

▷ Nursing the baby also promotes the release of **oxytocin,** a hormone that causes uterine contractions, which stop bleeding.

▷ Monitor for signs and symptoms of hypovolemic shock.

▷ Transport in a position of comfort.

▶PROBLEM SOLVING

Breech Presentation

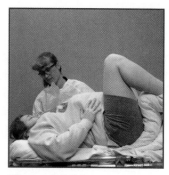

Figure 37.11

▷ Occurs when the baby's buttocks or feet present first instead of the head.

▷ Position mother head-down with pelvis elevated (Figure 37.11).

▷ Support body as delivery progresses.

▷ Provide high-flow oxygen to the mother.

▷ Rapid transport.

Limb Presentation

▷ Instead of head crowning, you may see an arm or leg.

▷ May be associated with a prolapsed cord. If so, follow prolapsed cord procedure.

▷ Position mother head-down with pelvis elevated.

▷ Provide high-flow oxygen to the mother.

▷ Rapid transport.

Prolapsed Cord

▷ Umbilical cord presents first instead of the head.

▷ As delivery progresses, cord will be caught between head and vaginal wall obstructing blood flow to the baby.

▷ Position mother head-down with pelvis elevated.

▷ Cover the exposed cord to maintain warmth.

▷ Insert several fingers into the vagina to keep pressure off umbilical cord.

▷ Provide high-flow oxygen to the mother.

▷ Rapid transport.

Meconium

▶ Meconium is amniotic fluid that is green, yellow, or brown in color. It is an indication of fetal distress.

▶ Suction infant aggressively before stimulation—mouth first, then nose.

▶ Monitor closely and provide resuscitation, if necessary.

Excessive Bleeding

▶ Vaginal bleeding is normal after delivery.

▶ Greater than 500 cc may be considered excessive.

▶ Massaging the uterus may reduce bleeding.

▶ Cup your hand over the uterus; kneading or circular motion seems to work best. The uterus should feel hard like a grapefruit.

▶ If the bleeding does not immediately stop, place the mother in the shock position and transport immediately.

▶CASE STUDY

You are transporting a 24-year-old female who is 34 weeks pregnant. Her contractions are less than 1 minute apart and they are regular. She also has a "bloody show," but there is no vaginal bleeding or crowning. Her airway is patent and respirations are even and unlabored at 16 per minute. Her pulse is 114, strong and regular. The patient states that she has had good prenatal care and that this is her first pregnancy.

While en route, the patient states that she feels as though she has to push. On inspection, you note that the patient is crowning. You immediately explain this to your partner, who pulls the ambulance over and comes into the back of the ambulance to assist in the delivery. As you are coaching the patient to push, the baby is slowly delivered.

After delivering the baby, you note that the baby has good color, is breathing on his own, and does not appear to be in distress. The patient, however, appears to be bleeding more heavily than usual. The patient's bleeding is cause for concern so you advise your partner to continue to the hospital. While en route, you attempt to control the bleeding and focus on keeping the baby warm.■

(continued)

REVIEW QUESTIONS

1. Which stage of labor begins with full dilation and ends with the delivery of the baby?
   a. first stage
   b. second stage
   c. third stage
   d. fourth stage

2. While evaluating your patient for impending delivery, you time the contractions. Delivery is imminent if contractions are:
   a. between 5 and 10 minutes apart.
   b. between 2 and 5 minutes apart.
   c. less than 2 minutes apart.
   d. less than 20 minutes apart.

3. As you assist with the delivery of the baby, you notice the amniotic fluid is greenish-brown in color. You should immediately suction the baby's:
   a. nose then mouth before stimulating the baby to breathe.
   b. nose then mouth after stimulating the baby to breathe.
   c. mouth then nose before stimulating the baby to breathe.
   d. mouth then nose after stimulating the baby to breathe.

SECTION 3
MEDICAL EMERGENCIES

QUESTION BANK

1. The administration site for an epinephrine auto-injector is the:
   - A. lateral lower leg midway between the knee and ankle.
   - B. lateral lower arm midway between the elbow and wrist.
   - C. lateral upper leg midway between the knee and waist.
   - D. lateral upper arm midway between the elbow and shoulder.

2. A medication used in some overdoses to bind with the unwanted substance and prevent or reduce absorption into the body is called:
   - A. nitroglycerin.
   - B. activated charcoal.
   - C. syrup of ipecac.
   - D. epinephrine.

3. What is the minimum number of people needed to restrain a patient?
   - A. 2
   - B. 3
   - C. 4
   - D. 5

4. Oral glucose is indicated for a diabetic patient with:
   - A. hyperglycemia.
   - B. hypoglycemia.
   - C. tachyglycemia.
   - D. bradyglycemia.

5. Which stage of labor goes from the complete dilation of the cervix until delivery of the baby?
   - A. first stage
   - B. second stage
   - C. third stage
   - D. fourth stage

6. The most significant problem associated with nitroglycerin is:
   - A. hypothermia.
   - B. hyperthermia.
   - C. hypotension.
   - D. hypertension.

7. Activated charcoal is indicated in patients who:
   - A. cannot swallow.
   - B. have ingested acids or alkalis.
   - C. are alert and swallow some pills.
   - D. took cyanide.

8. Which of the following is a shockable rhythm recognized by an AED?
   A. ventricular tachycardia
   B. ventricular fibrillation
   C. asystole
   D. both a and b

9. A nebulizer delivers medication by:
   A. topical absorption.
   B. oral ingestion.
   C. aerosolized mist.
   D. auto-injection.

10. While the AED is analyzing rhythms:
    A. compressions must stop but ventilations may continue.
    B. compressions and ventilations may continue.
    C. all patient contact must stop and you must "clear" the patient.
    D. compressions may continue but ventilations must stop.

11. Before administering an MDI, you should be sure the canister is:
    A. at room temperature and not shaken.
    B. at room temperature and shaken for at least 30 seconds.
    C. below room temperature and not shaken.
    D. below room temperature and shaken for at least 30 seconds.

12. What is the single most important link in the "chain of survival" for the adult cardiac arrest patient?
    A. early access
    B. early defibrillation
    C. early CPR
    D. early ALS

13. What liter flow is needed for most nebulizers to properly deliver the medication?
    A. 2 liters per minute
    B. 6 liters per minute
    C. 10 liters per minute
    D. 15 liters per minute

14. _____ occurs when the baby's buttocks or both feet present first.
    A. A limb presentation
    B. A prolapsed presentation
    C. A breech presentation
    D. A meconium presentation

15. All of the following are common bronchodilators *except*:
    A. albuterol (Proventil, Ventolin).
    B. metaproterenol (Metaprel, Alupent).
    C. naproxen (Naprosyn, Aleve).
    D. isoetharine (Bronchosol, Bronkometer).

16. The restrained patient should be secured to the ambulance cot in any of the following positions *except*:
    A. right lateral recumbent.
    B. left lateral recumbent.
    C. prone.
    D. supine.

17. If contractions are less than _____ minutes apart, you should prepare for imminent delivery.
    A. 2
    B. 5
    C. 8
    D. 12

18. Epinephrine causes:
    A. vasoconstriction and bronchiole dilation.
    B. vasoconstriction and bronchiole constriction.
    C. vasodilation and bronchiole dilation.
    D. vasodilation and bronchiole constriction.

19. Oral glucose is normally administered:
    A. under the tongue only.
    B. between the check and gum only.
    C. either between the check and gum or under the tongue.
    D. none of the above

20. Which of the following is not an indication for the administration of nitroglycerin?
    A. The patient complains of chest pain.
    B. The patient's systolic blood pressure is greater than 100.
    C. The patient's systolic blood pressure is less than 100.
    D. Medical direction, a standing medical order, or local protocol allows you to assist the patient with nitroglycerin administration.

SECTION 4
Trauma Emergencies

Trauma is the leading cause of death for persons aged 1 to 44 and the third leading cause of death in all age groups. Traumatic injuries are frightening, disfiguring, and often fatal. Rapid assessment and treatment by EMTs can minimize much of the death and damage caused by trauma in the prehospital setting.

The EMT will use the skills in this section when treating wounds that result from lacerations, punctures, fractures, and spinal injuries. Proper use of splints and spinal immobilization techniques will limit further damage to nerves and blood vessels and prevent potentially life-threatening hemorrhage and paralysis.

Remember that traumatic injuries can be gruesome to look at and, therefore, can distract the EMT from realizing that more serious, but less obvious injuries such as internal hemorrhage or shock have occurred. The EMT must use his assessment skills thoroughly to determine if and when the skills taught in this chapter should be utilized.

CHAPTER 38

Bleeding Control and Shock Management

KEY TERMS

Cravats

Exsanguination

Hemorrhage

Hypotension

Hypovolemic shock

Kling

Military anti-shock trousers
(MAST)

Pneumatic anti-shock
garment (PASG)

Proximal

Roller gauze

Shock management

Tachycardia

OBJECTIVE

The student will successfully control bleeding and administer shock management as needed.

INTRODUCTION

Bleeding is an interruption in circulation caused by blunt or penetrating forces. Insults to circulation should be identified in the initial assessment and management begun immediately if the bleeding is uncontrolled. Extensive bleeding can cause **hypovolemic shock.** Signs of shock include changes in mental status, **tachycardia,** cool and clammy skin, and **hypotension.** Left untreated, **hemorrhage** can lead to **exsanguination,** or bleeding to death.

►EQUIPMENT

You will need the following equipment:

- ► BSI equipment
- ► Absorbent material such as gauze pads for dressing
- ► Bandaging material such as **Kling, roller gauze, cravats,** or elastic bandages
- ► One or more rescuers

ASSESSMENT

Be sure to manage any scene hazards before engaging in this skill. The presence of blood and body fluids is assured on these types of calls, so the use of body substance isolation procedures is imperative.

Additionally, all threats to airway and breathing should be corrected before hemorrhage control is initiated. Once the bleeding is controlled, the physical exam can be completed and vital signs measured. However, providers should not rely on the very late sign of hypotension to determine if their patient is in shock from hemorrhage. Uncontrolled bleeding can be life threatening and should be controlled immediately.

PROCEDURE: Bleeding Control and Shock Management

1. Apply BSI precautions.
   Rationale: Gloves and goggles are required at minimum, and a gown may be necessary if large amounts of blood or fluid are present to prevent exposure to infectious diseases.
2. Expose the bleeding wound if possible.
   Rationale: It is easier to treat a wound that is visible.
3. Apply direct pressure to the wound with a gloved hand or dressing material (Figure 38.1).
   Rationale: Bleeding should be controlled as quickly as possible to prevent further blood loss.

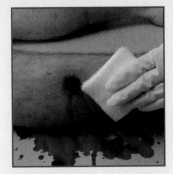   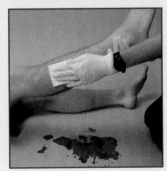

Figure 38.1   **Figure 38.2**

4. Elevate the injury to above the level of the heart (Figure 38.2).
   Rationale: This makes it harder for the heart to pump blood to the affected area.
5. If bleeding persists, apply additional dressing material and continue direct pressure.
   Rationale: Dressings should not be pulled away once placed on the injury site because doing so could dislodge a clot starting to form.

continued...

 PEDIATRIC NOTE:

Remember that blood is frightening to children, and care should be taken to cover a bleeding wound as soon as possible to calm the injured pediatric patient.

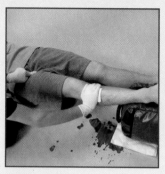

Figure 38.3

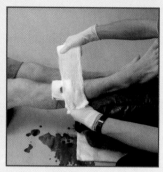

Figure 38.4

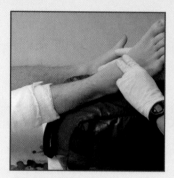

Figure 38.5

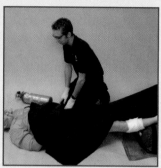

Figure 38.6

6. Locate the arterial pulse **proximal** to the injury site and apply firm pressure (Figure 38.3).

   Rationale: Pressure on the proximal pulse point will occlude blood flow to the injured area, minimizing bleeding from the wound.

7. Bandage the dressing in place with Kling, roller gauze, elastic bandages, triangular bandages, or cravats (Figure 38.4).

   Rationale: Without a bandage to hold the dressing in place, the dressing would fall away, possibly dislodging clots that had successfully formed.

8. Assess distal circulation to ensure the bandage was not applied too tightly (Figure 38.5).

   Rationale: The intent is to control the bleeding, not apply a tourniquet to the area.

9. Position the patient properly and begin transport.

10. Treat for shock if needed. **Shock management** includes administration of high-flow, high-concentration oxygen and prevention of body heat loss (Figure 38.6).

    Rationale: Some bleeding will be severe enough to cause hypotension and signs of shock. Treatment with oxygen and transport is imperative to the survival of the patient.

11. Document findings.

    Rationale: It is extremely important to document your findings in order to have a history of facts and events that occurred at the scene.

 GERIATRIC NOTE:

Elderly patients who have underlying cardiac problems may experience difficulty breathing when they are supine. Despite their hypoperfusion from extensive bleeding, geriatric patients may need to be placed in the semi-Fowler's position.

ONGOING ASSESSMENT

Reassess stable patients every 15 minutes and critical patients every 5 minutes, including vital signs and a physical exam. Be sure to manage all life threats before spending time bandaging wounds. It is inappropriate to carefully bandage a small wound if the patient is not breathing or has other, more serious injuries.

If bleeding persists through your bandage, apply additional dressings and a pressure bandage. Do not remove the soaked material because doing so may break away clots that have begun to form and heal the patient's wound.

▶PROBLEM SOLVING

▶ Bleeding from a neck or chest wound should be controlled with an occlusive dressing that prevents any air from entering the wound site. Occlusive material includes any nonbreathable substance such as petroleum-infused gauze.

▶ Active bleeding will cleanse many wounds. Debridement of the wound is not the responsibility of the EMT, but care should be taken to avoid further contamination.

▶ In the absence of appropriate dressing and bandaging material, any clean cloth will work. Look around you for materials such as sheets, towels, and even clothing.

▶ Some EMS systems allow the use of air splints and **MAST** or **PASG** for hemorrhage control because these devices use circumferential pressure to control bleeding.

▶CASE STUDY

You are called to respond to the local furniture factory where "a person is bleeding profusely." On arrival, the plant foreman meets you and advises you that the victim was using a saw to cut some boards and somehow he lost his balance and his left wrist fell into the saw blade's path. He states the plant's first response team is with him and he thinks that they have the situation under control.

On approaching the patient, you notice that his wrist is bandaged with Kling and there appears to be blood leaking through the bandage. On assessing the patient's ABCs, you note that he is speaking to you and has a patent airway with even and un-labored respirations. His pulse is 118 beats per minute, regular, and weak. One of the first responders states that he has already changed the dressing three times and each time, the bleeding comes through. You ask him how quickly the bleeding is occurring and he states that every time they open the dressing, the wound "shoots blood every-where." You determine that, based on the amount of blood the patient has potentially lost, you should delay no longer and begin transporting him to the emergency de-partment immediately.

While en route to the ambulance, you ask your partner to apply direct pressure to the bandage site. Once in the ambulance you apply a nonrebreather mask at 15 lpm. As soon as you begin transporting, your partner advises you that the wound is again bleeding through the dressing. You ask your partner to maintain direct pressure and to elevate the left arm above the level of the patient's heart while identifying and compressing a pulse pressure site. Your partner elevates the patient's arm and suc-cessfully applies pressure to the pulse point. As you continue transporting the patient, he complains of dizziness. You then have the patient lie flat and elevate his legs. The patient responds by stating that he feels better. You continue transport to the ED.■

(continued)

REVIEW QUESTIONS

1. Signs and symptoms of shock include all of the following *except*:
   a. bradycardia.
   b. altered mental status.
   c. cool, clammy skin.
   d. hypotension.

2. You are applying a dressing and direct pressure to a wound when you notice blood seeping through the dressing. You should:
   a. replace the bloody dressing with a clean one and continue direct pressure.
   b. apply additional dressings and continue direct pressure.
   c. apply additional dressings and apply a tourniquet proximal to the wound.
   d. none of the above

3. All of the following are early signs of shock *except*:
   a. anxiety.
   b. hypotension.
   c. cool, clammy skin.
   d. pale skin.

CHAPTER 39
Dressing and Bandaging

OBJECTIVE

The student will successfully demonstrate how to bandage various types of open wounds.

INTRODUCTION

Injuries that break the skin are considered **open wounds.** In addition to the likelihood of bleeding, open wounds create a risk of infection. All soft tissue injuries should have bleeding controlled and a bandage secured to limit further damage to internal structures such as blood vessels and nerves.

KEY TERMS

Amputation

Avulsion

Bandaging

Circumferential

Debridement

Dressing

Evisceration

Hemorrhage

Impaled object

Occlusive dressing

Open wounds

Pneumothorax

Sutures

▶EQUIPMENT LIST

You will need the following equipment:

▶ Gloves, goggles, mask or gown

▶ Absorbent dressing material such as gauze pads

▶ Bandaging material such as Kling, roller gauze, or elastic bandages

▶ Bulky material for securing **impaled objects**

▶ Occlusive material for neck and chest injuries

▶ Saline for **eviscerations**

▶ Tape

▶ One or more rescuers

ASSESSMENT

Be sure to manage any scene hazards before engaging in this procedure. The presence of blood and body fluids is assured on these types of calls, so the use of body substance isolation procedures is imperative. Additionally, all threats to airway and breathing should be corrected before attempting **hemorrhage** control. Once the bleeding is controlled, the physical exam can be completed and vital signs measured. Following hemorrhage control, **bandaging** can take place. An appropriate bandage is secured to keep dressing materials in place and limit further bleeding and nerve or muscle damage.

PROCEDURE: Dressing and Bandaging

1. Apply BSI precautions.

   Rationale: Gloves and eye protection are required at minimum, and a gown may be necessary if large amounts of blood or fluid are present to prevent exposure to infectious diseases.

2. Expose the wound if possible (Figure 39.1).

   Rationale: It is easier to treat wounds that are visible.

3. Use a bandage of absorbent material to control bleeding. Control bleeding with direct pressure, elevation, pressure **dressings,** and arterial pulse pressure as needed (Figure 39.2).

   Rationale: A bandage should not be placed over a dressing until bleeding has been controlled. Additional dressing material will need to be applied if blood soaks through the original dressing.

4. Secure the dressing in place with a bandage of Kling, roller gauze, elastic bandages, triangular

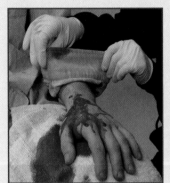
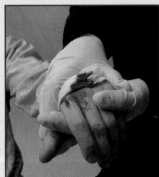

Figure 39.1   **Figure 39.2**

bandages, cravats, or other appropriate material. The bandage should be tight enough to secure the dressing, but not so tight as to compromise distal circulation. Loosen the bandage if circulation is compromised (Figure 39.3).

   Rationale: The objective is to control bleeding and hold the dressing in place, not to impede distal circulation.

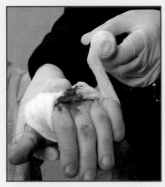

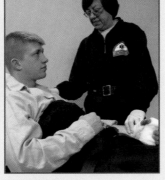

Figure 39.3 **Figure 39.4**

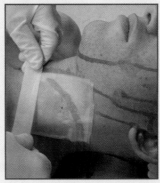

Figure 39.5 **Figure 39.6**

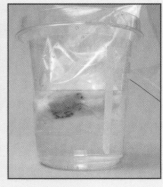

5. Position the patient properly and begin transport (Figure 39.4).

   Rationale: Patients who have been bleeding should be transported to the hospital for evaluation to determine risk of infection and need for **sutures.**

6. Document findings.

   Rationale: It is extremely important to document your findings in order to have a history of facts and events that occurred at the scene.

Figure 39.7

SPECIAL BANDAGING TECHNIQUES

Impaled objects: Do not remove the impaled object, unless it is through the cheek or mouth and is compromising the airway. Use care not to press downward on the object while trying to control bleeding. Have one rescuer stabilize the impaled object while another pads either side of the impalement with bulky dressings such as universal pads, sanitary napkins, roller gauze, or other material. The bulky dressings should hold the impaled object in place. Tape or tie the dressing in place (Figure 39.5).

Eye injuries: If an object is impaled in the eye, use bulky dressings to secure the object in the same fashion as other impaled objects. Fit a disposable paper cup or cone over the injured eye. Use roller gauze to secure the cup, then tape the cup in place. Bandage the uninjured eye as well to limit sympathetic eye movements.

Avulsions: Cleanse the wound surface and fold the skin back to its normal position if possible. Bandage as usual.

Amputations: Wrap completely avulsed or amputated parts in sterile dressing, then bag the part in plastic and label it. Keep the part cool by placing the sealed plastic bag in cool water. The part should not be allowed to get wet or freeze (Figure 39.6).

Neck wounds: Immediately place your gloved hand over the open wound to seal it. This prevents air from entering the neck veins. Replace your gloved hand with an **occlusive dressing.** Apply a dressing over the occlusive dressing. Bandage it in place, taking care to avoid compressing the neck veins and arteries. Be sure to consider the possibility of cervical spine injury based on the mechanism of injury (Figure 39.7).

> **GERIATRIC NOTE:**
>
> Elderly patients can be strongly affected by pressure on the carotid bodies of the neck, and can become hypotensive with stimulation of this area. For this reason, if pressure is to be applied to the neck, lay the patient supine to minimize the risk of syncope.

Open Chest Wounds: Open chest wounds place patients at risk of a **pneumothorax,** which occurs when air enters the pleural space but cannot escape the chest cavity. An occlusive dressing is used to seal the chest so that air cannot enter through the wound. A flutter valve is placed on the dressing to allow air to escape passively or with the assistance of the rescuer. Initially seal the wound with a gloved hand. Replace

continued...

the gloved hand with an occlusive dressing taped only on three sides. Periodically lift the edge of the dressing to allow air to escape the chest cavity (Figure 39.8).

Eviscerations: Place patient supine with legs flexed to release the pressure on the abdominal muscles. Soak a universal or other bulky dressing in sterile saline. Place the moist dressing on the eviscerated organs, and seal with a large occlusive dressing. Maintain warmth of the eviscerated organs by placing towels or a blanket over the abdomen. Secure the bandage in place.

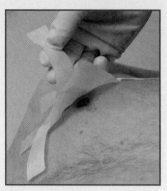

Figure 39.8

ONGOING ASSESSMENT

Reassess stable patients every 15 minutes and critical patients every 5 minutes, including vital signs and a physical exam. Be sure to manage all life threats before spending time bandaging wounds. It is inappropriate to carefully bandage a small wound if the patient is not breathing or has other, more serious injuries. If bleeding persists through your bandage, apply additional dressings and a pressure bandage. Do not remove the soaked material because doing so may break away clots that have begun to form and heal the patient's wound. If reassessment reveals compromised distal circulation, loosen the bandage until distal pulses return or skin color improves.

▶PROBLEM SOLVING

▷ Active bleeding will cleanse many wounds. **Debridement** of the wound is not the responsibility of the EMT, but care should be taken to avoid further contamination.

▷ In the absence of appropriate dressing and bandaging material, any clean cloth can work. Look around you for materials such as sheets, towels, and even clothing.

▷ Some EMS systems allow the use of air splints, MAST or PASG for hemorrhage control because these devices use **circumferential** pressure to control bleeding.

▷ Anytime a wound is cleansed with sterile saline, care must be taken that germs from the rescuer's gloves do not flow into the wound. Additionally, once a container of saline is opened, it is no longer considered sterile.

▷ If distal circulation is impeded by a bandage that is too tight, as evidenced by pain, numbness, tingling or discoloration of the fingers or toes, the bandage should immediately be loosened until distral circulation returns to normal.

►CASE STUDY

You are called to the scene to help a 17-year-old male who reportedly put his hand through a plate glass window. On arrival, the patient is seated next to the window with a towel on his arm. After determining that the patient has an intact airway and no deficits in his breathing or pulse, you move on to the assessment of the patient's arm.

After removing the towel from the patient's arm, you note several lacerations across his forearm. Blood is oozing from the wounds, but no arterial spurting is visualized. Your patient denies any other complaints. As you prepare to bandage the patient's wounds, you ask your partner to obtain a set of vital signs. The vital signs are as follows: Pulse is 110, strong, and regular; respirations are 20, even and unlabored; and his blood pressure is 126 over palp.

You then apply a 5 × 9 dressing to the patient's forearm and wrap it with Kling. After wrapping the extremity, you reassess the radial pulse in that extremity and compare it to the opposite arm. Pulses are strong and equal. You document the patient's vital signs and transport him to the emergency department. ■

(continued)

1. Which of the following should be used on an open neck wound?
   a. a gauze dressing
   b. an occlusive dressing
   c. a gauze dressing covered with an occlusive dressing
   d. an occlusive dressing covered with a gauze dressing

2. Which would NOT be acceptable bandaging material?
   a. paper towels
   b. clean sheet
   c. Kling
   d. roller gauze

3. Your patient was involved in a knife fight and his intestines are protruding through an abdominal wound. You should:
   a. replace the organs and cover the wound with a moist dressing then seal with an occlusive dressing.
   b. replace the organs and cover the wound with an occlusive dressing then seal with a moist dressing.
   c. not replace the organs, but cover the wound with a moist dressing then seal with an occlusive dressing.
   d. not replace the organs, but cover the wound with an occlusive dressing then seal with a moist dressing.

CHAPTER 40
Immobilizing a Long Bone

OBJECTIVE
The student will successfully demonstrate immobilization of an extremity.

INTRODUCTION

Signs of a possible dislocation or fracture of an extremity, such as pain, deformity, crepitus, or swelling, should be treated by **splinting** the **extremity.** Splinting the extremity immobilizes the limb and prevents further damage to soft tissue, nerves, and blood vessels. Effective splints always immobilize the adjacent joints and bone ends. Many types of commercial splinting devices exist, and they are categorized as **rigid, formable,** and **traction splints.** Traction splints are used specifically for femur fractures and will be addressed as a separate skill in Chapter 43.

KEY TERMS
Extremity

Formable splint

Immobilization

Rigid splint

Splinting

Tissue necrosis

Traction splint

▶EQUIPMENT

You will need the following equipment:

- ▶ Rigid or formable splints
- ▶ Cravats, roller bandage, or tape
- ▶ Padding
- ▶ Two or more rescuers

ASSESSMENT

Be sure to manage any scene hazards before engaging in this skill. Additionally, all threats to airway, breathing, or circulation should be managed, and a rapid trauma assessment or focused physical exam completed at this time. Only stable patients with minor or isolated injuries should have individual extremities splinted. Any unstable patient or any patient with life-threatening injuries should have his or her entire body immobilized on a long spine board and be transported without delay.

PROCEDURE: Immobilizing a Long Bone

1. Apply BSI precautions.

   Rationale: Gloves and eye protection are required at minimum, and a gown may be necessary if large amounts of blood or fluid are present to prevent exposure to infectious diseases.

2. Explain the splinting procedure to your patient, gaining her consent to perform the procedure.

   Rationale: Any kind of manipulation of the extremity may be painful. Prepare your patient for this temporary discomfort, assuring her that **immobilization** will minimize pain thereafter and prevent further injury.

3. Utilize a second rescuer to manually stabilize the bones above and below the injury site. If a deformity is present or distal circulation is absent, realign the bone ends until neutral alignment or return of circulation is achieved. Stop realignment if resistance is felt and splint in the position found (Figure 40.1).

   Rationale: Manual stabilization provides the most immediate protection against movement and further injury to unstable bone ends.

4. Assess the patient's sensory, motor, and circulatory status in the extremity prior to immobilization.

   Rationale: Lack of distal circulation is an indication that you need to attempt realignment of the extremity.

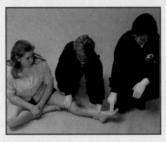

Figure 40.1

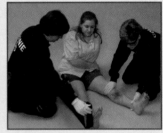

Figure 40.2

5. Measure the splint to several inches beyond both joints above and below the injury site. Measure the device on the opposite extremity if possible to avoid bumping and possibly further injuring the already injured extremity (Figure 40.2).

   Rationale: The splint must be long enough to immobilize adjacent joints in order to properly secure the injured bone.

PEDIATRIC NOTE:

Because the extremities of children are relatively small, nontraditional splinting devices may be utilized effectively. For example, an IV armboard might be used to immobilize a child's arm or infant's leg.

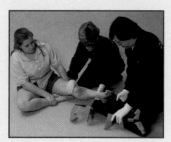

Figure 40.3

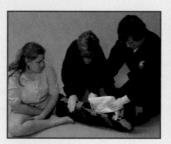

Figure 40.4

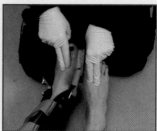

Figure 40.5

6. Lift the extremity while supporting the bone ends. Utilize a second rescuer to position the device on or under the extremity (Figure 40.3).

   Rationale: Support is needed whenever an injured extremity is moved to prevent further manipulation of the bone and additional injury.

7. Pad the splint when necessary. Gauze pads, towels, or other soft items can be used as padding.

   Rationale: Rigid splints need padding to avoid pressure points within the splint. Other splints may need padding in areas where voids exist.

 GERIATRIC NOTE:

Elderly patients are prone to degradation of soft tissue due to deteriorating integumentary systems. Padding is especially important to prevent **tissue necrosis** or pressure ulcers caused by splinting material.

8. Secure the splint in place with cravats, roller bandage, tape, or other fasteners. The device should be secure enough to prevent movement but not constrict distal circulation (Figure 40.4).

   Rationale: If splints are applied too tightly, distal circulation can be impeded and cause further injury to the extremity.

9. Reassess the patient's sensory, motor, and circulatory status noting any changes from your initial assessment (Figure 40.5).

   Rationale: Changes in distal circulation, sensation or movement can indicate that the splint was applied improperly, causing further damage to the injured extremity.

10. Document findings.

    Rationale: It is extremely important to document your findings in order to have a history of facts and events that occurred at the scene.

ONGOING ASSESSMENT

Once secured, and after every time the patient is moved, reassess circulatory, sensory, and motor function in the injured extremity.

▶PROBLEM SOLVING

▷ Assessment of the injured extremity often includes pain, pallor, paresthesia, pulses, and paralysis.

▷ Compound fractures should be covered with a sterile dressing prior to application of the splint to prevent further contamination of the wound. Bone ends should not be pushed back through the skin. However, when the extremity is moved, the bone ends may relocate themselves beneath the skin. Be sure to report this to the emergency department.

▷ A cold pack applied to the injury site may help reduce swelling.

- Rigid splints include wire ladder, cardboard, and padded board splints. The inflexibility of these devices may require padding in the voids to prevent movement of the extremity inside the splint.
- Formable splints can be molded to the position of the extremity and are often good for angulated or deformed extremities. Pillows, the SAM splint, and vacuum splints are considered formable splints.

▶CASE STUDY

You are sitting at your station when a woman approaches and states that she wants you to look at her arms because she just fell off of her bike and has a great deal of pain and difficulty in moving her hands. Your initial assessment reveals no deficits in her ABCs.

She explains to you that she was riding her bike and tried to stop too quickly and, as a result, she fell off of her bike. She tells you that as she began to fall, she stretched her arms forward to break her fall. On assessing her lower arms, you notice that she has gross angulation of both wrists. Fortunately, she has good feeling in her fingers and has a strong radial pulse in both wrists.

The decision is made to transport her to the emergency department. You tell your partner that you want to splint her wrists before you leave. He concurs with your decision and immediately supports her hand and elbow to stabilize the fracture while you immobilize it with the splint. After immobilizing the first fracture, he reassesses the patient's pulse, motor, and sensation (PMS). Her PMS are intact. You now move onto the second fracture and the process is repeated.

After reassessing the PMS on the second extremity, you realize that the patient no longer has a radial pulse. You remove the second splint and apply gentle traction to the patient's hand and ask your partner to assess for the return of the pulse after traction is applied. He states that he can palpate a strong radial pulse and you re-splint the extremity in the new traction position. After splinting this extremity, you again assess the PMS and note a strong radial pulse and good movement and sensation in the fingers. You document your findings and transport the patient to the emergency department. ■

1. Signs and symptoms of a possible musculoskeletal injury may include:
   a. pain.
   b. swelling.
   c. crepitus.
   d. all of the above

2. All of the following are formable splints *except:*
   a. pillows.
   b. a wire ladder splint.
   c. a SAM splint.
   d. a vacuum splint.

3. You should assess your patient's distal pulse, motor, and sensory status:
   a. before immobilizing.
   b. after immobilizing.
   c. before and after immobilizing.
   d. only during the initial assessment.

CHAPTER 41
Joint Immobilization

KEY TERMS

Crepitus

Deformity

Dislocation

Fracture

Swelling

OBJECTIVE

The student will successfully demonstrate immobilization of a suspected joint fracture or dislocation.

INTRODUCTION

Signs of a possible **dislocation** or **fracture** of a joint include pain, **deformity, crepitus,** and **swelling.** Splinting immobilizes the joint and prevents further damage to soft tissue, nerves, and blood vessels. Joint injuries should be treated by splinting the joint in the position found. Adjacent bones will need to be secured in the splinting device to minimze movement of the joint. Many types of commercial splinting devices exist, and they are broadly categorized as rigid, formable, and traction.

▶ EQUIPMENT

You will need the following equipment:

- ▶ Cravats, roller bandage, or tape
- ▶ Padding
- ▶ Two or more rescuers

ASSESSMENT

Be sure to manage any scene hazards before engaging in this skill. Additionally, all threats to airway, breathing, or circulation should be managed, and a rapid trauma assessment or focused physical exam completed at this time. Only stable patients with minor or isolated injuries should have splints applied. Any unstable patient or any patient with life-threatening injuries should have his or her entire body immobilized on a long spine board and be transported without delay.

PROCEDURE: Joint Immobilization

1. Apply BSI precautions.

   Rationale: Gloves and eye protection are required at minimum, and a gown may be necessary if large amounts of blood or fluid are present to prevent exposure to infectious diseases.

2. Explain the splinting procedure to your patient, gaining her consent to perform the procedure.

   Rationale: Any kind of manipulation of the joint may be painful. Prepare your patient for this temporary discomfort, assuring her that immobilization will minimize pain thereafter and prevent further injury.

3. Utilize a second rescuer to manually stabilize the bones adjacent to the injury site. If distal circulation is absent, realign the joint to the correct anatomical position or until return of circulation is achieved (Figure 41.1).

   Rationale: Manual stabilization will provide the most immediate protection against further injury from bone ends moving.

4. Assess the patient's sensory, motor, and circulatory status in the extremity prior to immobilization.

   Rationale: Lack of distal circulation is an indication that you need to attempt realignment of the joint.

5. If there is a pulse deficit, realign the joint following the long axis of the adjoining bones.

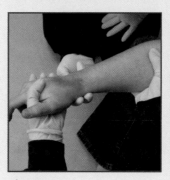

Figure 41.1

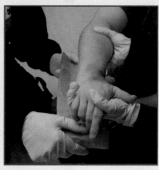

Figure 41.2

> ### PEDIATRIC NOTE:
>
> Small children may not be able to follow the commands typically used by an EMT to assess distal circulation, sensation, and movement. In this case, assess circulation by checking pulses and capillary refill. Assess movement by observing for spontaneous movement or withdrawal from mild painful stimuli.

6. Select appropriate splinting material (Figure 41.2).

   Rationale: Although there is no exact formula for choosing splinting material, some splints are better suited for certain types of injuries. For instance, formable splints and soft padding are usually required for joint injuries, given the precarious positions in which they present to the rescuer.

continued...

7. Provide manual stabilization of the joint while the splinting material is being prepared and placed. Utilize a second rescuer to position the device on or under the extremity.

   Rationale: Manual stabilization prevents further injury from movement of bone ends.

8. Pad the splint when necessary. Gauze pads, towels, or other soft items can be used as padding.

   Rationale: Rigid splints need padding to avoid pressure points within the splint. Other splints may need padding in areas where there are voids, especially around joint angles.

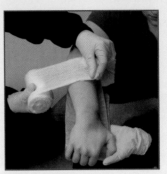
Figure 41.3

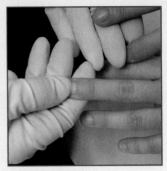
Figure 41.4

 GERIATRIC NOTE:

Elderly patients' tissue breaks down naturally as they age. These changes to the soft tissue will begin to cause tissue necrosis in as few as 20 minutes if a splint is not padded properly to avoid pressure points.

9. Secure the splint in place with cravats, roller bandage, tape, or other fasteners (Figure 41.3).

   Rationale: The device should be secure enough to prevent movement but not constrict distal circulation.

10. Reassess the patient's sensory, motor, and circulatory status, noting any changes from your initial assessment (Figure 41.4).

    Rationale: Any change in distal circulation, sensation, or movement can indicate further injury or improper application of the splint.

11. Document findings.

    Rationale: It is extremely important to document your findings in order to have a history of facts and events that occurred at the scene.

ONGOING ASSESSMENT

Once secured, and after every time the patient is moved, reassess circulatory, sensory, and motor function in the extremity. Reassess often to be sure the splint has not become too tight secondary to any swelling from the injury.

▶ PROBLEM SOLVING

▷ Assessment of the injured extremity often includes pain, pallor, paresthesia, pulses, and paralysis.

▷ Compound fractures should be covered with a sterile dressing prior to application of the splint to prevent further contamination of the wound. Bone ends should not be pushed back through the skin. However, when the extremity is moved, the bone ends may relocate themselves beneath the skin. Be sure to report this to the emergency department.

▷ A cold pack applied to the injury site may help reduce swelling.

- Rigid splints include wire ladder, cardboard, and padded board splints. The inflexibility of these devices may require padding in the voids to prevent movement of the extremity inside the splint.

- Formable splints can be molded to the position of the extremity and are often good for angulated or deformed extremities. Pillows, the SAM splint, and vacuum splints are considered formable splints.

▶CASE STUDY

Your squad has been called to a local school to aid a 16-year-old female who stated that she lost her balance and felt her knee give out after landing wrong while playing volleyball. On inspection, you note the patient's foot to be turned inward and she is unable to flex or extend her knee.

Your partner brings the splint bag to you and you explain to the patient that you will have to remove her shoe to check the pulses in her foot. After explaining the procedure to the patient, your partner manually stabilizes the knee and you remove her shoe. After removing the shoe, you check the patient's pulse, motor, and sensation (PMS). You are unable to find either a pedal or a posterior tibial pulse and the patient is complaining of a loss of sensation in her foot. Your partner continues to stabilize the knee while you apply a splint. After the splint is applied, PMS remain unchanged. You check her pulse at the dorsalis pedis because it is farthest from the injury and receive a pulse. You immediately transport her to the emergency department. ■

(continued)

1. The purpose of splinting is to prevent further damage to:
   a. soft tissues.
   b. blood vessels.
   c. nerves.
   d. all of the above

2. All of the following are rigid splints *except*:
   a. cardboard splints.
   b. wire ladder splints.
   c. SAM splints.
   d. padded board splints.

3. Checking capillary refill to evaluate distal circulation is a reliable method in all of the following patients *except* a:
   a. 6-year-old who injured her leg while roller skating.
   b. 5-year-old who fell off the jungle gym at school.
   c. 34-year-old who fell off a ladder, injuring his arm and leg.
   d. 3-year-old who was involved in a motor vehicle crash.

CHAPTER 42
Sling and Swathe Immobilization

OBJECTIVE
The student will successfully demonstrate immobilization of the shoulder girdle using a sling and swathe device.

INTRODUCTION

Signs of a possible dislocation or fracture of the bones of the **shoulder girdle,** including the **humerus, clavicle,** and **scapula,** include pain, deformity, crepitus, swelling, and a "dropped" appearance of the injured shoulder. A suspected shoulder injury should not be **reduced,** but should be treated by splinting with a **sling and swathe.** Splinting all bones of the shoulder girdle immobilizes the bones and joints, limits anterior/posterior movement, and prevents further damage to soft tissue, nerves, and blood vessels.

KEY TERMS
Clavicle

Humerus

Reduced

Scapula

Shoulder girdle

Sling and swathe

▶EQUIPMENT

You will need the following equipment:

- ▶ Two triangular bandages or cravats
- ▶ Padding
- ▶ Two or more rescuers

ASSESSMENT

Be sure to manage any scene hazards before engaging in this skill. Additionally, all threats to airway, breathing, or circulation should be managed, and a rapid trauma assessment or focused physical exam completed at this time. Only stable patients with minor or isolated injuries should have individual extremities splinted. Any unstable patient or any patient with life-threatening injuries should have his or her entire body immobilized on a long spine board and be transported without delay.

PROCEDURE: Sling and Swathe Immobilization

1. Apply BSI precautions.

   Rationale: Gloves and eye protection are required at minimum, and a gown may be necessary if large amounts of blood or fluid are present to prevent exposure to infectious diseases.

2. Explain the splinting procedure to your patient, gaining her consent to perform the procedure.

   Rationale: Any kind of manipulation of the shoulder girdle may be painful. Prepare your patient for this temporary discomfort, assuring her that immobilization will minimize pain thereafter and prevent further injury.

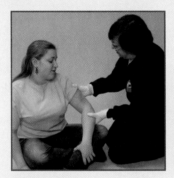 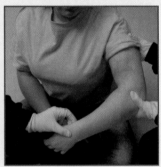

Figure 42.1   **Figure 42.2**

 PEDIATRIC NOTE:

Children are likely to be especially frightened by an extremity injury. Take an extra moment to prepare them for the pain they may experience, assuring them it is only temporary.

3. Utilize a second rescuer to manually stabilize the bones above and below the injury site. If deformity is present or distal circulation is absent, realign the bone ends until neutral alignment or return of circulation is achieved. Stop realignment if resistance is felt and splint in the position found (Figure 42.1).

   Rationale: Manual stabilization is the quickest way to prevent further movement of the bone ends.

4. Assess the patient's sensory, motor, and circulatory status in the extremity prior to immobilization (Figure 42.2).

   Rationale: Lack of distal circulation is an indication that you need to attempt realignment of the extremity.

5. Position the sling across the patient's chest, aligning the top corner at the uninjured shoulder and the other sling corner at the hip on the

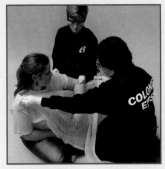
Figure 42.3

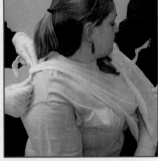
Figure 42.4

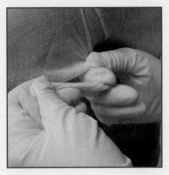
Figure 42.5

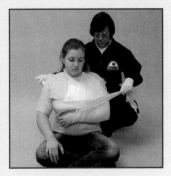
Figure 42.6

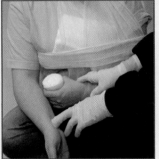
Figure 42.7

injured side. Lie the patient's injured arm across the sling and chest (Figure 42.3).

Rationale: The sling reduces gravity's painful effects on the injured shoulder joint.

 PEDIATRIC NOTE:

Triangular bandages come as a standard size, and may be too large for a child's small shoulder. The bandages can simply be folded in half to create a smaller triangle, or cut along the long edge of the triangle to make a bandage half the original size.

6. Draw up the end of the triangular bandage that was at the hip on the injured side. Bring the end around and behind the patient's neck. Draw up the ends of the bandage until the patient's hand is several inches above the level of the elbow. Tie the two ends of the triangular bandage in a knot (Figure 42.4).

Rationale: Keeping the hand several inches above the elbow will reduce strain on the joint, minimizing pain.

7. Reassess the patient's sensory, motor, and circulatory status, noting any changes from your initial assessment.

Rationale: It is important to ensure that the splint has helped, not hurt, the patient in any way.

8. Draw up, twist, or pin the excess fabric at the elbow to make a pocket for the elbow (Figure 42.5).

Rationale: Twisting up the extra fabric prevents the patient from catching it on something, possibly causing further injury and pain.

9. A swathe is made with another triangular bandage tied around the injured arm and chest of the patient. Do not include the uninjured arm in the swathe (Figure 42.6).

Rationale: The swathe further minimizes movement of the shoulder girdle and upper extremity.

10. Reassess the patient's sensory, motor, and circulatory status, noting any changes from your initial assessment (Figure 42.7).

11. Document findings.

Rationale: It is extremely important to document your findings in order to have a history of facts and events that occurred at the scene.

ONGOING ASSESSMENT

Once secured, and after every time the patient is moved, reassess circulatory, sensory, and motor function in the extremity. Avoid covering the fingertips of the patient within the sling to facilitate the reassessment of distal circulation, sensation, and movement.

▶PROBLEM SOLVING

▷ Assessment of the injured extremity often includes pain, pallor, paresthesia, pulses, and paralysis.

▷ A cold pack applied to the injury site may help reduce swelling.

▷ If a second triangular bandage is unavailable, tape or cravats could be used to secure the arm in a sling to the torso.

▷ A small pillow or other padding laid across the chest will give comfort to some shoulder girdle injuries.

▷ Patients with suspected spinal injuries should not have a sling tied around the neck.

▷ Fractures of the humerus alone can also be immobilized with a sling and swathe. Proximal fractures are treated exactly like the immobilization procedure for the shoulder girdle injury. However, fractures of the distal end of the humerus are drawn up level with the elbow, not several inches above.

▷ Compound fractures should be covered with a sterile dressing prior to application of the splint to prevent further contamination of the wound. Bone ends should not be pushed back through the skin. However, when the extremity is moved, the bone ends may relocate themselves beneath the skin. Be sure to report this to the emergency department.

▶CASE STUDY

Your squad is dispatched to help a 19-year-old male who is complaining of pain in his left shoulder after diving into the water. The patient states that he has a dislocated shoulder and has had this injury occur several times in the past. He is standing upright with a noticeable drop in his left shoulder. He states that movement of his arm causes him an extreme amount of pain.

You make the decision to immobilize his extremity using a sling and swathe. After determining that the patient has intact pulses distal to the injury, you decide to move forward with the splinting. The patient's arm is moved into a 90-degree angle and the sling is placed under his arm and secured in place. After applying the sling, a swathe is applied across the patient's chest and the patient is assessed for pain response and pulse, motor, and sensory response.

The patient is transported to the emergency department in an upright position on the cot. On arrival at the ED, care is turned over to the charge nurse.■

1. All of the following are signs and symptoms of a dislocated shoulder *except:*
   a. pain.
   b. "raised" appearance.
   c. deformity.
   d. swelling.

2. Your patient has a possible fracture to the distal end of the humerus. You should immobilize the lower arm:
   a. several inches above the elbow.
   b. at the same level as the elbow.
   c. several inches below the elbow.
   d. either above, below, or at the same level as the elbow.

3. Used in conjunction with a sling, the swathe helps immobilize the extremity by limiting:
   a. distal/proximal movement.
   b. superior/inferior movement.
   c. anterior/posterior movement.
   d. none of the above

CHAPTER 43

Applying a HARE Traction Splint

KEY TERMS

Ankle hitch

Ischial strap

Ischium

HARE traction splint

Manual traction

Midshaft femur

Vascular compromise

OBJECTIVE

The student will successfully demonstrate immobilization of a femur using correct application of the HARE traction splint.

INTRODUCTION

Signs of a possible dislocation or fracture of an extremity, such as pain, deformity, crepitus, and swelling, should be treated by splinting the extremity. Splinting the extremity immobilizes the limb and prevents further damage to soft tissue, nerves, and blood vessels. Effective splints always immobilize the adjacent joints and bone ends. Many types of commercial splinting devices exist, and they are categorized as rigid, formable, and traction. Traction splints are used specifically for **midshaft femur** fractures. The traction splint is contraindicated for fractures involving the knee or hip joints.

▶ EQUIPMENT

You will need the following equipment:

- ▶ **HARE traction splint**
- ▶ **Ankle hitch**
- ▶ Splint straps or cravats
- ▶ Long spine board
- ▶ Two or more rescuers

ASSESSMENT

Be sure to manage any scene hazards before engaging in this skill. Additionally, all threats to airway, breathing, or circulation should be managed, and a rapid trauma assessment or focused physical exam completed at this time. Because the femur fracture can cause life-threatening blood loss, it is considered a serious injury. Proper immobilization with a traction splint can reduce the incidence of further **vascular compromise** or nerve damage. However, any unstable patient or any patient with threats to airway, breathing, or circulation should have his or her entire body immobilized on a long spine board and be transported without delay.

 GERIATRIC NOTE:

Pelvic injuries are common in the elderly, but because they involve either the pelvic bones themselves or the proximal head of the femur, hip injuries should not be splinted using a traction splint. Only midshaft femur fractures should be splinted with traction splints.

 PROCEDURE: Applying a HARE Traction Splint

1. Apply BSI precautions.

   Rationale: Gloves and eye protection are required at minimum, and a gown may be necessary if large amounts of blood or fluid are present to prevent exposure to infectious diseases.

2. Explain the splinting procedure to your patient, gaining her consent to perform the procedure.

   Rationale: Any kind of manipulation of the extremity may be painful. Prepare your patient for this temporary discomfort, assuring her that immobilization will minimize pain thereafter and prevent further injury. Many patients report feeling much better after traction is applied to a femur fracture.

3. Utilize a second rescuer to manually stabilize the bones above and below the injury site. If deformity is present or distal circulation is absent,

   realign the bone ends until neutral alignment or return of circulation is achieved.

   Rationale: Manual stabilization is the most efficient way to prevent any further manipulation of the bone ends.

4. Direct another rescuer to apply **manual traction** to the extremity by pulling gently on the ankle in line with the body (Figure 43.1).

   Rationale: Manual traction will provide immediate relief to the patient as the bone ends realign.

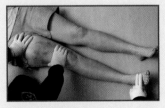

Figure 43.1

continued...

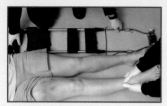
Figure 43.2

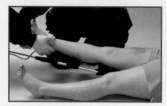
Figure 43.3

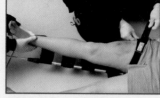
Figure 43.4

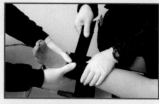
Figure 43.5

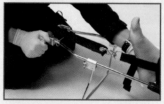
Figure 43.6

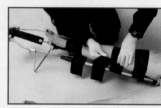
Figure 43.7

5. Assess the patient's sensory, motor, and circulatory status in the extremity prior to immobilization (Figure 43.1).

   Rationale: Lack of distal circulation is an indication that you need to attempt realignment of the extremity.

6. Place the HARE traction splint at the level of the **ischium** and measure the splint to 8 to 10 inches beyond the foot. Measure the device on the opposite extremity if possible (Figure 43.2).

   Rationale: Measuring the splint on the opposite extremity will prevent bumping the leg and possibly further injuring the already injured extremity.

 PEDIATRIC NOTE:

   An adult HARE should not be used for pediatric patients. A specialized, smaller HARE exists for children.

7. Position the splint in line with the injured leg. Have the rescuers who are holding manual stabilization and traction lift the extremity while you place the splint under the injured leg. Lay the leg down onto the splint, while maintaining the previously established traction (Figure 43.3).

   Rationale: Proper positioning requires that the splint be adjusted high into the pelvis until it meets the ischium.

8. Apply the proximal securing device, or **ischial strap** (Figure 43.4).

   Rationale: This strap will keep the splint in place when traction is applied at the opposite end.

9. Apply the distal securing device or ankle hitch. Remove the sock if one is present to prevent the ankle hitch from moving (Figure 43.5).

   Rationale: The ankle hitch is the device to which mechanical traction is applied.

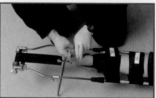
Figure 43.8

10. Apply mechanical traction using the hand crank on the device until relief is felt (Figure 43.6).

    Rationale: Mechanical traction can be secured for long periods of time, whereas manual traction is reduced or changed given the fatigue of the rescuer.

11. Secure the device, using the straps provided, on the proximal and distal lower extremity. Do not place straps over the injury site (Figure 43.7).

    Rationale: The straps should hold the splint in place while still allowing assessment of the injury.

12. Reassess the patient's sensory, motor, and circulatory status, noting any changes from your initial assessment (Figure 43.8).

    Rationale: Traction splinting causes significant manipulation of the bone ends. Reassessment of PMS (pulses, motor function, and sensation) will ensure that the splint has improved circulation, rather than impeded it.

13. Move and secure patient to a long spine board for transport.

    Rationale: Placing a patient on a long spine board assists in moving the patient while maintaining immobilization of the extremity.

14. Document findings.

    Rationale: It is extremely important to document your findings in order to have a history of facts and events that occurred at the scene.

Once secured, and after every time the patient is moved, reassess circulatory, sensory, and motor function in the extremity. It is important to maintain traction once it is applied. Additional traction may be necessary after re-evaluation because the quadriceps muscles may have begun to relax. Watch for hemorrhage from the femoral artery, which could cause noticeable bruising and swelling of the femur or thigh.

▶ PROBLEM SOLVING

▶ Assessment of the injured extremity often includes pain, pallor, paresthesia, pulses, and paralysis.

▶ Compound fractures should be covered with a sterile dressing prior to application of the splint to prevent further contamination of the wound. Bone ends should not be pushed back through the skin. However, when the extremity is moved, the bone ends may relocate themselves beneath the skin. Be sure to report this to the emergency department.

▶ A cold pack applied to the injury site may help reduce swelling.

▶ If the ankle hitch is lost, fasten one out of cravats or roller gauze.

▶ Hemorrhage from the femoral artery is possible and could cause noticeable bruising and swelling of the femur or thigh.

▶ CASE STUDY

You respond to the scene of a single-car collision at which a 25-year-old female is complaining of left upper leg pain. She is awake, alert, and oriented. The patient states that she was leaning down to change her CD and lost control of her vehicle. The vehicle has a small amount of damage to the front driver's side quarter panel. The patient tells you that she can remember all aspects of the accident.

First responders have obtained vital signs as follows: Pulse is 118, strong and regular; respirations are 22, even and unlabored; and her blood pressure is 106/70. Upon further assessment of the patient, aside from the left leg injury, she has no other injuries and no other complaints. Your assessment reveals gross deformity of the patient's left femur. Pulse, motor, and sensory exams are intact in the patient's left foot.

The first responders successfully extricate the patient to a long spine board without event. Once on the spine board, the patient is transferred to the ambulance. Once in the ambulance, the patient's leg and distal neurovascular status are reassessed. The patient's pulse is very weak compared to your initial exam. You decide to apply a HARE traction splint. You ask your partner to take manual control of the patient's lower extremity as you fit her to the splint. After manual control is achieved, you apply the traction splint. After applying the splint, you reassess the patient's pulse, motor, and sensory response. The patient's pulse is stronger and she still has good movement and sensation in her left leg and foot. ■

(continued)

1. Traction splints are only used for:
   a. dislocations of the knee.
   b. fractures of the hip.
   c. dislocations of the hip.
   d. fractures of the midshaft femur.

2. Signs and symptoms often associated with an extremity injury include:
   a. pain.
   b. paralysis.
   c. paresthesia.
   d. all of the above

3. When using the HARE traction splint, how do you know when enough mechanical traction has been applied?
   a. You have applied traction equivalent to 10 percent of the patient's body weight.
   b. The patient's pain is relieved.
   c. The bone ends realign.
   d. The patient's injured leg is as long as the uninjured leg.

CHAPTER 44

Applying a Sager Traction Splint

OBJECTIVE

The student will successfully demonstrate immobilization of a femur using correct application of the Sager traction splint.

KEY TERMS

Ischium

Manual traction

Midshaft femur

Sager traction splint

INTRODUCTION

Signs of a possible dislocation or fracture of an extremity, such as pain, deformity, crepitus, and swelling, should be treated by splinting the extremity. Splinting the extremity immobilizes the limb and prevents further damage to soft tissue, nerves, and blood vessels. Effective splints always immobilize the adjacent joints and bone ends. Many types of commercial splinting devices exist, and they are categorized as rigid, formable, and traction. Traction splints are used specifically for **midshaft femur** fractures. The traction splint is contraindicated for fractures involving the knee or hip joints.

►EQUIPMENT

You will need the following equipment:

- ► **Sager traction splint**
- ► Splint straps or cravats
- ► Long spine board
- ► Two or more rescuers

ASSESSMENT

Be sure to manage any scene hazards before engaging in this skill. Additionally, all threats to airway, breathing, or circulation should be managed, and a rapid trauma assessment or focused physical exam completed at this time. Because the femur fracture can cause life-threatening blood loss, it is considered a serious injury. Proper immobilization with a traction splint can reduce the incidence of further vascular compromise or nerve damage. However, any unstable patient or any patient with threats to airway, breathing, or circulation should have his or her entire body immobilized on a long spine board and be transported without delay.

> **GERIATRIC NOTE:**
>
> Hip fractures and dislocations are common injuries in the elderly population. These injuries involve either the bones of the pelvis or the proximal head of the femur. Therefore, Sager traction splints are usually not indicated in the elderly patient with a hip injury.

PROCEDURE: Applying a Sager Traction Splint

1. Apply BSI precautions.

    Rationale: Gloves and eye protection are required at minimum, and a gown may be necessary if large amounts of blood or fluid are present to prevent exposure to infectious diseases.

2. Explain the splinting procedure to your patient, gaining his consent to perform the procedure. Next, expose the injury site.

    Rationale: Any kind of manipulation of the extremity may be painful. Prepare your patient for this temporary discomfort, assuring him that immobilization will minimize pain thereafter and prevent further injury. Many patients report feeling much better after traction is applied to a femur fracture (Figure 44.1).

3. Utilize a second rescuer to manually stabilize the bones above and below the injury site. If deformity is present or distal circulation is absent,

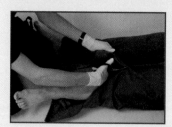

Figure 44.1

realign the bone ends until neutral alignment or return of circulation is achieved.

Rationale: Manual stabilization is the most efficient way to prevent any further manipulation of the bone ends.

4. Direct another rescuer to apply **manual traction** to the extremity by pulling gently on the ankle in line with the body (Figure 44.2).

    Rationale: Manual traction will provide immediate relief to the patient as the bone ends realign.

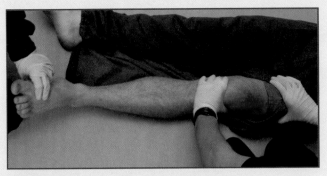
Figure 44.2

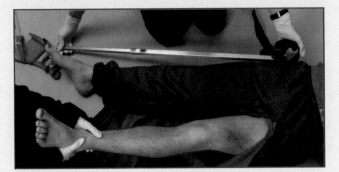
Figure 44.3

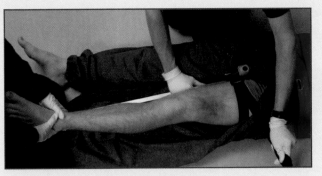
Figure 44.4

9. Apply the distal securing device or ankle hitch. Remove the sock if one is present to prevent the ankle hitch from moving (Figure 44.5).

   Rationale: The ankle hitch is the device to which mechanical traction is applied.

10. Apply mechanical traction by pulling on the distal end of the device until relief is felt or you have applied traction equivalent to 10 percent of the patient's body weight (Figure 44.6).

    Rationale: This formula provides enough traction to realign the bone ends without causing further separation.

5. Assess the patient's sensory, motor, and circulatory status in the extremity prior to immobilization (Figure 44.2).

   Rationale: Lack of distal circulation is an indication that you need to attempt realignment of the extremity.

6. Place the Sager traction splint at the level of the **ischium** and measure the splint to 8 to 10 inches beyond the foot. Measure the device on the opposite extremity if possible (Figure 44.3).

   Rationale: Measuring the splint on the opposite extremity will prevent bumping the leg and possibly further injuring the already injured extremity.

> **PEDIATRIC NOTE:**
>
> The standard size Sager is not appropriate for most children. Pediatric sized splints will be required.

7. Position the splint in-line with the injured leg.

   Rationale: Proper positioning requires that the splint be adjusted high into the pelvis until it meets the ischium.

8. Apply the proximal securing device, or ischial strap (Figure 44.4).

   Rationale: This strap will keep the splint in place when traction is applied at the opposite end.

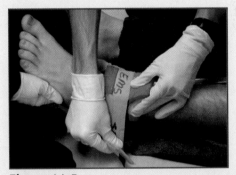
Figure 44.5

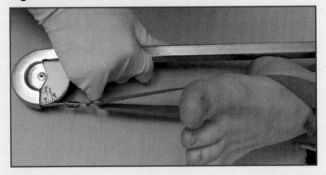
Figure 44.6

continued...

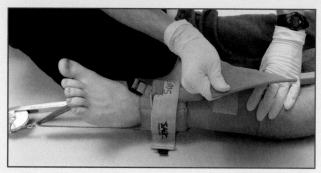

Figure 44.7

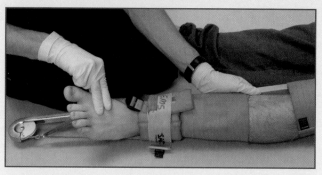

Figure 44.8

11. Secure the device, using the straps provided, on the proximal and distal lower extremity (Figure 44.7). The legs may then be tied together to further immobilize the leg.

Rationale: Securing the legs will prevent the splint from moving.

12. Reassess the patient's sensory, motor, and circulatory status, noting any changes from your initial assessment (Figure 44.8).

Rationale: Ensure the splinting procedure has improved, not damaged, the patient's distal PMS.

13. Move and secure patient to a long spine board for transport. Be sure the splint itself is secured to the board to prevent movement and further injury during transport.

14. Document findings.

Rationale: It is extremely important to document your findings in order to have a history of facts and events that occurred at the scene.

ONGOING ASSESSMENT

Once secured, and after every time the patient is moved, reassess circulatory, sensory, and motor function in the extremity. It is important to maintain traction once it is applied. Additional traction may be necessary after re-evaluation because the quadriceps muscles may have begun to relax. Additionally, hemorrhage from the femoral artery is possible and could cause noticeable bruising and swelling of the femur or thigh.

▶ PROBLEM SOLVING

▷ Assessment of the injured extremity often includes pain, pallor, paresthesia, pulses, and paralysis.

▷ Compound fractures should be covered with a sterile dressing prior to application of the splint to prevent further contamination of the wound. Bone ends should not be pushed back through the skin. However, when the extremity is moved, the bone ends may relocate themselves beneath the skin. Be sure to report this to the emergency department.

▷ A cold pack applied to the injury site may help reduce swelling.

►CASE STUDY

You respond to a call for assistance with a 28-year-old restrained female driver who was reported as unconscious on the arrival of the police officers. On your arrival, the patient is awake, alert, and oriented and states that she cannot feel anything from the waist down. The patient states that she is not sure how the collision occurred and does not know what is wrong with her. The vehicle has extensive front-end damage.

First responders have obtained vital signs and they are as follows: Pulse is 128, strong and regular; respirations are 16, even and unlabored; and her blood pressure is 100/68. Upon further assessment of the patient, you note that in addition to her right leg injury, she also has a large laceration on her forehead as well as some bruising on her chest. Your partner bandages her head and advises you that her chest is stable and that there are no open wounds on her chest. Assessment of the patient's right femur reveals gross deformity. Pulse in the right foot is absent and the patient still has no sensation below her waist.

The patient is extricated to a long spine board without event. Once on the spine board, the patient is transferred to the ambulance. Once in the ambulance, the patient's leg and distal neurovascular status are reassessed. The patient's pulse is still absent and she still has no sensation from the waist down. You decide to apply your Sager traction splint. After you fit her to the splint, you apply the traction splint. After applying the splint, you reassess the patient's pulse, motor, and sensory response. You regain a pedal pulse but there is no change in the patient's ability to move her lower extremities or feel anything. You transport her to the ED.■

(continued)

1. Your patient was hit by a car and has an obvious open fracture to her left, mid-femoral shaft. She is bleeding profusely and has a rapid pulse, rapid respirations, and a low blood pressure. You should support:

    a. the airway and breathing, control bleeding, apply a traction splint, immobilize to a long board, and provide rapid transport.

    b. the airway and breathing, control bleeding, immobilize to a long board, and provide rapid transport.

    c. the airway and breathing, apply a traction splint, immobilize to a long board, and provide rapid transport.

    d. the airway and breathing, immobilize to a long board, and provide rapid transport.

2. To help reduce swelling, you should:

    a. apply a hot pack to the injury site.

    b. apply a cold pack to the injury site.

    c. do not apply a hot or cold pack to the injury site.

    d. apply a hot pack for the first 30 minutes, then a cold pack.

3. When using a Sager traction splint, how do you know when enough mechanical traction has been applied?

    a. You have applied traction equivalent to 10 percent of the patient's body weight.

    b. The patient's pain is relieved.

    c. The bone ends realign.

    d. The patient's injured leg is as long as the uninjured leg.

CHAPTER 45
Applying a Cervical Collar

OBJECTIVE

The student will successfully demonstrate application of a properly sized cervical collar.

INTRODUCTION

Spinal immobilization should be considered any time the patient has sustained an injury of significant mechanism; is complaining of head, neck, or back pain; has a penetrating injury, laceration, or contusion to the head or scalp; has an altered level of consciousness; or is unconscious for unknown reasons. Spinal immobilization begins with manual immobilization of the cervical spine and continues with application of a **cervical collar** and some form of cervical immobilization device. The cervical collar supports the head and neck, maintains neutral alignment of the cervical spine, and reminds the patient to keep from moving his or her head and neck. Spinal immobilization is not complete until the patient is secured to a spine board, with a cervical collar and cervical immobilization device in place.

▶EQUIPMENT

You will need the following equipment:

▶ Cervical collar

▶ Two rescuers

ASSESSMENT

Be sure to manage any scene hazards before engaging in this skill. Additionally, all threats to airway, breathing, or circulation should be managed concurrently or prior to application of the cervical collar. The neck and throat should be examined prior to application of the collar because **inspection** and **palpation** are difficult once the collar is in place. Whenever possible, apply the cervical collar prior to moving the patient onto a spine board because the collar provides support for the cervical vertebrae during lifting and moving of the patient.

PROCEDURE: Applying a Cervical Collar

1. Apply BSI precautions.

   Rationale: Gloves and eye protection are required at minimum, and a gown may be necessary if large amounts of blood or fluid are present to prevent exposure to infectious diseases.

2. Approach the patient from his front side, introduce yourself, and instruct him not to move (Figure 45.1).

   Rationale: Approaching from the front minimizes the likelihood that your patient will turn his head to view you, compromising his neck and spine.

3. Have the second rescuer hold manual cervical stabilization with one hand on either side of the patient's head and neck (Figure 45.2).

   Rationale: Manual stabilization provides immediate neutral alignment of the spine.

 GERIATRIC NOTE:

Manual and mechanical stabilization should keep the patient's head and neck in a neutral position. Elderly patients often suffer from kyphosis and degenerative changes in the spine that may cause them to hunch forward. Rescuers should hold the head of the elderly patient in place without forcing the head into a position that is unnatural for the patient.

4. Explain the need for and steps involved in application of the cervical collar to the patient, gaining his consent to perform the procedure.

   Rationale: Cervical collar application can be uncomfortable.

5. Evaluate circulation, sensation, and movement in all extremities. Do this by palpating radial and pedal pulses and by assessing grip strength and flexion, extension of the feet, and perceived sensation while touching the patient's extremities (Figure 45.3).

   Rationale: It is important to establish a baseline pulse, motor, and sensory (PMS) level in potentially spine-injured patients because any change in this level can indicate serious spinal injury and possible permanent disability.

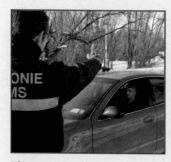

Figure 45.1

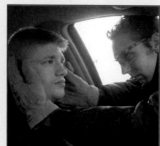

Figure 45.2

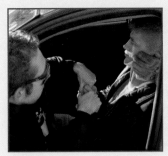

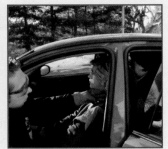

Figure 45.3   **Figure 45.4**

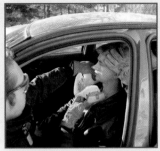

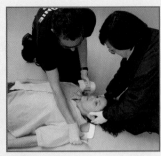

Figure 45.5   **Figure 45.6**

6. Determine the proper size of cervical collar needed by measuring the distance between the trapezius muscle and angle of the jaw. Use your finger width as a guide. Correlate this distance to the distance on the cervical collar between the bottom of the rigid plastic and the sizing post (Figure 45.4).

   Rationale: Improperly sized cervical collars can occlude the airway, causing aspiration.

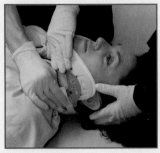

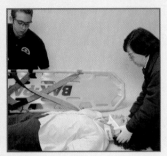

Figure 45.7   **Figure 45.8**

 PEDIATRIC NOTES:

   Children will not fit into adult cervical collars. Collars that are too large will force the neck into a hyperextended position. Pediatric cervical collars should be used, when available. If properly sized equipment is not available, then blanket or towel rolls should be used in lieu of a collar.

7. Place the collar around the neck and secure in place. The collar should rest on the clavicles and mandible of the patient. For seated patients, slide the collar up the sternum until it is in position under the jaw. Then, wrap the collar around the back of the neck, securing it in place (Figure 45.5).

   For supine patients, first slide the back of the collar in place under the patient's head and neck. Then, wrap the front of the collar around until it sits in place (Figure 45.6).

   Rationale: These methods avoid pulling the hair.

8. Ensure the collar is fitted and applied properly (Figure 45.7).

   Rationale: The collar should not hyperextend the neck or fit so snugly that it constricts the airway or impedes breathing.

9. Maintain manual cervical stabilization until the patient is secured to a spine board (Figure 45.8).

   Rationale: Cervical collars merely minimize movement of the head and neck; they do not prevent it. Manual stabilization is required to fully prevent movement of the head and neck.

10. Reassess the patient's circulation, sensation, and movement in all four extremities, noting any changes from your initial assessment.

   Rationale: Changes can indicate a significant spinal injury and even permanent disability.

11. Move the patient to a spine board for further movement or transport. Movement of the head can be further minimized by placing head blocks or towel rolls on either side of the head before taping the head to the board.

   Rationale: Padding around the head takes up the voids and stabilizes the head on the spine board.

12. Document findings.

   Rationale: It is extremely important to document your findings in order to have a history of the facts and events that occurred at the scene.

ONGOING ASSESSMENT

Once immobilized, and after every time the patient is moved, reassess circulatory, sensory, and motor function (CSM) in all four extremities. Additionally, document any changes in mental status. CSM compromise is a significant finding in the spine-injured patient and can indicate permanent disability.

Be aware of the patient's breathing and airway status. Your spinal immobilized patient will not be able to sit up to cough or vomit. Should your patient need to vomit, roll him or her to the side and have suction ready to prevent aspiration of stomach contents.

►PROBLEM SOLVING

► As soon as you identify that a patient has head, neck, or back pain or other trauma; has an altered mental status, is unconscious, is intoxicated; or has suffered a significant mechanism of injury, the spine should immediately be manually immobilized without any further manipulation.

► Earrings, necklaces, hoods, and collars may need to be removed before application of the cervical collar to prevent further injury and ensure neutral alignment can be achieved.

► Do not include the soft foam in your finger-width measurement of the collar. The foam provides no support and will compress when in place around the patient's neck.

► Avoid catching the patient's hair in the adhesive of the collar. Lift the hair out of the way during application of the collar.

►CASE STUDY

Miss Emily, a favorite elderly neighbor, had gotten up during the night and gone into the kitchen for a glass of water. As she approached the sink, she stumbled on a throw rug and fell toward the cabinet, striking her chin violently on the countertop as she fell to the floor. Dazed and confused, she got up and made her way back to the bedroom.

Her nephew arrives early the next morning and finds her in bed complaining of severe neck pain, tingling in her shoulders and arms, and difficulty moving her upper extremities. He notices a bruise on her chin and calls 911.

During the initial assessment, EMS personnel recognize the need for cervical spine stabilization and immobilization. As they continue their assessment and prepare for full immobilization and transport, they explain the procedure to Miss Emily and her nephew. The medic determines the proper size of cervical collar needed and carefully places the collar around her neck. Circulation, sensation, and movement of all four extremities are evaluated before and after immobilization to the long spine board.

After full immobilization has been completed, Miss Emily is transported to the emergency department where she is found to have a fracture of her cervical vertebrae and compression of the spinal cord, resulting in the neurological impairment. ■

1. Manual stabilization must be maintained until:
   a. a proper cervical collar is applied.
   b. a proper cervical immobilization device is applied.
   c. proper collar and immobilization devices have been applied.
   d. proper collar and immobilization devices have been applied and the patient is secured to a long spine board.

2. To properly measure for cervical collar size, you measure from the:
   a. trapezius muscle to the angle of the jaw.
   b. trapezius muscle to the base of the occipital.
   c. trapezius muscle to the ear canal.
   d. none of the above

3. All of the following are indications of an improper cervical collar fit *except:*
   a. the head is hyperextended.
   b. the head is hypoextended.
   c. the head is in a neutral position.
   d. impaired airway or breathing.

CHAPTER 46

Spinal Immobilization with a Kendrick Extrication Device

KEY TERMS

Kendrick Extrication Device
(KED)

Neutral alignment

Tidal volume

OBJECTIVE

The student will successfully demonstrate spinal immobilization of the seated patient utilizing the Kendrick Extrication Device.

INTRODUCTION

This skill is indicated for patients injured while seated. Spinal immobilization of the seated patient can be accomplished with either a short backboard or a **Kendrick Extrication Device (KED).** However, it is also common for injured victims to be assisted to a seated position to "rest" while awaiting rescue personnel. For instance, the victim of a motor vehicle collision may get out of the vehicle to assess the damage, then return to the driver position to await the ambulance. Or, a patient may fall at home, then climb into a chair to rest, later finding that the pain in his neck or back requires medical attention. Both of these instances, and many others, would require spinal immobilization of the seated patient.

▶EQUIPMENT

You will need the following equipment:

- ▶ Kendrick extrication device
- ▶ Long spine board
- ▶ Cervical collar
- ▶ Head blocks or towel rolls
- ▶ 2- or 3-inch tape
- ▶ Backboard straps
- ▶ Three rescuers

ASSESSMENT

Be sure to manage any scene hazards before engaging in this skill. Additionally, all threats to airway, breathing, or circulation should be managed, and a rapid trauma assessment or focused physical exam completed at this time. The KED is applied to stable patients determined to have neck or back pain. Unstable patients, or those with vital sign abnormalities, should have rapid extrication performed rather than the KED (see Chapter 50).

PROCEDURE: Spinal Immobilization with a Kendrick Extrication Device

1. Apply BSI precautions.

   Rationale: Gloves and eye protection are required at minimum, and a gown may be necessary if large amounts of blood or fluid are present to prevent exposure to infectious diseases.

2. Approach the patient from her front side, introduce yourself, and instruct her not to move (Figure 46.1).

   Rationale: Approaching from the front minimizes the likelihood that your patient will turn her head to view you, compromising her neck and spine.

3. Hold manual cervical stabilization with one hand on either side of the patient's head and neck.

   Rationale: Manual stabilization is the most immediate way to protect the spine while appropriate immobilization devices are being selected.

4. Explain the spinal immobilization procedure to your patient, gaining her consent to perform the procedure (Figure 46.2).

   Rationale: Spinal immobilization can be uncomfortable.

5. Instruct a partner to place a properly fitted cervical collar on the patient's neck after

Figure 46.1

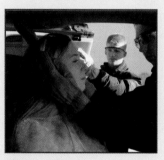

Figure 46.2

continued...

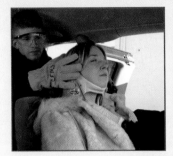

Figure 46.3

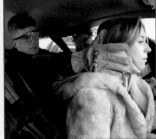

Figure 46.4

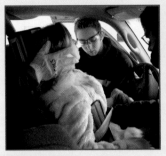

Figure 46.5

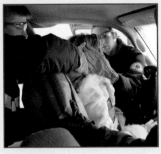

Figure 46.6

palpation and inspection of the cervical vertebrae (Figure 46.3).

Rationale: The cervical collar will assist in supporting the head and neck during application of the KED.

6. Assess the patient's sensory, motor, and circulatory status in all four extremities prior to immobilizing her.

Rationale: Lack of PMS (pulses, motor function, and sensation) can indicate a neurological deficit and further support the decision to use the KED.

7. Lean the patient slightly forward while another rescuer inserts the KED behind the patient's back. Reposition the patient against the KED. *Pull the leg straps, which are often secured behind the head of the device, down NOW to ensure access to the straps later* (Figure 46.4).

Rationale: If the leg straps are not accessed at this point, additional movement and manipulation of the patient may be required to get to the leg straps later in the procedure.

8. Secure the torso to the board using the colored straps of the KED. Fasten the leg straps to ensure the pelvis is immobilized. Be sure none of the straps prevent adequate chest excursion or otherwise limit **tidal volume** (Figure 46.5).

Rationale: In an effort to secure the device, the straps can be applied too tightly, making it difficult for the patient to breathe.

9. Place padding behind the head if necessary to ensure **neutral alignment** (Figure 46.6). Secure the head to the board using tape or the straps provided with the KED.

Rationale: The shoulders of some patients will require padding behind the patient's head in order to attain neutral alignment of the spine.

10. Reassess the patient's circulation, sensation, and movement in all four extremities, noting any changes from your initial assessment.

Rationale: Any change after the KED is applied or the patient moved can indicate an insult to the central nervous system.

11. Use the handles of the KED to move the patient as a unit to a long spine board for further immobilization (Figure 46.7).

Rationale: Use of the handles minimizes the need to use the patient's extremities or clothing to move the patient. Pulling on the patient's arms or legs can cause further injury.

12. Release the leg straps so that the patient can lie supine (Figure 46.8).

Rationale: The leg straps, when fastened, hold the patient in a seated position, making it uncomfortable to lie supine.

13. Secure the patient's body and the KED to the long spine board with straps, binders, or tape, placing straps close to or across the bony prominences of the shoulders, hips, and ankles (Figure 46.9).

Rationale: The body should be secured before the head because it weighs more and will pull the spine out of alignment if secured in reverse order.

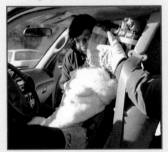

Figure 46.7

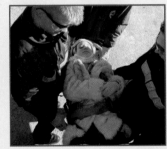

Figure 46.8

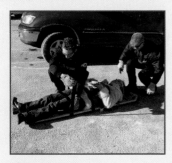

Figure 46.9

14. Place padding behind the head if necessary to ensure neutral alignment. Place headblocks or blanket rolls on either side of the head, securing the chin and forehead in place with tape.

    Rationale: Padding on either side of the head prevents the head of the KED from moving, causing further injury to the patient.

15. Secure the arms of the patient to prevent injury. The arms can either be restrained with backboard straps or tape. Lift the patient to the stretcher (Figure 46.10).

    Rationale: Unrestrained extremities can fall off the board, potentially causing injury to patient or rescuers.

16. Reassess the patient's circulation, sensation, and movement in all four extremities, noting any changes from your initial assessment.

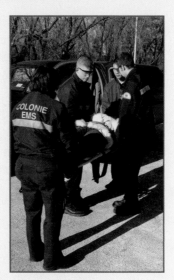

Figure 46.10

Rationale: The standard of care calls for PMS to be reassessed after every time the patient is moved when a spinal injury is suspected. Any change can indicate exacerbation of a spinal injury.

17. Document findings.

    Rationale: It is extremely important to document your findings in order to have a history of facts and events that occurred at the scene.

ONGOING ASSESSMENT

Once secured, and after every time the patient is moved, reassess circulatory, sensory, and motor function in all four extremities. Additionally, document any changes in mental status.

Be aware of the patient's breathing and airway status. Your spinal immobilized patient will not be able to sit up to cough or vomit. Should your patient need to vomit, roll him or her to the side on the spine board and have suction ready to prevent aspiration of stomach contents.

Patient's placed in spinal immobilization may need additional positioning. The head of the board may be raised for head injury patients in an effort to decrease intracranial pressure. The foot of the board may be elevated for patients with hypotension or poor perfusion. Pregnant patients may need the board tilted to the left to reduce pressure on the inferior vena cava from the weight of the baby. Accomplish all of these with toweling, blankets, or other padding beneath the board.

▶PROBLEM SOLVING

▶ The most common problem with spinal immobilization of the seated patient is that it is not performed when indicated often enough. Too often, the patient is encouraged to walk to the ambulance or over to the stretcher and lie down on the backboard. As soon as you identify the patient has head, neck, or back pain or other trauma; has an altered mental status, is unconscious, is intoxicated; or has suffered a significant mechanism of injury, the spine should immediately be immobilized without any further manipulation.

▶ The KED is often used to remove patients from vehicles following traffic collisions, but can also be used when a patient is found seated at the curb, in a chair, or even in the bathtub.

▶ Pregnant mothers late in gestation may be too large to fit in the KED. If the straps of the device will not buckle, then the KED should not be used. Spinal immobilization with a short spine board and longer straps, cravats, or tape may better serve the patient.

▶ Obese patients may not fit in the KED. Because the KED is one size, if the straps do not close across the chest or abdomen of the patient, then the KED should not be used. Consider, instead, immobilization using the short spine board and cravats, tape, or longer straps.

 GERIATRIC NOTE:
Some EMS systems teach application of the KED for immobilization of the pelvis when a hip fracture is suspected. This is an alternate application technique not necessarily supported by the manufacturer.

 PEDIATRIC NOTE:
The KED is sized for an average adult. Many children will be too small for proper application of the KED. In this case, use a short spine board or pediatric immobilization device instead of the KED.

▶CASE STUDY

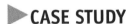

You are called to respond to a motor vehicle collision with injuries. You arrive on scene to find a small car struck by an SUV. The 21-year-old female in the front seat of the small car is complaining of neck and back pain. She was restrained by a safety belt and did not strike the windshield or steering wheel. Because you suspect that the patient could have sustained a neck injury, you decide to extricate the patient using the Kendrick extrication device. You explain the device to her as you and your partner prepare to secure her to the KED and remove her from the car. She continues to complain of pain as your partner applies in-line stabilization. You place the device and begin securing the straps around the torso. After securing the leg straps, you secure the device around her head. You go to prepare the cot and backboard. After returning to the vehicle, you and your partner extricate the patient. As you place her on the backboard, you release the leg straps and allow her legs to rest flat on the board. You secure the patient to the backboard and begin transport.

You complete the transport without any changes in the patient's condition. En route, you notify the emergency department of the patient's condition. You transfer the patient to the ED staff. It was later determined that she had no fractures, but the pain in her neck and shoulders was a result of overstretching and tearing of the muscles during her hyperextension injury. She was released from the hospital the next day and has resumed her normal daily routines. ■

1. The Kendrick Extrication Device is best used for which of the following?
   a. securing a patient who is supine on the ground, complaining of neck pain only
   b. instead of a backboard for securing a patient who has no complaints of neck or back pain
   c. to secure a stable seated patient who is complaining of neck and back pain
   d. to secure a patient with multiple traumatic injuries who requires rapid treatment

2. Cervical spine immobilization with the KED is best accomplished by:
   a. placing a cervical collar on the patient prior to positioning the KED.
   b. placing a cervical collar on the patient after securing the patient in the KED.
   c. using padding instead of a cervical collar due to the design of the KED.
   d. the KED adequately securing the cervical spine without the need for a cervical collar.

3. A patient who is secured in a KED needs:
   a. additional stabilization below the waist.
   b. full immobilization to a long spine board.
   c. no additional immobilization because the KED extends the length of the spine.
   d. to be removed from the KED prior to being secured to a long backboard.

CHAPTER 47

Spinal Immobilization of a Supine Patient

KEY TERMS

Aspiration

Mechanism of injury

Supine

OBJECTIVE

The student will successfully demonstrate spinal immobilization of the supine patient.

INTRODUCTION

Spinal immobilization of the **supine** patient should be considered any time the patient has sustained an injury of significant mechanism or is complaining of head, neck, or back pain. Penetrating injuries, lacerations, or contusions to the head or scalp are also indications of potential spinal injury. Additionally, when a patient is unconscious for unknown reasons, spinal precautions should be taken. Patients requiring spinal immobilization can have many **mechanisms of injury,** which include, but are not limited to, traffic collisions, boating accidents, sporting injuries, falls, and assaults.

▶EQUIPMENT

You will need the following equipment:

▶ Long spine board
▶ Cervical collar
▶ Head blocks or towel rolls
▶ 2- or 3-inch tape
▶ Backboard straps
▶ Four rescuers

ASSESSMENT

Be sure to manage any scene hazards before engaging in this skill. Additionally, all threats to airway, breathing, or circulation should be managed, and a rapid trauma assessment or focused physical exam completed before beginning this procedure. In some cases if the patient begins to deteriorate, spinal immobilization will be initiated before all assessments are completed.

PROCEDURE: Spinal Immobilization of a Supine Patient

1. Apply BSI precautions.

   Rationale: Gloves and eye protection are required at minimum, and a gown may be necessary if large amounts of blood or fluid are present to prevent exposure to infectious diseases.

2. Approach the patient from her front side, introduce yourself, and instruct her not to move (Figure 47.1).

   Rationale: Approaching from the front minimizes the likelihood that your patient will turn her head to view you, compromising her neck and spine.

3. Hold manual cervical stabilization with one hand on either side of the patient's head and neck (Figure 47.2).

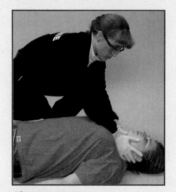

Figure 47.2

   Rationale: Manual stabilization is the most immediate way to protect the spine while immobilization equipment is being gathered and assessments being completed.

4. Explain the need for and steps involved in spinal immobilization, gaining her consent to perform the procedure.

   Rationale: Spinal immobilization can be uncomfortable.

5. Evaluate circulation, sensation, and movement in all extremities. Do this by palpating radial and pedal pulses and by assessing grip strength and flexion, extension of the feet, and perceived

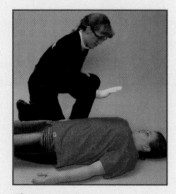

Figure 47.1

continued...

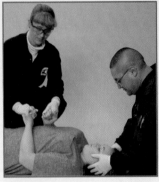
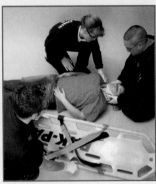

Figure 47.3   **Figure 47.4**

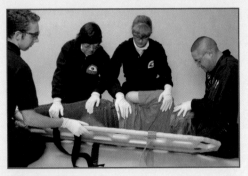

Figure 47.6

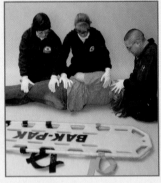
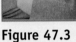

Figure 47.5

sensation while touching the patient's extremities (Figure 47.3).

Rationale: Lack of CSM can indicate a neurological deficit. CSM will be measured repeatedly during the procedure to ensure that worsening of the spinal injury does not occur.

6. Instruct a partner to place a properly fitted cervical collar on the patient's neck after palpation and inspection of the cervical vertebrae. Next, align the spine board parallel to the patient (Figure 47.4).

Rationale: The cervical collar will assist in keeping the patient's head and neck in the neutral position during the movement required of a spinal immobilization procedure.

7. With one rescuer supporting the head, another at the shoulder and hip, and the third at the hip and lower extremities, roll the patient toward the rescuers (Figure 47.5). The rescuer at the patient's head calls for all patient movement. While the patient is on her side, expose, inspect, and

palpate the posterior torso and buttocks for any injuries.

Rationale: Rescuers are positioned as described to ensure that the spine is kept still and supported during the movement required of the spinal immobilization procedure.

8. Have a fourth rescuer slide the spine board parallel to the patient. Roll the patient back down onto the spine board. The verbal instructions are again given by the rescuer at the patient's head (Figure 47.6).

Rationale: Using a fourth rescuer to slide the board into place ensures that the rescuers supporting the patient do not lose contact with the patient, causing manipulation of the spine.

9. Pad any voids between the patient and board with towels, blankets, or bandages. Voids may exist under the neck, under the lumbar spine, under knees, or at the feet (Figure 47.7).

Rationale: Padding is required to support parts of the spine not in direct contact with the spine board.

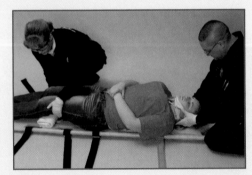

Figure 47.7

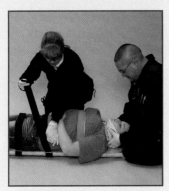

Figure 47.8

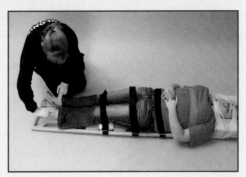

Figure 47.9

10. Secure the patient's body to the spine board with straps, binders, or tape, placing straps close to or across the bony prominences of the shoulders, hips, and ankles (Figure 47.8).

    Rationale: The body should be secured before the head because it weighs more and will pull the spine out of alignment if secured in reverse order.

11. Place padding behind the head if necessary to ensure neutral alignment. Place headblocks or blanket rolls on either side of the head, securing the chin and forehead in place with tape.

    Rationale: Padding on either side of the head prevents the head from moving about on the board.

12. Secure the arms of the patient to prevent injury. The arms can either be restrained with backboard straps or tape.

    Rationale: Unrestrained extremities can fall off the board, potentially causing injury to patient or rescuers.

13. Reassess the patient's circulation, sensation and movement in all four extremities, noting any changes from your initial assessment (Figure 47.9).

    Rationale: The standard of care calls for PMS (pulses, motor function, sensation) to be reassessed before and after any splint is applied, including a spine board, and after each time the patient is moved. Any changes in PMS can indicate a neurological deficit caused by spinal cord injury.

14. Document findings.

    Rationale: It is extremely important to document your findings in order to have a history of facts and events that occurred at the scene.

ONGOING ASSESSMENT

Once secured, and after every time the patient is moved, reassess circulatory, sensory, and motor function in all four extremities. Additionally, document any changes in mental status.

Be aware of the patient's breathing and airway status. Your spinal immobilized patient will not be able to sit up to cough or vomit. Should your patient need to vomit, roll him or her to the side on the spine board and have suction ready to prevent **aspiration** of stomach contents.

Patient's placed in spinal immobilization may need additional positioning. The head of the board may be raised for head injury patients in an effort to decrease intracranial pressure. The foot of the board may be elevated for patients with hypotension or poor perfusion. Pregnant patients may need the board tilted to the left to reduce pressure on the inferior vena cava from the weight of the baby. Accomplish all of these with toweling, blankets, or other padding beneath the board.

▶ PROBLEM SOLVING

▶ As soon as you identify the patient has head, neck, or back pain or other trauma; has an altered mental status, is unconscious, is intoxicated; or has suffered a significant mechanism of injury, the spine should immediately be immobilized without any further manipulation.

▶ A common problem of spinal immobilization is pushing or pulling on sections of the body in an effort to position the patient on the board. The patient must be moved as a unit, using at least three rescuers, to prevent manipulation of the spine.

▶ If a fourth rescuer is not available to pull the spine board into place underneath the patient, then this simple task can be accomplished by the rescuer at the hip pulling the board into place.

▶ When tape is used on the chin to secure the head in place on the board, care should be taken to place the tape straight across and not up from ear-to-ear, which can prevent the mouth from opening and, hence, prevent the patient from being able to talk or vomit as needed.

▶ CASE STUDY

Tom, a 46-year-old home owner, had decided to take advantage of a clear Saturday afternoon to clean the gutters around his single-story home. As he twisted the top off of his third beer, he dragged the ladder out from under the porch and waved to his wife as she pulled out of the driveway on her way to the market. Guzzling the last of the beer, he extended the ladder, braced it against the side of the house, and climbed toward the roof. As he neared the edge of the roof, he lost his footing and shifted his weight quickly to one side. Tom let out a loud yelp as he and the ladder fell noisily to the ground. His neighbor saw the fall and ran across the yard to Tom's side, instructing Tom not to move while he yelled for his wife to call 911.

Upon arriving at the scene, you find a middle-aged male in pain, but not distress. The neighbor tells you what he saw, so your partner immediately goes to the head of the patient. You approach the patient from the front and introduce yourself. You warn him that he is going to feel someone's hands on his head, but not to move. Your partner then applies manual in-line stabilization of the cervical spine. At this point, Tom is alert and oriented, has a patent airway, is breathing without difficulty, and has strong pulses. You complete a rapid trauma assessment and find no apparent life threats. You also look to see the distance of the fall, which appears to be less than 15 feet. You prepare the long spine board and cervical immobilization device (CID) as your partner obtains a SAMPLE history. You return and apply a cervical collar, check circulation, motor function, and sensation, and then log roll the patient to the board. After securing the patient's torso, you apply the CID, recheck circulation, motor function, and sensation, and move the patient to the cot.

En route to the emergency department, you complete a detailed physical exam and find that Tom is only complaining of lower back pain. You notify the ED and continue without any further changes. At the ED, you transfer care to the emergency staff, and tell Tom you hope that he feels better soon. ■

1. Why is it important to check for circulation, motor function, and sensation every time you move the patient?
   a. as a reminder so that you at least check it once
   b. to ensure that you have not caused any further injuries by moving the patient onto the board
   c. to make sure that the patient's status has not deteriorated
   d. to get a rough estimate on the blood pressure without actually taking one

2. Why is it important to immobilize the torso prior to immobilizing the head?
   a. because the torso is larger than the head and weighs more
   b. so that the patient can be moved easily if needed
   c. because immobilizing the torso acts as a restraint
   d. you should immobilize the head first to free up a rescuer

3. What is the most appropriate way to approach a supine patient who is in need of spinal immobilization?
   a. You should approach from the front to prevent the patient from turning his or her head.
   b. You should approach from the side so that you do not startle the patient.
   c. You should approach from the head so that you can stabilize the head before the patient can move.
   d. You should approach from the head so that the patient will not move his or her head side to side.

CHAPTER 48
Spinal Immobilization of a Standing Patient

KEY TERMS
Ambulatory

Standing takedown

Synchronous

OBJECTIVE
The student will successfully demonstrate spinal immobilization of the standing patient utilizing the standing takedown method.

INTRODUCTION

Spinal immobilization of the standing patient is accomplished with a maneuver known as the **standing takedown.** This skill may be necessary if the victim of a traumatic incident presents **ambulatory** at the scene or standing while calling for help, inspecting a vehicle for damage, or wandering about due to confusion or disorientation. The standing takedown is used to immediately provide manual stabilization of the head and neck while immobilizing the spine to a long spine board. The maneuver prevents the patient from making any further movements or manipulations of the spine and secures him or her to the board while easing the patient to the supine position.

►EQUIPMENT

You will need the following equipment:

- ► Long spine board
- ► Cervical collar
- ► Head blocks or towel rolls
- ► 2- or 3-inch tape
- ► Backboard straps
- ► Three rescuers

ASSESSMENT

Be sure to manage any scene hazards before engaging in this skill. Additionally, all threats to airway, breathing, or circulation should be managed, and a rapid trauma assessment or focused physical exam completed at this time. In some cases, the rescuer may feel it is necessary for the patient to be supine before assessing him or her. In this case, the standing takedown procedure can be performed first, and the assessments completed once the patient is on the board at the scene or in the back of the ambulance.

PROCEDURE: Spinal Immobilization of a Standing Patient

1. Apply BSI precautions.

   Rationale: Gloves and eye protection are required at minimum, and a gown may be necessary if large amounts of blood or fluid are present to prevent exposure to infectious diseases.

2. Approach the patient from his front side, introduce yourself, and instruct him not to move.

   Rationale: Approaching from the front minimizes the likelihood that your patient will turn his head to view you, compromising his neck and spine.

3. Hold manual cervical stabilization with one hand on either side of the patient's head and neck (Figure 48.1).

   Rationale: Manual stabilization is the most immediate way to protect the spine while appropriate immobilization equipment is being assembled.

4. Explain the standing takedown procedure to your patient, gaining his consent to perform the procedure.

   Rationale: The sensation that one is falling backward can be frightening to an unprepared patient.

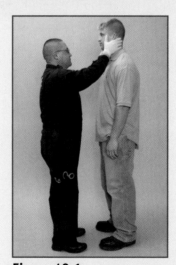

Figure 48.1

5. Have the second rescuer assume manual stabilization of the head and neck by replacing his hands with yours from behind the patient.

   Rationale: He should be standing behind the backboard with his hands in a position to rotate as the board is lowered.

continued...

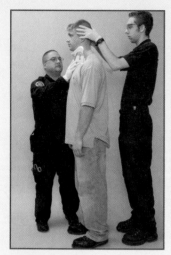

Figure 48.2

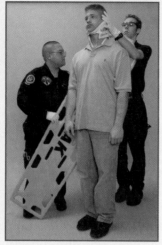

Figure 48.3

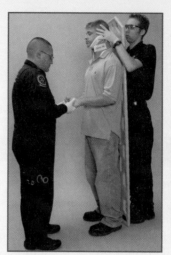

Figure 48.4

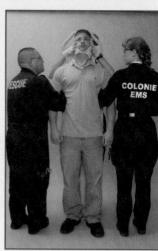

Figure 48.5

6. Instruct a partner to place a properly fitted cervical collar on the patient's neck after palpation and inspection of the cervical vertebrae (Figure 48.2).

   Rationale: The cervical collar will assist in supporting the head and neck during the standing takedown procedure.

7. Align the backboard behind the patient, parallel to the patient's spine (Figure 48.3).

   Rationale: The board is positioned behind the patient so that he can be lowered directly onto it.

8. Assess the patient's sensory, motor, and circulatory status in all four extremities prior to immobilizing him (Figure 48.4).

   Rationale: Changes in PMS (pulses, motor function, sensation) can indicate a serious spinal injury. Initial measurement of PMS establishes a baseline against which subsequent measurements can be compared.

9. You and a third rescuer should stand on either side, facing the patient. Grasp the board from underneath the patient's arm. Use your arm and shoulder to anchor the patient to the board (Figure 48.5).

   Rationale: No straps are used to secure the patient at this point, so the patient must be "pinned" to the board by the bodies of the rescuers to prevent movement as he is lowered to the ground on the spine board.

10. Lower the patient to the ground on the board by taking **synchronous** steps forward and

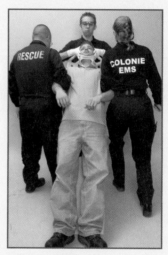

Figure 48.6

straightening your arm at the same time. Take three steps forward with your eyes straight ahead. Use your free arm for balance. Be sure to keep your abdominal muscles taut and your back straight. At this time, the rescuer holding manual stabilization of the head should ensure that the head remains in a neutral position to the board, rather than flexed or extended, by rotating his hands (Figure 48.6).

Rationale: The body position of rescuers is essential to the safety of the rescuers. The rescuers will be strongest and safest when facing straight ahead. Side stepping encourages twisting of the spine, potentially causing injury to rescuers.

11. Secure the patient's body to the spine board with straps, binders, or tape, placing straps across the bony prominences of the shoulders, hips, and ankles.

    Rationale: The body should be secured before the head because it weighs more and will pull the spine out of alignment if secured in reverse order.

12. Place padding behind the head if necessary to ensure neutral alignment. Place headblocks or blanket rolls on either side of the head, securing the chin and forehead in place with tape.

    Rationale: Padding on either side of the head prevents movement of the head on the board.

13. Reassess the patient's sensory, motor, and circulatory status in all four extremities, noting any changes from your initial assessment (Figure 48.7).

    Rationale: Any change in PMS can indicate that a spinal injury has been exacerbated by movement.

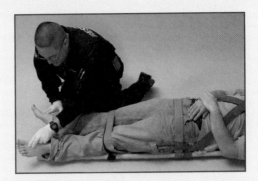

Figure 48.7

This assessment of PMS should be compared to the baseline assessment taken earlier.

14. Document findings.

    Rationale: It is extremely important to document your findings in order to have a history of facts and events that occured at the scene.

ONGOING ASSESSMENT

Once secured, and after every time the patient is moved, reassess circulatory, sensory, and motor function in all four extremities. Additionally, document any changes in mental status.

Be aware of the patient's breathing and airway status. Your spinal immobilized patient will not be able to sit up to cough or vomit. Should your patient need to vomit, roll him or her to the side on the spine board and have suction ready to prevent aspiration of stomach contents.

Patient's placed in spinal immobilization may need additional positioning. The head of the board may be raised for head injury patients in an effort to decrease intracranial pressure. The foot of the board may be elevated for patients with hypotension or poor perfusion. Pregnant patients may need the board tilted to the left to reduce pressure on the inferior vena cava from the weight of the baby. Accomplish all of these with toweling, blankets, or other padding beneath the board.

▶ PROBLEM SOLVING

▶ The most common problem with the standing takedown procedure is that it is not performed often enough when indicated. Too often, the patient is encouraged to walk to the ambulance or over to the stretcher and to lay down on the backboard. As soon as you identify the patient has head, neck, or back pain or other trauma; has an altered mental status, is unconscious, is intoxicated; or has suffered a significant mechanism of injury, the spine should immediately be immobilized without any further manipulation.

▶ Occasionally, when the patient is laid supine, he will not be in proper position on the board. The patient can be adjusted on the board using the "Z-drag" method of keeping the patient moving along the long axis of the body. In no case should his or her shoulders or hips be pushed laterally to move the patient to the center of the board.

▶ When taping the head down, be sure the tape on the chin does not act as a fulcrum, preventing opening of the mouth, which is necessary for speaking or vomiting as needed. Instead, place the tape straight across the chin and be sure padding or headblocks are used as well.

 GERIATRIC NOTE:

Geriatric patients may have significant deformities of the neck and spine. Extensive padding may be needed to achieve neutral alignment.

 PEDIATRIC NOTE:

Standing takedown should not be attempted on pediatric patients using an adult-sized long spine board. Instead, a short board or pediatric-sized spine board should be used.

▶CASE STUDY

You are dispatched to aid a person injured during an assault. Upon arrival, you see a local law enforcement officer speaking with a young female in the parking lot who has obvious blunt trauma to her face and neck. As you approach, you observe that her face and eyes are severely swollen and bruised. You hear a hoarse voice crying and the woman is complaining of pain to her head and neck. The police officer informs you that the assault occurred several hours earlier and this scene is safe.

Your partner quickly returns to the ambulance to collect necessary equipment, and the police officer agrees to help you with stabilization of the cervical spine as you continue your assessment. Your partner arrives with oxygen and immobilization equipment and you explain to the patient that you will need to immobilize her from a standing position because you don't want to risk any additional movement of her head or neck. She reluctantly agrees if you promise to be careful and not drop her.

Your partner places a cervical collar and then relieves the police officer, maintaining cervical immobilization. You slide the board behind the patient and take immobilization from your partner. Your partner than advises the officer on how to lower the patient to the ground. You assess distal circulation, motor function, and sensation. You continue to calm the patient as she is lowered to the ground. Once she is supine, your partner applies the backboard straps and then the cervical immobilization device. After securing the patient, you reassess the distal circulation, motor function, and sensation. You load the patient onto the cot and proceed to the local emergency department. En route, you notify the ED. Upon arrival at the ED, you transfer care to the emergency staff. ■

1. Which of the following best describes the reason for using the standing take-down procedure?

   a. Any unnecessary movement by the patient can aggravate a suspected injury.

   b. It allows you to more easily secure the patient to the long backboard.

   c. It allows you to place the patient directly on the cot.

   d. It prevents you from having to bend all the way to the ground to lift the patient.

2. When utilizing the standing takedown, at which point should the patient be secured to the backboard?

   a. before lowering the backboard to the ground to prevent any movement

   b. before lowering the backboard to the ground because it is easier

   c. after lowering the backboard to the ground because the patient may need to be repositioned

   d. after lowering the patient to the ground so that any patient movement is prevented

3. Which of the following is the appropriate method for lowering the patient to the ground?

   a. Secure the torso with straps to prevent excessive movement.

   b. Manually stabilize the patient with your arms to prevent excessive movement.

   c. Fully immobilize the patient with straps and cervical immobilization device (CID) to prevent any injuries.

   d. The patient should not be secured at all to prevent further injuries.

CHAPTER 49
Helmet Removal

KEY TERMS

Mandible

Occiput

OBJECTIVE

The student will successfully demonstrate helmet removal from an injured patient without compromising the neck or spine.

INTRODUCTION

Helmets are no longer found only on motorcycle riders. Many sporting activities encourage helmet use such as bicycling, in-line skating, skiing, and hockey. Helmet removal may be necessary when the helmet is ill fitting or impedes assessment and management of airway and breathing. However, the helmet can be left in place when all of the following criteria are met: (1) it is form fitted enough that no movement of the head is possible within the helmet, (2) all injuries can be managed with the helmet in place, (3) there is no risk for hyperextension or flexion of the neck resulting from the helmet's position on the **occiput** of the head, and (4) airway and breathing can be assessed and managed with the helmet in place.

►EQUIPMENT

You will need the following equipment:

- ► Cervical collar
- ► Headblocks or towel rolls
- ► 2- or 3-inch tape
- ► Long spine board
- ► Backboard straps
- ► Two to four rescuers

ASSESSMENT

Be sure to manage any scene hazards before engaging in this skill. If the airway is accessible, manage all threats to airway, breathing, and circulation before removing the helmet. Many helmet face masks are removable; if you can remove the face mask, you might not have to remove the helmet entirely. Should treatment of an injury be impeded by the helmet, or the airway cannot be managed with the helmet in place, quickly remove the helmet before engaging in any other assessment or treatment activities.

PROCEDURE: Helmet Removal

1. Apply BSI precautions.

   Rationale: Gloves and eye protection are required at minimum, and a gown may be necessary if large amounts of blood or fluid are present to prevent exposure to infectious diseases.

2. Approach the patient from her front side, introduce yourself, and instruct her not to move (Figure 49.1).

   Rationale: Approaching from the front minimizes the likelihood that your patient will turn her head to view you, compromising her neck and spine.

3. Hold manual cervical stabilization with one hand on either side of the patient's head and helmet (Figure 49.2).

   Rationale: It will be difficult to hold the head directly with the helmet in place. If need be, hold onto the helmet to remind the patient to hold her head still.

4. Explain the need for and steps involved in helmet removal, gaining her consent to perform the procedure.

   Rationale: You should prepare your patient for any discomfort that might be experienced when removing the helmet.

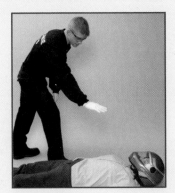

Figure 49.1

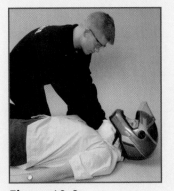

Figure 49.2

continued...

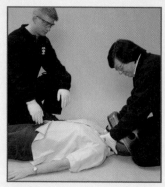

Figure 49.3

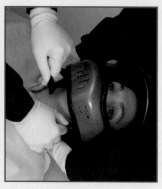

Figure 49.4

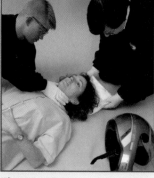

Figure 49.7

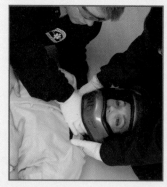

Figure 49.5

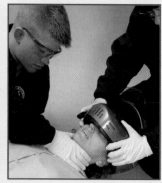

Figure 49.6

5. Manual spinal immobilization will now be assumed by the second rescuer who can hold the head secure between the occipital region and **mandible.** Evaluate circulation, sensation, and movement in all extremities. Do this by palpating radial and pedal pulses and by assessing grip strength and flexion, extension of the feet, and perceived sensation while touching the patient's extremities (Figure 49.3).

   Rationale: Lack of PMS can indicate a spinal injury and should be noted as the baseline assessment at this time.

6. Remove the chin strap (Figure 49.4).

   Rationale: This will make the helmet easier to remove.

7. Place one hand on the occiput behind the patient's head, and the other on the mandible. (Figure 49.5).

   Rationale: Support of the occiput will later prevent the head from falling to the ground when the space between the head and ground is no longer filled by the bulk of the helmet.

8. The second rescuer can now pull outward on the sides of the helmet to avoid pulling on the ears. She then tilts the face of the helmet up to avoid contact with the nose, and then rotates the helmet forward to clear the back of the head (Figure 49.6).

9. The second rescuer can set aside the helmet and get a cervical collar (Figure 49.7).

   Rationale: Do not discard the helmet as damage to the helmet can be a predictor of mechanism of injury. The emergency room physician will likely want to examine the helmet.

10. A cervical collar should be placed and the patient secured to a long spine board when possible.

    Rationale: Any injury significant enough to warrant removal of the helmet will likely have a high index of suspicion for neck or back injuries and should be fully immobilized.

11. Maintain manual cervical stabilization until the patient is secured to a spine board.

    Rationale: The spine is not fully protected until the patient is secured to a long spine board.

12. Reassess the patient's circulation, sensation, and movement in all four extremities, noting any changes from your initial assessment.

    Rationale: Any change in CSM could indicate that a spinal injury has been exacerbated.

13. Document findings.

    Rationale: It is extremely important to document your findings in order to have a history of facts and events that occurred at the scene.

ONGOING ASSESSMENT

Once immobilized, and after every time the patient is moved, reassess circulatory, sensory, and motor function in all four extremities. Additionally, document any changes in mental status.

Be aware of the patient's breathing and airway status. Your spinal immobilized patient will not be able to sit up to cough or vomit. Should your patient need to vomit, roll him or her to the side on the spine board and have suction ready to prevent aspiration of stomach contents.

▶PROBLEM SOLVING

▷ As soon as you identify the patient has head, neck, or back pain or other trauma; has an altered mental status is unconscious, is intoxicated; or has suffered a significant mechanism of injury, the spine should immediately be manually immobilized without any further manipulation.

▷ If shoulder pads are worn by the patient when helmet removal is accomplished, the pads will also need to be removed or padding will need to be placed behind the head to compensate for the space created by the pads and decrease the likelihood of hyperextension of the neck.

▷ To perform the helmet removal procedure safely, at least two rescuers are required.

PEDIATRIC NOTE:

Remember that a child's head is larger in proportion to the rest of his body. Even without a helmet, the head of a pediatric patient is disproportionately large and will require padding behind the shoulders in order to achieve neutral alignment of the spine. If the helmet is left in place, an inordinate amount of padding could be required.

GERIATRIC NOTE:

Some providers mistakenly believe that they will never have to remove a helmet from a geriatric patient, but many geriatric patients remain active long into their senior years. It is not uncommon to have to remove a bike, motorcycle, or ski helmet from a geriatric patient.

►CASE STUDY

You are called to a scene where a motorcycle has crashed into a car. Upon arriving on scene, you find a 30-year-old male patient lying supine on the ground. The patient is conscious and breathing, however, he is confused. You walk up to the patient from the front while your partner proceeds to the top of the head. You advise the patient that your partner is going to hold his head still until you can secure him to the backboard.

During the initial assessment, you notice that the patient is having increasing difficulty breathing and is becoming more confused. Your partner advises you that the patient's head is flexed forward. You decide to remove the patient's helmet to prevent flexion of the neck and to allow for better access to the patient's airway. You assess distal circulation, motor function, and sensation. You take over manual stabilization from your partner and he proceeds to remove the helmet from the patient. After removing the helmet, you reassess distal circulation, motor function, and sensation.

You place the head and neck in a neutral position and the patient's breathing improves. You apply high-flow, high-concentration oxygen and then secure the patient to the long spine board and then to the cot. En route to the emergency department you notify them of the patient's condition. During the transport, the patient's level of consciousness improves, and by the time you arrive at the ED, the patient is alert and oriented to person, place, and time. You transfer the patient to the ED bed and give your report to the emergency staff.■

1. It may not be necessary to remove the helmet on which of the following patients?
    a. a 16-year-old football player complaining of numbness in the lower extremities
    b. a 32-year-old bicyclist with neck and back pain and a half helmet
    c. a 3-year-old roller skater who has a helmet and is complaining of difficulty breathing
    d. a 55-year-old motorcyclist who fell from the bike and has shallow respirations

2. Which of the following is the most appropriate manner to maintain in-line cervical spine immobilization during helmet removal?
    a. You should stabilize the head by facing the patient and resting a hand on either side of the patient's neck.
    b. You should stabilize the head by facing the patient and placing your thumbs on the patient cheeks and fingers behind the ears.
    c. You should place one hand on the back of the patient's neck and the other hand on the patient's lower jaw.
    d. You should place one hand at the base of the skull and the other hand on the patient's lower jaw.

3. It is important to pad the voids between the patient and the backboard because:
    a. padding prevents movement of the patient from side to side.
    b. padding supports areas of the spine not in direct contact with the backboard.
    c. padding of the patient prevents the patient from sliding up and down on the backboard.
    d. padding prevents the neck from being flexed in the adult patient.

CHAPTER 50
Rapid Extrication

KEY TERMS

Kendrick Extrication Device

Rapid extrication

OBJECTIVE

The student will successfully demonstrate rapid extrication of a patient from a vehicle when a danger or life threat exists to the patient or rescuers.

INTRODUCTION

Rapid extrication from a vehicle should be used only when a patient must be removed from a vehicle expediently due to a threat to airway, breathing, or circulation or to a scene hazard such as a fire. Most patients who present in the vehicle complaining of neck or back pain should be removed using the standard of care for a stable patient, which is a short spine board or **Kendrick Extrication Device.** Only a small percentage of patients will be in critical condition that requires rapid extrication with a long spine board and the procedure discussed in this chapter.

▶ **EQUIPMENT LIST**

You will need the following equipment:

▶ Long spine board
▶ Cervical collar
▶ Four rescuers

ASSESSMENT

Attempt to manage or avoid scene hazards such as fire, vehicle instability, or hazardous materials whenever possible. Additionally, attempt to intervene and correct any patient life threats to airway, breathing, or circulation by opening the airway, assisting ventilations with a bag-valve-mask unit, or controlling hemorrhage with direct pressure. When attempts to make the scene safe or correct life threats fail, ensure the safety of you and your crew and begin rapid extrication.

PROCEDURE: Rapid Extrication

1. Apply BSI precautions.

   Rationale: Gloves and eye protection are required at minimum, and a gown may be necessary if large amounts of blood or fluid are present to prevent exposure to infectious diseases.

2. Do attempt to correct or avoid any scene hazards.

   Rationale: Scene hazards are actually an indication for this skill.

3. Direct a rescuer to the backseat to apply manual cervical spinal immobilization (Figure 50.1).

   Rationale: Manual immobilization of the spine provides immediate protection for the patient while spinal immobilization equipment is being assembled.

4. Apply a properly sized cervical collar. One rescuer remains in the backseat to hold manual stabilization (Figure 50.2).

   Rationale: A cervical collar will assist in supporting the patient's head and neck during the rapid extrication procedure.

5. Position rescuers on either side of the patient, one in the vehicle, one out (Figure 50.3).

   Rationale: The rescuers on either side of the patient are going to work together to both support the patient's spine and maneuver him out of the vehicle.

6. Position an additional rescuer outside of the vehicle holding the long spine board.

   Rationale: The patient will be moved onto the board for removal from the vehicle.

7. Lift the patient vertically as a unit until the patient can be effectively slid onto the spine board placed between the patient and the seat. The rescuer in the backseat, who is in control of the head, may command the team (Figure 50.4).

   Rationale: It will be easier to turn the patient when he is on the smooth surface of the spine board rather than on the upholstery of the car seat.

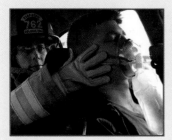
Figure 50.1

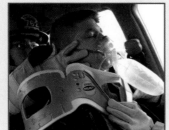
Figure 50.2

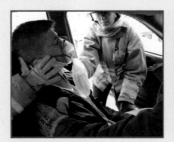
Figure 50.3

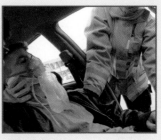
Figure 50.4

continued...

8. As a unit, turn the patient a one-quarter turn until the back-seat rescuer is unable to turn any further while properly holding the head (Figure 50.5).

   Rationale: The backseat rescuer will run into the B-post, preventing further turning of the patient.

9. Transfer immobilization of the head and neck to the rescuer outside of the vehicle and complete another quarter turn until the patient is in line with the spine board. The backseat rescuer can now come around to the front of the outside of the vehicle to assist with moving the patient's torso (Figure 50.6).

   Rationale: Now that the patient's shoulders are out of the vehicle, the majority of the weight will be as well.

10. Lay the patient supine onto the spine board. Be sure to maintain manual immobilization of the head and neck (Figure 50.7).

    Rationale: The head is not fully protected until it has been secured to the spine board with tape. Manual stabilization will be required until the body is secured, then the head.

11. Slide the patient into position for full immobilization onto the spine board (Figure 50.8).

12. Carefully move the patient on the spine board to a safe location to fully assess and immobilize. Take extra caution if the patient is not fully strapped to the backboard.

    Rationale: The patient should not be lowered to the ground next to the vehicle if a scene hazard was the indication for rapid extrication. Both patient and rescuers should be safe during patient care.

13. Document findings.

    Rationale: It is extremely important to document your findings in order to have a history of facts and events that occurred at the scene.

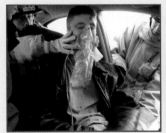

Figure 50.5

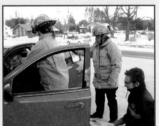

Figure 50.6

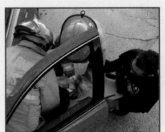

Figure 50.7

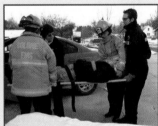

Figure 50.8

ONGOING ASSESSMENT

Now that the patient has been moved to safety, repeat the initial assessment. Correct any threats to airway, breathing, or circulation. Consider moving the patient directly to the ambulance and initiating transport if the patient's condition was life threatening enough to warrant rapid extrication.

Once secured, and after every time the patient is moved, reassess circulatory, sensory, and motor function in all four extremities. Additionally, document any changes in mental status.

Be aware of the patient's breathing and airway status. Your spinal immobilized patient will not be able to sit up to cough or vomit. Should your patient need to vomit, roll him or her to the side on the spine board and have suction ready to prevent aspiration of stomach contents.

▶PROBLEM SOLVING

▶ The most common problem associated with rapid extrication is too frequent utilization. Commonly, a patient is over-triaged and the rapid extrication technique is used when the patient is not critical. The standard of care for a stable patient complaining of neck and back pain is careful removal using a short board or Kendrick Extrication Device.

▶ Because the rapid extrication technique will be used when a scene hazard exists, rescuers are often in a hurry to move away from the vehicle. Often, the rescuers will forego strapping the patient to the spine board in the interest of time. However, the straps left dangling present a hazard to the rescuers who may trip over them, causing a fall for other rescuers and presenting the potential to drop the patient.

 PEDIATRIC NOTE:

Children who present to rescuers in a car seat should be left in the car seat and removed as a unit from the vehicle when a scene hazard exists. However, a booster seat for larger children usually does not provide any spinal protection. When a child is in a booster seat, rapid extrication should be performed when indicated as described in this chapter.

 GERIATRIC NOTE:

Because geriatric patients often have extensive medical histories, be sure to determine the cause of the accident. It is possible that a medical condition such as a heart attack, stroke, or seizure caused the accident to which you have responded.

▶CASE STUDY

You are called to the scene of a motor vehicle collision. Upon arrival you see that the vehicle impacted with a bridge support. You also see smoke coming from the engine compartment, but there are no flames. You and your partner decide to perform a rapid extrication after your dispatcher informs you that the fire department is still about four minutes away. You see that there is only one occupant inside the vehicle. Your partner is able to gain entry into the vehicle through the passenger-side rear door. You approach the patient from the front and, after calling out, realize that the patient is unresponsive. Your partner takes in-line immobilization as you retrieve immobilization equipment from the ambulance. Your partner advises you that the patient has a patent airway and is breathing normally. You quickly apply a cervical collar as the fire department arrives on scene. You direct one of the firefighters to assist you in extrication.

Another firefighter comes over to support the spine board and cot while the others attempt to locate the source of the smoke. Your partner directs you and the firefighter to lift the patient as the other firefighter slides the spine board between the patient and the seat. After placing the patient on the spine board, you rotate the patient 45 degrees. You then wait as the other rescuer exits the vehicle and takes over in-line immobilization. When your partner is ready, the other rescuer directs you to rotate the patient the rest of the way so that he is in the proper position to be secured.

The rescuer then directs you to lay the patient supine and then move the patient toward the head of the spine board. After the patient is properly positioned on the backboard, you quickly secure the torso in place. The firefighter continues to maintain cervical spine immobilization as you slide the spine board onto the cot.

As soon as everyone is ready, you move the cot to your ambulance and finish immobilizing the patient. You assess circulation, motor function, and sensation. Your patient has good distal pulses, but you have no response to motor function or sensation. You load the patient in the ambulance and immediately begin to repeat the initial assessment. En route to the trauma center, you complete the rapid trauma assessment and find no obvious life threats. You notify the emergency department of the patient and they advise you that they will alert the trauma team. You continue to monitor and reassess the patient until you arrive at the ED and transfer patient care to the trauma team. ■

1. When would it be appropriate to begin the rapid extrication of a patient?
    a. after all threats to safety of the crew and the patient have been located and corrected
    b. after all the life threats have been corrected
    c. as soon as the transport vehicle has arrived on the scene
    d. when it is safe to enter the vehicle, but some hazards remain that cannot be corrected quickly

2. When rapid extrication is indicated, which of the following is the lowest priority?
    a. placing a cervical collar prior to extricating the patient to a spine board
    b. correcting life threats found on the initial assessment prior to moving the patient
    c. assessing for circulation, motor function, and sensation prior to moving the patient
    d. making sure that the scene is free of hazards that will prevent you from safely extricating the patient

3. During the rapid extrication, it is acceptable to do all of the following except:
    a. risk your own safety to remove the patient from the vehicle more quickly.
    b. forgo trying to correct scene hazards that will make you and your partner safe.
    c. move the patient on the spine board prior to adequately securing him.
    d. forgo correcting apparent life threats until the patient is in a safe environment.

TRAUMA EMERGENCIES

QUESTION BANK

1. A traction splint should be used only on a:
   - A. pelvic fracture.
   - B. knee injury.
   - C. midshaft femur fracture.
   - D. proximal femur fracture.

2. A dressing designed to prevent air movement at the wound site is a(n):
   - A. trauma dressing.
   - B. burn dressing.
   - C. occlusive dressing.
   - D. wet (saline) dressing.

3. Manual cervical spine stabilization may be released:
   - A. when a properly fitting cervical collar is in place.
   - B. when the patient is placed on a long spine board, before securing.
   - C. when the patient is placed on a long spine board and the head and body are properly secured to the board.
   - D. before placing the cervical collar if patient denies pain.

4. You should check for distal pulse, motor, and sensory functions:
   - A. before immobilization.
   - B. during immobilization.
   - C. after immobilization.
   - D. before and after immobilization.

5. The maneuver to immobilize the spine of a standing patient is called a:
   - A. vertical takedown.
   - B. vertical immobilization.
   - C. standing takedown.
   - D. none of the above

6. Signs of a possible dislocation or fracture of an extremity include:
   - A. deformity.
   - B. crepitus.
   - C. swelling.
   - D. any of the above

7. When applying a swathe you should:
   - A. include only the injured arm under the swathe.
   - B. include only the uninjured arm under the swathe.
   - C. include both arms under the swathe.
   - D. use it to secure the shoulder, not the arms.

8. In what order do you secure the straps while immobilizing a patient in a KED?

    A. head, torso, legs

    B. torso, legs, head

    C. legs, torso, head

    D. torso, head, legs

9. To help reduce the swelling of a joint injury, you can apply a:

    A. hot pack.

    B. cold pack.

    C. wet dressing.

    D. none of the above

10. When using a sling and swathe for a shoulder injury, you should position the patient's hand:

    A. no risk of hypertension or flexion exists.

    B. above the level of the elbow.

    C. at the same level as the elbow.

    D. any of the above

11. A helmet can be left in place if:

    A. all injuries can be managed.

    B. the airway and breathing can be assessed and managed.

    C. it fits properly allowing no movement of the head.

    D. all of the above

12. Any patient with musculoskeletal injuries and life-threatening injuries should have his:

    A. musculoskeletal injuries splinted individually.

    B. entire body immobilized on a long spine board.

    C. body transported with manual stabilization only.

    D. none of the above

13. How should you remove a stable patient complaining of neck and back pain from a vehicle?

    A. using rapid extrication with a long spine board without cervical collar

    B. using a cervical collar, short spine board or KED, and long spine board

    C. using rapid extrication with cervical collar and long spine board

    D. using a short spine board or KED, without a cervical collar, and long spine board

14. To determine the proper cervical collar size, you measure the distance from the:

    A. trapezius muscle to the angle of the jaw.

    B. trapezius muscle to the ear canal.

    C. trapezius muscle to the bottom of the earlobe.

    D. trapezius muscle to the base of the occiput.

15. All of the following are rigid splints *except:*

    A. wire ladder splint.

    B. SAM splint.

    C. cardboard splint.

    D. padded board splint.

16. Mechanisms of injury that require spinal immobilization include:

    A. traffic collisions.

    B. assaults.

    C. boating accidents.

    D. all of the above

17. Appropriate bandaging should be secured:

    A. to keep dressing materials in place.

    B. to limit further bleeding.

    C. to limit nerve or muscle damage.

    D. all of the above

18. Your patient has a deformed extremity and absent distal pulse; you should:

    A. immobilize in position found.

    B. leave in position found, but do not immobilize.

    C. realign and immobilize when circulation has been restored.

    D. realign until circulation has been restored, but do not immobilize.

19. Signs of shock include all of following *except:*

    A. changes in mental status.

    B. tachycardia.

    C. cool and clammy skin.

    D. hypertension.

20. When sealing an open chest wound, you should:

    A. use a nonocclusive dressing and seal on only three sides.

    B. use a nonocclusive dressing and seal on all four sides.

    C. use an occlusive dressing and seal on only three sides.

    D. use an occlusive dressing and seal, on all four sides.

ANSWER KEY

Chapter 1
1. b
2. b
3. c

Chapter 2
1. b
2. a
3. c

Chapter 3
1. a
2. b
3. d

Chapter 4
1. b
2. c
3. d

Chapter 5
1. d
2. b
3. c

Chapter 6
1. c
2. b
3. d

Chapter 7
1. c
2. a
3. d

Chapter 8
1. b
2. d
3. a

Chapter 9
1. c
2. d
3. b

Chapter 10
1. c
2. b
3. d

Chapter 11
1. b
2. d
3. a

Chapter 12
1. d
2. c
3. b

Chapter 13
1. c
2. b
3. b

Chapter 14
1. c
2. b
3. d

Chapter 15
1. c
2. b
3. d

Chapter 16
1. b
2. a
3. d

Chapter 17
1. d
2. c
3. b

Chapter 18
1. b
2. a
3. c

Chapter 19
1. c
2. b
3. a

Chapter 20
1. a
2. c
3. c

Chapter 21
1. b
2. d
3. d

Chapter 22
1. c
2. d
3. b

Chapter 23
1. c
2. b
3. d

Chapter 24
1. c
2. c
3. c

Chapter 25
1. b
2. a
3. d

Chapter 26
1. b
2. d
3. a

Chapter 27
1. a
2. c
3. b

Chapter 28
1. b
2. c
3. c

Chapter 29
1. c
2. c
3. b

Chapter 30
1. d
2. b
3. c

Chapter 31

1. d
2. b
3. a

Chapter 32

1. b
2. c
3. a

Chapter 33

1. d
2. c
3. d

Chapter 34

1. d
2. b
3. a

Chapter 35

1. d
2. c
3. b

Chapter 36

1. d
2. b
3. c

Chapter 37

1. b
2. c
3. c

Chapter 38

1. a
2. b
3. b

Chapter 39

1. c
2. a
3. c

Chapter 40

1. d
2. b
3. c

Chapter 41

1. d
2. c
3. c

Chapter 42

1. b
2. b
3. c

Chapter 43

1. d
2. d
3. b

Chapter 44

1. b
2. b
3. a

Chapter 45

1. d
2. a
3. c

Chapter 46

1. c
2. a
3. b

Chapter 47

1. b
2. c
3. a

Chapter 48

1. a
2. c
3. b

Chapter 49

1. a
2. d
3. b

Chapter 50

1. d
2. c
3. a

Review Questions

Section 1

1. d

RATIONALE: A nonrebreather face mask will provide concentrations of oxygen ranging from 80 to 100 percent.

2. d

RATIONALE: The Combitube® is the primary backup airway in most ALS systems. The device offers several major advantages. First, it is a "blind technique" that does not require visualization of the trachea. Second, the Combitube® may prevent vomit from entering the trachea, thus protecting the airway. Third, the Combitube® allows for rapid intubation of the patient independent of the patient's position. This is especially helpful for trauma patients who require limited movement of the cervical spine.

3. c

RATIONALE: Children's and infant's ventilations should be delivered over 1 to 1.5 seconds and the rate of ventilations should be at least one breath every 3 seconds.

4. b

RATIONALE: A soft catheter is inserted down the ET tube beyond the tip to the level of the carina, the branching point of the trachea.

5. c

RATIONALE: On E-size cylinders, or smaller, the pressure regulator is secured to the cylinder valve assembly by a yoke assembly. This is called a pin-index safety system. This system prevents an oxygen delivery system from being connected to a cylinder containing a gas other than oxygen because the pin position varies for different gases. Cylinders larger than the E size have a valve assembly with a threaded outlet. The inside and outside diameters of the threaded outlets vary according to the gas in the cylinder. This is to prevent an oxygen regulator from being connected to a cylinder containing a different gas such as helium or nitrogen.

6. b

RATIONALE: Use of an oral airway should be considered in any patient who is not breathing or who is unresponsive and a gag reflex is not present.

7. b

RATIONALE: A nasogastric tube may be used to help relieve gastric distension, a common problem with ventilating a nonintubated patient. Such distension occurs when the procedure's high pressures cause air to become trapped in the stomach.

8. b

RATIONALE: The jaw-thrust maneuver should be considered in a patient who needs his airway opened and has a suspected head and/or spinal injury.

9. b

RATIONALE: If mucus is too thick to suction, and the materials are available to you, consider injecting 3 to 5 cc of normal saline through the stoma to break up the plug and aid in its removal.

10. b

RATIONALE: When using a pulse oximeter, keep in mind that readings will not be accurate in all patients. For example, patients exposed to carbon monoxide (CO), including chronic cigarette smokers, may have falsely high readings because CO binds to hemoglobin, producing the red color read by the device. Anemic patients and patients who have ingested certain kinds of poisons may also have falsely high SpO_2 readings. Hypoperfused patients, including patients in shock or hypothermic patients, do not have enough blood flowing through their capillaries to provide accurate readings. False readings can also result if the probe is placed on the patient's injured extremity.

11. c

RATIONALE: A flowmeter is used to regulate the flow of oxygen in liters per minute. It is connected to the pressure regulator and most services keep the flowmeter permanently attached to it. The three major types of flowmeters are the Bourdon gauge flowmeter (useful for most portable units), constant flow selector valve (useful with any size oxygen cylinder), and pressure-compensated flowmeter (useful for fixed delivery systems).

12. c

RATIONALE: Never suction for more than 15 seconds at a time. Do not suction more than 5 seconds in children and infants.

13. c

RATIONALE: Ideally, once you have applied Sellick's maneuver, you must maintain it until endotracheal intubation is confirmed and personnel are ready to suction the oropharynx or place a nasogastric tube to decompress the stomach.

14. c

RATIONALE: Insertion of an endotracheal tube is the preferred technique for maintaining the airway of an unconscious patient. Although the ET is usually used in situations where the patient does not have a gag reflex, patients may be given a medication to remove the gag reflex.

15. d

RATIONALE: EMT-Basics must become familiar with several types of tanks. Portable cylinders for the field include D cylinders, which contain about 350 liters of oxygen, and E cylinders, which contain about 625 liters of oxygen. Onboard cylinders include M cylinders, which contain about 3,000 liters of oxygen; G cylinders, which contain about 5,300 liters of oxygen; and H cylinders, which contain about 6,900 liters of oxygen.

16. b
RATIONALE: A nasal cannula provides low concentrations of oxygen, ranging from 24 to 44 percent.

17. a
RATIONALE: The head-tilt/chin-lift maneuver opens the airway by tilting the head back while simultaneously lifting the chin forward. This movement brings the tongue forward, thus opening the air passage.

18. b
RATIONALE: The amount of volume generated by the BVM is directly related to the abilities of the EMS provider. If the BVM is attached to oxygen, the amount of volume needed to ventilate the average size adult patient is 500 mL delivered over 1 to 2 seconds.

19. c
RATIONALE: The cricoid cartilage is located inferior to the thyroid cartilage, or Adam's apple. To find it, palpate the thyroid cartilage with the tip of your finger until you find a slight depression. This depression is the cricothyroid membrane. Just inferior to the cricothyroid membrane is the solid ring of cartilage known as the cricoid cartilage.

20. a
RATIONALE: Gently pushing the tip of the nose upward, insert the airway with the bevel (angled portion at the tip) pointing toward the base of the nostril or toward the septum (wall that separates nostrils).

Section 2

1. d
RATIONALE: After ensuring scene safety, the initial assessment is performed and any life-threatening problems identified and treated. The initial assessment includes forming a general impression of the patient, condition, and MOI/NOI; assessing mental status using the AVPU mnemonic; assessing airway, breathing, and circulation and treating any life-threatening problems; and determining the priority for transport.

2. b
RATIONALE: During the detailed physical exam, the EMT systematically inspects and palpates each part of the body for abnormalities including deformities, contusions, abrasions, punctures and penetrations, burns, tenderness, lacerations, or swelling.

3. c
RATIONALE: High-priority conditions that require immediate transport include poor general impression, unresponsive, responsive but not following commands, difficulty breathing, shock, complicated childbirth, chest pain with systolic blood pressure less than 100, uncontrolled bleeding, and severe pain.

4. c
RATIONALE: Instead of a physical exam focused just on the area of injury, the patient with a significant mechanism of injury receives a complete, head-to-toe, rapid trauma assessment.

5. d
RATIONALE: BSI personal protective equipment includes protective latex or vinyl gloves, eye protection shields, masks, and gowns.

6. d
RATIONALE: If properly sized equipment is not available, then blood pressures may not have been taken for small children. Perfusion can be assessed and reassessed using distal pulses, skin color, and capillary refill instead.

7. b
RATIONALE: Assess mental status using the AVPU mnemonic, which stands for *Alert, Verbal, Painful,* and *Unresponsive.*

8. c
RATIONALE: Rocking the pelvis to assess for stability is no longer acceptable. Gentle pressure lateral to medial and anterior to posterior is appropriate and will identify most pelvic injuries without compromising the spine.

9. b
RATIONALE: Provide manual cervical stabilization upon first contact for any patient suspected of having a neck or spinal injury.

10. b
RATIONALE: The *baseline vitals*—the first readings that you record—will give you a foundation on which to make health care decisions and to judge the impact of these decisions. As you retake vital signs, the *serial vital signs,* you will compare the readings to your previous findings. Serial vital sign assessments allow you to note trends in the patient's condition, such as a declining blood pressure or increasing respiratory rate.

11. b
RATIONALE: Proper body mechanics for lifting include positioning feet on a firm surface, shoulder width apart; using legs, not back, to lift by bending at the knees and keeping head up; keeping back straight; keeping patient's weight close to body; not twisting while lifting; not reaching more than 20 inches in front of your body; pushing, rather than pulling, an object when possible; keeping elbows bent and arms close to sides; and using the power lift and power grip whenever possible.

12. d

RATIONALE: The ongoing assessment begins with reassessment of the initial assessment. Interruptions in airway, breathing, or circulation should be treated without delay. Vital signs will be reassessed and changes noted. It is during the ongoing assessment that serial vital signs are established. The focused physical exam should be repeated to determine if any further treatment is needed. Or, if a detailed physical exam was conducted, this should be repeated now. Overall, you should be able to report to the hospital any changes in the patient's condition and whether or not your interventions helped the patient.

13. d

RATIONALE: For a trauma patient, first conduct a physical exam to assess injuries. Next, assess baseline vitals and take a SAMPLE history.

14. c

RATIONALE: Vital signs should be reassessed every 5 minutes for critical patients and every 15 minutes for stable patients. All patients should have an initial or baseline set of vital signs taken, as well as at least one more set taken prior to arrival at the hospital or transfer of care to another agency or unit.

15. d

RATIONALE: Check the neck for injuries, plus jugular venous distension and crepitation of the cervical spine bones. This should be done before a cervical collar is placed. Careful assessment of the neck can prevent serious injuries that can result in paralysis.

16. b

RATIONALE: Significant mechanisms of injury include ejection from a vehicle, death in the same passenger compartment, falls of more than 15 feet or three times the patient's height, rollover of vehicle, high-speed vehicle collision, vehicle-pedestrian collision, motorcycle crash, unresponsive or altered mental status, and penetrations of the head, chest, or abdomen, for example, stab and gunshot wounds. Additional significant mechanisms of injury for children include falls from more than 10 feet, bicycle collisions, and medium-speed vehicle collisions.

17. b

RATIONALE: Both HEPA and N-95 masks filter out small particulates and are approved for use in reducing transmission of tuberculosis.

18. c

RATIONALE: Assess the chest for DCAP-BTLS, plus crepitation, paradoxical motion, and breath sounds.

19. a

RATIONALE: In contrast to the trauma patient assessment, which relies heavily on the physical exam to identify life-threatening injuries, the medical patient assessment requires a thorough history taking. The past medical history and history of present illness are easily obtained from the conscious medical patient. For the unconscious medical patient, however, the history may have to be pieced together from items found on scene, bystanders, and findings of the physical examination.

20. c

RATIONALE: The initial assessment, formerly referred to as the primary assessment, is aimed at identifying any life-threatening problems. Abnormal findings in the initial assessment should be treated immediately, before proceeding with any further assessment.

Section 3

1. c

RATIONALE: Place auto-injector device on the lateral thigh midway between the knee and the waist. This area has a large amount of muscle mass that allows for good absorption of epinephrine.

2. b

RATIONALE: Activated charcoal is not an antidote, that is, a substance that neutralizes a poison or its effects. It works through absorption, the process in which one substance becomes attached to the surface of another. Activated charcoal has been manufactured to have many cracks and crevices, thereby increasing the surface area to which poisons might bind.

3. c

RATIONALE: At least four people are required to restrain a patient. Each person should be preassigned a limb to restrain. Rescuers should act all at once to overwhelm the patient.

4. b

RATIONALE: Glucose can reverse a diabetic patient's potentially life-threatening hypoglycemic or low blood sugar condition.

5. b

RATIONALE: Labor is divided into three stages. The first stage is when contractions start and the cervix becomes fully dilated. The second stage ends when the baby is delivered. Finally, the third stage ends with the delivery of the placenta.

6. b

RATIONALE: The most significant problem associated with nitroglycerin is the possibility of causing a hypotensive event. Usually you can relieve this condition by placing the patient in a supine position and raising the legs slightly.

7. c

RATIONALE: Keep in mind the several groups of patients in which activated charcoal is generally contraindicated. Patients who cannot swallow obviously cannot take activated charcoal. Patients with an altered mental status might choke when swallowing the slurry and aspirate the substance into their lungs. Patients who have ingested acids or alkalis should not swallow activated charcoal; the caustic materials may have damaged the mouth, throat, and esophagus and swallowing the slurry might cause further injury. Also, patients who have been poisoned by cyanide, organic solvents, iron, ethanol, and methanol should not be given activated charcoal because, again, swallowing the slurry might cause further injury.

8. d
RATIONALE: The device has the ability to recognize ventricular fibrillation (VF) or ventricular tachycardia (VT) as a shockable rhythm without the need for interpretation by the user. The device can also interpret rhythms that are not VF or VT as nonshockable rhythms. Because these devices interpret the rhythm, they do not require the expertise of rhythm recognition by the manual defibrillator.

9. c
RATIONALE: A nebulizer is a device that is used to aerosolize medications into a mist for delivery directly to the lungs. Medication is then absorbed from the lower airways and the lungs to the bloodstream.

10. c
RATIONALE: While the AED is analyzing, all patient contact must stop. You should visually check the area and state loudly and clearly "stand clear." In some EMS systems they require you to say the following: "I'm clear, you're clear, everyone clear."

11. b
RATIONALE: For the medication to be properly dosed, the inhaler should be at room temperature or warmer. Shake the canister vigorously for at least 30 seconds. The shaking of the canister mixes the medication and the propellant to a specific metered dose. Without shaking, a wrong dose can be administered.

12. b
RATIONALE: The single most important link in the "chain of survival" in the cardiac arrest patient is the successful use of the defibrillator. Studies show that time to defibrillation may be even more important than CPR.

13. b
RATIONALE: Attach the oxygen-connecting tubing from the nebulizer to the oxygen source. Adjust oxygen to 6 lpm. You should be able to see a mist coming out of both the flex tube and the mouthpiece.

14. c
RATIONALE: A breech presentation occurs when the baby's buttocks or both feet present first instead of the head.

15. c
RATIONALE: The most common bronchodilators include albuterol (Proventil, Ventolin), metaproterenol (Metaprel, Alupent), and isoetharine (Bronchosol, Bronkometer).

16. c
RATIONALE: The patient should be secured on the ambulance gurney in a supine or lateral position.

17. a
RATIONALE: If contractions are less than 2 minutes apart, prepare for imminent delivery.

18. a
RATIONALE: In the patient with a severe reaction, it will constrict blood vessels and will dilate the bronchioles. The actions will assist with the patient suffering from hypotension and/or shortness of breath.

19. c
RATIONALE: Insert tongue depressor with glucose into the patient's mouth and apply between the cheek and the gum. Or apply it under the patient's tongue without using the tongue depressor. In some cases the patient can self-administer the glucose by directly squeezing the glucose into his own mouth.

20. c
RATIONALE: To assist a patient with nitro, all of the following indications must be met: The patient complains of chest pain; the patient has a history of cardiac problems; the patient's physician has prescribed nitro; the patient has the medication with him or her; the patient's systolic blood pressure is greater than 100 systolic; and medical direction, a standing medical order, or local protocol allows you to assist the patient with nitro.

Section 4

1. c
RATIONALE: Pelvic injuries commonly involve either the pelvic bones themselves or the proximal head of the femur. Hip injuries should not be splinted using a traction splint. Only midshaft femur fractures should be splinted with traction splints.

2. c
RATIONALE: An occlusive dressing is a dressing that prevents any air from entering the wound site. Occlusive material may include any nonbreathable substance.

3. c

RATIONALE: Ensure the collar is fitted and applied properly. The collar should not hyperextend the neck or fit so snugly that it constricts the airway or impedes breathing. Maintain manual cervical stabilization until the patient is secured on a spine board. Move the patient to a spine board for further movement or transport. Movement of the head can be further minimized by placing headblocks or towel rolls on either side of the head before taping the head to the board.

4. d

RATIONALE: Assess the patient's sensory, motor, and circulatory status in the extremity prior to immobilization. Lack of distal circulation is an indication that you need to attempt realignment of the joint. Reassess the patient's sensory, motor, and circulatory status in the extremity after immobilizations. Any change in distal circulation, sensation, or movement can indicate further injury or improper application of the splint.

5. c

RATIONALE: Spinal immobilization of the standing patient is accomplished with a maneuver known as the standing takedown. This skill may be necessary if the victim of a traumatic incident presents ambulatory at the scene or standing while calling for help, inspecting a vehicle for damage, or wandering about due to confusion or disorientation. The standing takedown is used to immediately provide manual stabilization of the head and neck while immobilizing the spine to a long spine board. The maneuver prevents the patient from further movement or manipulation of the spine and secures him to the board while easing the patient to the supine position.

6. d

RATIONALE: Signs of a possible dislocation or fracture of an extremity, such as pain, deformity, crepitus, and swelling, should be treated by splinting the extremity.

7. a

RATIONALE: A swathe is made with another triangular bandage tied around the injured arm and chest of the patient. Do not include the uninjured arm in the swathe. The swathe further minimizes movement of the shoulder girdle and upper extremity.

8. b

RATIONALE: Secure the torso to the board using the straps of the KED. Fasten the leg straps to ensure the pelvis is immobilized. Be sure the straps do not prevent adequate chest excursion or otherwise limit tidal volume. Place padding behind the head if necessary to ensure neutral alignment. Secure the head to the board using tape or the straps provided with the KED.

9. b

RATIONALE: A cold pack applied to the injury site may help reduce swelling.

10. b

RATIONALE: Draw up the ends of the bandage until the patient's hand is several inches above the level of the elbow. Tie a knot using both ends of the triangular bandage. Keeping the hand several inches above the elbow will reduce strain on the joint, thus minimizing pain.

11. d

RATIONALE: The helmet can be left in place when it is form fitted enough that no movement of the head exists within the helmet, all injuries can be managed with the helmet in place, and airway and breathing can be assessed and managed with the helmet in place. Helmet removal may be necessary when the helmet is ill fitting or impedes assessment and management of airway and breathing.

12. b

RATIONALE: Any unstable patient or any patient with life-threatening injuries should have his or her entire body immobilized on a long spine board and transported without delay.

13. b

RATIONALE: The standard of care for a stable patient complaining of neck and back pain is careful removal using a short board or Kendrick extrication device.

14. a

RATIONALE: Determine the proper size of cervical collar needed by measuring the distance between the trapezius muscle and the angle of the jaw. Use your finger width as a guide. Correlate this distance to the distance on the cervical collar between the bottom of the rigid plastic and the sizing post. Do not include the soft foam in your finger-width measurement of the collar. The foam provides no support and will compress when in place around the patient's neck.

15. b

RATIONALE: Rigid splints include wire ladder, cardboard, and padded board splints. Pillows, SAM splints, and vacuum splints are considered formable splints.

16. d

RATIONALE: Patients requiring spinal immobilization have many mechanisms of injury, which include, but are not limited to, traffic collisions, boating accidents, sporting injuries, falls, and assaults.

17. d

RATIONALE: Following hemorrhage control, an appropriate bandage can be secured to keep dressing materials in place and limit further bleeding, nerve, or muscle damage.

18. c

RATIONALE: If deformity is present or distal circulation is absent, realign the bone ends until neutral alignment or return of circulation is achieved.

19. d

RATIONALE: Signs of shock include changes in mental status, tachycardia, cool and clammy skin, and hypotension. Left untreated, hemorrhage can lead to exsanguination (bleeding to death).

20. c

RATIONALE: An occlusive dressing is used to seal the chest so that air cannot enter through the wound. A flutter valve is placed on the dressing to allow air to escape passively or with the assistance of the rescuer. Initially seal the wound with a gloved hand. Replace the gloved hand with an occlusive dressing taped on only three sides.

GLOSSARY

Abrasions scratches or scrapes.

Absorption passage of a substance through skin or mucous membranes upon contact.

Acetone wipe a cleaning agent containing a chemical solvent.

Activated charcoal a powder, usually premixed with water, that will absorb some poisons and will prevent them from being absorbed by the body.

Agonal respiration a gasping-type respiration that has no pattern and occurs very infrequently; a sign of impending cardiac or respiratory arrest. *Also called* agonal breathing.

Airborne particles particles transported by air.

Alkali a strong base, especially the metallic hydroxides. Alkalis combine with acids to form salts, combine with fatty acids to form soap, neutralize acids, and turn litmus paper blue.

Altered level of consciousness situation where a patient is in a questionable mental state, ranging from sleep to a coma.

Altered mental status a condition in which the patient displays a change in his normal mental state ranging from disorientation to complete unresponsiveness.

Ambulatory able to walk; not confined to bed.

Amniotic sac the "bag of waters" that surrounds the developing fetus.

Amputation the surgical removal or traumatic severing of a body part, usually an extremity.

Anatomical disturbances body-related abnormalities.

Anemia when blood lacks red blood cells, hemoglobin, or total volume.

Angina pain in the chest, occurring when blood supply to the heart is re-duced and a portion of the heart muscle is not receiving enough oxygen.

Angle of the jaw the angle formed by the junction of the posterior edge of the ramus of the mandible and the lower surface of the body of the mandible.

Ankle hitch traction device that slides over and stabilizes the ankle.

Antecubital fossa triangular area lying anterior to and below the elbow, bounded medially by the pronator teres and laterally by the brachioradialis muscles.

Anterior-axillary line a vertical skin fold along the anterior axillary fold; crease of the underarm.

Antidote substance that will neutralize the poison or its effects.

Apnea absence of breathing.

Artificial ventilation forcing air or oxygen into the lungs when a patient has stopped breathing or has inadequate breathing. *Also called* positive pressure ventilation.

Aspiration breathing a foreign substance into the lungs.

Auscultate Listen. A stethoscope is used to auscultate for characteristic body sounds.

Automated external defibrillator (AED) a device that can analyze the electrical activity or rhythm of a patient's heart and deliver an electrical shock (defibrillation) if appropriate.

Avulsion the tearing away or tearing off of a piece or flap of skin or other soft tissue. This term also may be used for an eye pulled from its socket or a tooth dislodged from its socket.

Bag-valve-mask ventilation artificial ventilation to a patient via squeezing a handheld device with a face mask and self-refilling bag. Can deliver air from the atmosphere or oxygen from a supplemental oxygen supply system.

Bandage any material used to hold a dressing in place.

Baseline mental status a control measurement used for comparisons when determining altered mental states.

Baseline vital signs the first set of vital signs measurements to which subsequent measurements can be compared.

Biphasic energy levels defibrillation shocks that are first administered in one direction, and then another.

Body mechanics the proper use of the body to facilitate lifting and moving and prevent injury.

Brachial pulse the pulse felt in the upper arm; the pulse checked during infant CPR.

Brachycardia a heart rate less than 60 beats per minute.

Bronchioles smaller branches of the bronchi that continue to branch and get smaller, eventually leading into alveolar sacs.

Bronchodilator therapy use of a medicine to enlarge constricted bronchial tubes, making breathing easier.

Bronchodilators drugs that relax the smooth muscle of the bronchi and bronchioles and reverse bronchoconstriction.

BSI equipment body substance isolation equipment, consisting of gloves, masks, goggles, used to prevent the spread of disease through pathogens.

BSI precautions steps taken to prevent the spread of disease through bloodborne or airborne pathogens.

Burns tissue injury resulting from excessive exposure to thermal, chemical, electrical, or radioactive agents.

Carbon monoxide poisoning toxicity that results from inhalation of small amounts of carbon monoxide over a long period or from large amounts inhaled for a short time.

Carina the fork at the lower end of the trachea where the two mainstem bronchi branch.

Carotid pulse the pulse felt along the large carotid artery on either side of the neck.

Caustic solutions an agent that burns or dissolves organic tissue through chemical action.

Caustic substance an agent, particularly an alkali, that destroys living tissue.

Cervical collar device placed around the neck to stabilize the spinal column in the event of a suspected injury.

Chief complaint in emergency medicine, the reason EMS was called, usually in the patient's own words.

Childbirth the physiological process by which the fetus is expelled from the uterus into the vagina and then to the outside of the body. *Also called* labor.

Chronic pulmonary disease umbrella term used to describe pulmonary diseases such as emphysema or chronic bronchitis.

Circumferential encircling a body area; e.g., arm, leg, or chest.

Clavicle the collarbone.

Constipation a decrease in a person's normal frequency of defecation accompanied by difficult or incomplete passage of stool and/or passage of excessively hard, dry stool.

Contraction a shortening or tightening, as of a muscle; a shrinking or reduction in size.

Contusions bruises; in brain injuries, a bruised brain caused when the force of a blow to the head is great enough to rupture blood vessels.

Cravat a band or scarf worn around the neck.

Crepitation the grating sound or feeling of broken bones rubbing together. *Also called* crepitus.

Crepitus the sound or feel of broken fragments of bone grinding against each other.

Cricoid cartilage the ring-shaped structure that circles the trachea at the lower end of the larynx.

Cross-finger technique a technique in which the thumb and index finger are crossed, with the thumb on the lower incisors and the index finger on the upper incisors. The fingers are moved in a snapping or scissor motion to open the mouth.

Crowning when part of the baby is visible through the vaginal opening.

Cyanide a rapid-acting agent that disrupts the ability of the cell to use oxygen, leading to severe cellular hypoxia and eventual death.

Cyanosis a blue or gray color resulting from lack of oxygen in the body.

Debridement the removal of foreign material and dead or damaged tissue, especially in a wound.

Defibrillation electrical shock or current delivered to the heart through the patient's chest wall to help the heart restore a normal rhythm.

Deformity alteration in the natural form of a part or organ; distortion of any part or general disfigurement of the body. It may be acquired or congenital. If present after injury, deformity usually implies the presence of fracture, dislocation, or both. It may be due to extensive swelling, extravasation of blood, or rupture of muscles.

Diabetes *also called* "sugar diabetes," the condition brought about by decreased insulin production or the inability of the body cells to use insulin properly. The person with this condition is a diabetic.

Diastolic blood pressure the pressure remaining in the arteries when the left ventricle of the heart is relaxed and refilling.

Dislocation the disruption or "coming apart" of a joint.

Distal farther away from the torso. *Opposite of* proximal.

Do not recuscitate (DNR) order a legal document, usually signed by the patient and his physician, which states that the patient has a terminal illness and does not wish to prolong life through resuscitative efforts.

Dorsalis pedal pulse pulse taken at the artery supplying blood to the foot, lateral to the large tendon of the big toe.

Dressing any material (preferably sterile) used to cover a wound that will help control bleeding and help prevent additional contamination.

Dysrhythmia a disturbance in heart rate and rhythm.

Edema swelling resulting from buildup of fluid in the tissues.

Endotracheal (ET) intubation placement of a tube down the trachea to facilitate air flow into the lungs and aid in breathing.

Endotracheal (ET) tube a tube designed to be inserted into the trachea. Oxygen, medication, or a suction catheter can be directed into the trachea through an endotracheal tube.

Epiglottis a leaf-shaped structure that prevents food and foreign matter from entering the trachea.

Epinephrine auto-injector a syringe with a spring-loaded needle that administers epinephrine to patients who are susceptible to severe allergic reactions.

Esophageal Tracheal Combitube® (ETC) a double lumen airway where the two lumens are separated by a partition wall; used on unconscious patients over five feet tall.

Esophagus the tube that leads from the pharynx to the stomach.

Evisceration an intestine or other internal organ protruding through a wound in the abdomen.

Exsanguination massive bleeding.

Extremity the portions of the skeleton that include the clavicles, scapulae, arms, wrists, and hands (upper extremities) and the pelvis, thighs, legs, ankles, and feet (lower extremities).

Extubation the removal of a tube.

Eye protection personal protective equipment such as goggles use to prevent illness or injury from affecting the eyes.

Femoral pulse pulse found in the major artery supplying the leg; can be found in the crease between the abdomen and groin.

Field impression evaluation of the environment to ascertain if a patient is in further danger because of location.

Flowmeter a valve that indicates the flow of oxygen in liters per minute.

Focused history the step of patient assessment that follows the initial assessment and includes the patient history, physical exam, and vital signs.

Fontanelle the "soft spot" on the top of an infant's head where the plates of the skull have not yet formed together.

Formable splint splints that can be molded to different angles, and therefore allow considerable movement.

Fracture any break in a bone.

French (unit of measure) a European term for a size of tubing equivalent to about .013 thousandths of an inch; the larger the number, the larger the catheter.

Gag reflex vomiting or retching that results when something is placed in the back of the pharynx.

Gastric distension inflation of the stomach.

Gastric extension enlargement of the stomach.

General impression impression of the patient's condition that is formed on first approaching the patient, based on the patient's environment, chief complaint, and appearance.

Glottic opening the opening to the trachea.

Gloves a protective covering for the hand. In medical care, the glove is made of a flexible, impervious material that permits full movement of the fingers. Gloves are used to protect both the operative site from contamination with organisms from the health care worker and the health care worker from contamination with pathogens from the patient.

Glucose monitoring process whereby people with diabetes determine the level of glucose in the blood, which dictates how much insulin should be taken.

Gown a coverall worn in an operating room

Handheld nebulizer portable device capable of emitting a fine spray.

HARE traction splint splint used for femur fractures that helps immobilize the leg during transport.

Head-tilt/chin-lift maneuver a means of corrrecting blockage of the airway by the tongue by tilting the head back and lifting the chin. Used when no trauma, or injury, is suspected. *See also* jaw-thrust maneuver.

Hemodynamically unstable situation where abnormalities exist in the circulation of the blood.

Hemoglobin a complex protein molecule found on the surface of the red blood cell that is responsible for carrying a majority of oxygen in the blood.

Hemorrhage bleeding, especially severe bleeding.

High-priority conditions situations that require immediate attention; include unresponsive, difficult breathing, shock, uncontrolled bleeding, severe pain, or complicated childbirth.

Humerus the bone of the upper arm, between the shoulder and the elbow.

Hydrocarbon a compound made up primarily of hydrogen and carbon.

Hydrochloric acid an aqueous solution of hydrogen chloride that is a strong corrosive irritating acid, is normally present in dilute form in gastric juice and is widely used in industry and in the laboratory.

Hyperextension extreme or abnormal extension.

Hyperventilate to provide ventilations at a higher rate than normal.

Hyperventilation increased minute volume ventilation, which results in a lowered carbon dioxide level. It is a frequent finding in many disease processes such as asthma, metabolic acidosis, pulmonary embolism, and pulmonary edema, and also in anxiety-induced states.

Hypoglycemia low blood sugar.

Hypoperfusion shock; inadequate perfusion of the cells and tissues of the body caused by insufficient flow of blood through the capillaries. *See also* perfusion.

Hypotension a deficiency in tone or tension; a decrease of the systolic and diastolic blood pressure to below normal. This occurs, for example, in shock, hemorrhage, dehydration, sepsis, Addison's disease, and in may other diseases and conditions.

Hypoventilation reduced rate and depth of breathing that causes an increase in carbon dioxide.

Hypovolemic shock shock resulting from blood or fluid loss.

Hypoxia an insufficiency of oxygen in the body's tissues.

Immobilization the making of a part or limb immovable.

Impaled object an object embedded in an injury to the body.

Index of suspicion awareness that there may be injuries.

Infection control plan a written policy required of all agencies that details the steps to follow in the event of exposure to infectious substances.

Infectious diseases illnesses spread by contact with patients carrying viruses or bacteria; minimized through the use of personal protective equipment.

Inferior away from the head; usually compared with another structure that is closer to the head (e.g., the lips are inferior to the nose). *Opposite of* superior.

Initial assessment the first element in assessment of a patient; steps taken for the purpose of discovering and dealing with any life-threatening problems. The six parts of initial assessment are: forming a general impression, assessing mental status, assessing airway, assessing breathing, assessing circulation, and determining the priority of the patient for treatment and transport to the hospital.

In-line immobilization bringing the patient's head into a neutral position in which the nose is lined up with the navel and holding it there manually.

Inspection visual examination of the external surface of the body as well as of its movements and posture.

Intercostal space between the ribs.

Intubation insertion of a tube.

Ischial strap device used for support of the ischium, or posterior portion of the pelvis.

Ischium the lower, posterior portions of the pelvis.

Jaundiced skin yellowness of the skin.

Jaw-thrust maneuver a means of correcting blockage of the airway by moving the jaw forward without tilting the head or neck. Used when trauma, or injury, is suspected to open the airway without causing further injury to the spinal cord in the neck. *See also* head-tilt/chin-lift maneuver.

Kendrick extrication device (KED) a vest-type immobilizer designed to limit movement of the cervical and thoracic spine in seated patients with suspected spinal cord injuries.

Kinematics the branch of biomechanics concerned with description of the movements of segments of the body without regard to the forces that caused the movement to occur.

Kling soft, flexible roller-gauze used in dressing and bandaging.

Lacerations cuts; in brain injuries, a cut to the brain.

Laryngectomy a surgical procedure in which a patient's larynx is removed. A stoma is created for the patient to breathe through.

Laryngoscope an illuminating instrument that is inserted into the pharynx to permit visualization of the pharynx and larynx.

Lateral position to the side; away from the midline of the body.

Level of consciousness varying stages of patient awareness.

Level of distress evaluation of the amount of pain or distress within the patient.

Life threats situation in which a patient is in need of immediate action for survival.

Lifting devices equipment used to elevate patients from the ground.

Low-flow oxygen method of delivering oxygen to a patient through nasal cannulas inserted in the nose.

Mandible the lower jaw bone.

Manual defibrillation older defibrillation method where an operator reviews a patient's heart rhythm, decides it is shockable, lubricates two paddles, and delivers a shock to the patient's chest.

Manual traction the process of applying tension to straighten and realign a fractured limb before splinting. *Also called* tension.

Mask a covering for the face that serves as a protective barrier.

MAST medical anti-shock trousers.

Mechanism of injury (MOI) a force or forces that may have caused injury.

Metered-dose inhaler (MDI) device consisting of a plastic container and a canister of medication that is used to inhale an aerosolized medication.

Midclavicular line the line through the center of each clavicle.

Midshaft femur thick portion of the lower leg bone.

Monophasic energy levels sending energy in one direction.

Mucous plugs clots of mucous built up in the lungs, which can block the airway if coughed up.

Myocardial infarction the loss of living heart muscle as a result of coronary artery occlusion.

Nares the nostrils.

Nasal cannula a device that delivers low concentrations of oxygen through two prongs that rest in the patient's nostrils.

Nasogastric (NG) tube a tube designed to be passed through the nose, nasopharynx, and esophagus. It is used to relieve distention of the stomach in an infant or child patient.

Nasopharyngeal airway (NPA) a flexible breathing tube inserted through the patient's nose into the pharynx to help maintain an open airway.

Nasopharynx the airway directly posterior to the nose.

Nature of the illness what is medically wrong with a patient.

Nebulizer chamber an apparatus for producing a fine spray or mist. This may be done by rapidly passing air through a liquid or by vibrating a liquid at a high frequency so that the particles produced are extremely small.

Neutral alignment the position of bones in anatomical position, without excessive extension, flexion, or rotation.

Neutrally aligned position the position of bones in anatomical position, without excessive extension, flexion, or rotation.

Nitroglycerin a drug that helps to dilate the coronary vessels that supply the heart muscle with blood.

Nitroglycerin patch adhesive-backed material that administers nitroglycerin through the skin (dermal administration) several times a day.

Nonmetallic surface area that does not contain the chemical properties of a metal.

Nonrebreather mask a face mask and reservoir bag device that delivers high concentrations of oxygen. The patient's exhaled air escapes through a valve and is not rebreathed.

Nonurgent moves patient moves made when no immediate threat to life exists.

Nostril one of the external apertures of the nose.

Occiput the back part of the skull.

Occlusive dressing any dressing that forms an airtight seal.

One-way valve valve that allows movement in only one direction, such as the valve that prevents blood from being forced back up the atrium.

Ongoing assessment a procedure for detecting changes in a patient's condition. It involves four steps: repeating the initial assessment, repeating and recording vital signs, repeating the focused assessment, and checking interventions.

Open wounds an injury in which the skin is interrupted, exposing the tissue beneath.

Oral glucose a form of glucose (a kind of sugar) given by mouth to treat an awake patient (who is able to swallow) with an altered mental status and a history of diabetes.

Orbits the bony structures around the eyes; the eye sockets.

Organic solvents naturally occurring compound used to dissolve or disperse other substances.

Oropharyngeal airway (OPA) a curved device inserted through the patient's mouth into the pharynx to help maintain an open airway.

Oxygen regulator a device connected to an oxygen cylinder that reduces pressure to a safe level for the patient to intake.

Oxygen saturation percentage the ratio of the amount of oxygen present in the blood to the amount that could be carried, expressed as a percentage.

Oxytocin a pituitary hormone that stimulates the uterus to contract, thus inducing parturition. It also acts on the mammary gland to stimulate the release of milk.

Pacemaker in cardiology, a specialized cell or group of cells that automatically regenerates impulses that spread to other regions of the heart. The normal cardiac pacemaker is the sinoatrial node, a group of cells in the right atrium near the entrance of the superior vena cava. A generally accepted term for artificial cardiac pacemaker.

Painful stimulus an agent that causes extreme discomfort for the patient.

Palpated blood pressure procedure where the radial or brachial pulse is felt with the fingertips to determine blood pressure; not as accurate as auscultated blood pressure, but is sometimes used when there is too much noise for a stethoscope to be effective.

Palpation touching or feeling. A pulse or blood pressure may be palpated with the fingertips.

Paradoxical motion movement of a part of the chest in the opposite direction to the rest of the chest during respiration.

PASG pneumatic anti-shock garment.

Past medical history record of previous medical issues and procedures that may be used to help the physician with diagnosis or treatment.

Pathogens the organisms that cause infection, such as viruses and bacteria.

Penetrations injuries caused by an object that passes through the skin or other body tissues.

Perfusion the supply of oxygen to and removal of wastes from the cells and tissues of the body as a result of the flow of blood through the capillaries. *See also* hypoperfusion.

Pharyngeal relating to or located or produced in the region of the pharynx.

Pharynx the area directly posterior to the mouth and nose. It is made up of the oropharynx and the nasopharynx.

Pin-index safety system a means by which anesthesiologists prevent misconnection to the wrong yoke.

Placenta the organ of pregnancy where exchange of oxygen, foods, and wastes occurs between a mother and fetus.

Pneumonia infection of the lungs, usually from a bacterium or virus.

Pneumothorax air in the chest cavity, outside the lungs.

Pocket mask a device, usually with a one-way valve, to aid in artificial ventilation. A rescuer breathes through the valve when the mask is placed over the patient's face. Also acts as a barrier to prevent contact with a patient's breath or body fluids. Can be used with supplemental oxygen when fitted with an oxygen inlet.

Positional asphyxia death of a person due to a body position that restricts breathing for a prolonged period of time.

Posterior the back of the body or body part. *Opposite of* anterior.

Power grip gripping with as much hand surface as possible in contact with the object being lifted, all fingers bent at the same angle, hands at least 10 inches apart.

Power lift a lift from a squatting position with weight to be lifted close to the body, feet apart and flat on the ground, body weight on or just behind balls of feet, back locked in. The upper body is raised before the hips. *Also called* the squat-lift position.

Presenting problem the illness or injury for which the patient is seeking medical attention.

Proximal closer to the torso. *Opposite of* distal.

Pulse the rhythmic beats felt as the heart pumps blood through the arteries.

Pulse oximeter an electronic device for determining the amount of oxygen carried in the blood, and the oxygen saturation or SpO_2.

Punctures open wounds that tear through the skin and destroy underlying tissues. A *penetrating puncture wound* can be shallow or deep. A *perforating puncture wound* has both an entrance and an exit wound.

Radial pulse the pulse felt at the wrist.

Rales crackles.

Rapid extrication a technique using manual stabilization rather than application of an immobilization device for the purpose of speeding extrication when the time saved will make the difference between life and death.

Rapid trauma assessment a rapid assessment of the head, neck, chest, abdomen, pelvis, extremities, and posterior of the body to detect signs and symptoms of injury.

Reasonable force the minimum amount of force required to keep a patient from injuring himself or others.

Reduce to restore to usual relationship, as the ends of a fractured bone. To weaken, as a solution. To diminish, as bulk or weight.

Reservoir bag a container that can hold air in a breathing apparatus.

Respiration breathing.

Rigid splint splint made of cardboard, wood, or pneumatic devices that requires the limb to be moved to the anatomical position, which provides the greatest support.

Roller gauze a strip of muslin or other cloth rolled up in cylinder form for surgical use. A roller bandage.

Sager traction splint unipolar traction splint that continuously shows the amount of traction being applied.

Scapula the shoulder blade.

Sellick's maneuver pressure applied to the cricoid cartilage to compress the esophagus. *Also called* cricoid pressure.

Septum a wall dividing two cavities.

Serial vital signs an ongoing monitoring of body systems.

Severe allergic reaction an allegic reaction where the patient has either respiratory distress or indications of shock.

Shock management treatment procedures to assist a patient in shock; includes maintaining an open airway, providing oxygen, elevating the legs, and protecting the patient from heat loss.

Shoulder girdle the two scapulae and two clavicles attaching the bones of the upper extremities to the axial skeleton.

Sling and swathe a support for an injured upper extremity.

Soft restraints items such as leather cuffs and belts that can be used to hold patients while minimizing the chance for soft-tissue injury.

Soft suction catheter a dilatation and curettage device designed to minimize trauma under certain conditions.

Sphygmomanometer the cuff and gauge used to measure blood pressure.

Splint any device used to immobilize a body part.

Spontaneous respirations automatic process of bringing oxygen into the body and distributing it throughout the body.

Standing takedown process of carefully but rapidly taking a standing patient down to the supine position to prevent spinal injury.

Stoma a permanent surgical opening in the neck through which the patient breathes.

Stridor a harsh, high-pitched sound heard on inspiration that indicates swelling of the larynx.

Stylet a long, thin, flexible metal probe.

Suction use of a vacuum device to remove blood, vomitus, and other secretions or foreign materials from the airway.

Supine position lying on the back. *Opposite of* prone.

Supplemental oxygen additional oxygen that is forced into a patient's lungs during periods of inadequate or absent breathing; accomplished through oxygen cylinders, pressure regulators, and a delivery device.

Sutures thread, wire, or other material used to stitch parts of the body together. The seam or line of union formed by surgical stitches.

Swelling an abnormal transient enlargement, especially one appearing on the surface of the body. Ice applied to the area helps to limit swelling.

Synchronous occurring simultaneously.

Systolic blood pressure the pressure created when the heart contracts and forces blood out into the arteries.

Tachycardia a rapid heart rate; any pulse rate above 100 beats per minute.

Tachypnea a breathing rate that is faster than the normal rate.

Tenderness pain in response to palpation.

Thermoregulatory pertaining to the regulation of temperature, especially body temperature.

Thyroid cartilage the bulky, shield-like structure, commonly known as the Adams's apple, that forms the anterior surface of the larynx.

Tidal volume the volume of air breathed in and out during one respiration.

Tissue necrosis tissue death.

Tongue blade a thin instrument rounded at the ends used to depress the tongue to inspect the mouth and throat; also called a tongue depressor.

Traction splint a splint that applies constant pull along the length of a lower extremity to help stabilize the fractured bone and to reduce muscle spasm in the limb. Traction splints are used primarily on femoral shaft fractures.

Trendelenburg positioning a position in which the patient's feet and legs are higher than the head. *Also called* shock position.

Trimester a three-month period.

Tripod positioning a position in which the patient sits upright, leans slightly forward, and supports the body with the arms in front and elbows locked. This is a common position found in respiratory distress.

T-tube tube inserted into the thoracic cavity.

Umbilical cord the fetal structure containing the blood vessels that carry blood to and from the placenta.

Unresponsive patient person who does not react to a stimulus or treatment.

Unresponsiveness a condition of not reacting to a stimulus or treatment.

Upper airway the portion of the respiratory system that extends from the nose and mouth to the larynx.

Urgent moves patient moves made because there is an immediate threat to life due to the patient's condition and the patient must be moved quickly for transport.

Uvula the free edge of the soft palate that hangs at the back of the throat above the root of the tongue; it is made of muscle, connective tissue, and mucous membrane.

Vascular compromise trauma or disruption of the circulatory system.

Vasodilator a nerve or drug that dilates blood vessels.

Vegetative state a state of severe mental impairment where only involuntary functions are sustained.

Ventricular fibrillation (VF) a condition in which the heart's electrical impulses are disorganized, preventing the heart muscle from contracting normally.

Ventricular tachycardia (VT) a condition in which the heartbeat is quite rapid; if rapid enough, ventricular tachycardia will not allow the heart's chambers to fill with enough blood between beats to produce blood flow sufficient to meet the body's needs.

Water-soluble lubricant material used to reduce friction that dissolves in water.

Wheezing the production of whistling sounds during difficult breathing such as occurs in asthma, coryza, croup, and other respiratory disorders.

Xiphoid process the inferior portion of the sternum.

INDEX

A

Abrasions, 121, 127

Absorption, 170

Acetone wipes, 84

Activated caharcoal, **170–174**

Adam's apple, 63

Administration of medicine. *See*
Medical emergencies

AED (automated external
defibrillation), **202–208**

Agonal respirations, 81

Airborne particles, 92

Airway management and
ventilation, 1–90

  bag-valve-mask ventilation,
15–20

  endotracheal intubation, 66–70

  esophageal tracheal combitube
(ETC), 71–77

  ET tube, 36–40

  head-tilt/chin-lift maneuver,
2–5

  jaw-thrust maneuver, 6–9

  nasal cannula, 51–55

  nasogastric intubation, 56–61

  nasopharyngeal airway (NPA),
26–30

  nonrebreather mask, 46–50

  oral suctioning, 31–35

  oropharyngeal airway (OPA),
21–25

  oxygen tank assembly, 41–45

  pocket mask, 10–14

  pulse oximetry, 83–87

  review questions, 88–90

  Sellick's maneuver, 62–65

  stoma breather, 78–82

Albuterol, 180

Alkali, 170

Altered level of consciousness, 2

Altered mental status, 159, 160

Alupent, 180

Ambulatory, 280

Amniotic sac, 216

Amputations, 233

Anatomical disturbances, 56

Anemic patients, 84

Angina, 186

Angle of the jaw, 7, 12, 22

Ankle hitch, 253

Antecubital fossa, 109

Anterior-axillary line, 204

Antidote, 170

Apnea, 107

Artificial ventilation, 56, 79

Aspiration/aspirate

  activated charcoal, 170

  endotracheal intubation, 66

  nasogastric intubation, 56

  NPA, 27

  OPA, 22

  oral suctioning, 31

  pocket mask, 11

  Sellick's maneuver, 62

  spinal immobilization of supine
patient, 277

Assembling the oxygen tank, **41–45**

Assessment. *See* Patient assessment

Auscultate, 74

Automated external defibrillation
(AED), **202–208**

Automatic AED (auto-AED), 202

AVPU

  assessment of responsive
patient, 138

  assessment of unresponsive
patient, 146

  initial assessment, 116

  trauma—no significant MOI,
153

  trauma—significant MOI, 160

Avulsions, 233

B

Bag-valve-mask ventilation, **15–20**

Bandaging, **231–236.** *See also*
Dressing and bandaging

Baseline mental status, 117

Baseline vital signs, 104

Biphasic energy levels, 202

Blanket drag, 101

Bleeding control, **226–230**

Blood pressure, 109–110

Bloody show, 216

BMV (bag-valve-mask) ventilation,
15–20

Body mechanics, 98

Body substance isolation (BSI)
precautions. *See* BSI
precautions

Bourdon gauge flowmeter, 42

Brachial pulse, 106

Brachycardia, 105

Breathing (respiration), 107–108

Breech presentation, 218

Bronchioles, 180, 192

Bronchodilator, 180

Bronchodilator therapy, 84

Bronchosol, 180

Bronkometer, 180

BSI equipment, 3

BSI precautions, **92–97**

  BMV ventilation, 16

  jaw-thrust maneuver, 7

  NPA, 27

  OPA, 22

  oral suctioning, 32

  pocket mask, 11

Burns, 122, 127

C

Cannula, nasal, **51–55**

Capillary refill, 161

Carbon monoxide poisoning, 111

Carina, 36

Carotid pulse, 106

Carries (lifting), 100–101

Caustic solutions, 56

Caustic substance, 72

Cervical collar, **263–267**

Chest wounds, 233–234

Chief complaint, 117, 138

Childbirth, 214–220

  breech presentation, 218

  contractions, 214

  crowning, 215

  excessive bleeding, 219

  limb presentation, 218

  meconium, 219